A Contemporary Nursing Process

The (Un)Bearable Weight of Knowing in Nursing

Rozzano C. Locsin, RN, PhD, FAAN

Rozzano C. Locsin, RN; PhD, FAAN is Professor of Nursing at Florida Atlantic University's Christine E. Lynn College of Nursing in Boca Raton, Florida. He holds a masters degree from Silliman University, and a Doctor of Philosophy in Nursing from the University of the Philippines. Understanding "life transformations and transitions in the human health experience" defines his nursing research, articulating knowing persons as whole through technology, caring, and nursing. Dr. Locsin published his middle-range theory entitled, *Technological Competency as Caring in Nursing* in 2005. *Advancing Technology, Caring and Nursing* published in 2001 and *Technology and Nursing Practice* published in 2007 are his two other books. Dr. Locsin's international work includes program developments in nursing education in Uganda, Thailand, and the Philippines. His national and international projects are on the topics of holistic nursing, care of older persons, and alternative and complementary therapies. He was a Fulbright Scholar to Uganda, a recipient of Fulbright Alumni Initiative Award and is a Fulbright Senior Specialist in Global Health and International Development. In 2003 he received the prestigious *Edith Moore Copeland Excellence in Creativity Award* from Sigma Theta Tau International Honor Society of Nursing. In 2006, he was elected Fellow of the American Academy of Nursing.

Marguerite J. Purnell, RN, PhD, AHN-BC

Marguerite J. Purnell, RN; PhD is Assistant Professor of Nursing at Florida Atlantic University's Christine E. Lynn College of Nursing. She holds a masters degree from Florida Atlantic University and a Doctor of Philosophy in Nursing from the University of the Miami, Miami, Florida. She is board certified in Holistic Nursing. Dr. Purnell's program of research is centered on intentionality, caring, and energetic healing in nursing practice. Her current leading edge research focuses on the creation of optimal healing environments with stored intention. An expert nurse educator, Dr. Purnell has published broadly on the topics of caring in Nursing, particularly on the valuing of caring in nursing education. Her *Model of Online Nursing Education* was designed for virtual environments and is grounded in caring intention as the organizing framework. She has published widely on other topics on nursing including the influences of technologies in Nursing. As co-editor of this book, Dr. Purnell declares her passion for communicating nursing in quintessential ways for the education of contemporary nurses, and for developing the ontologic thread of informed caring to support and affirm nurses of the future.

A Contemporary Nursing Process

The (Un)Bearable Weight of Knowing in Nursing

Rozzano C. Locsin, RN, PhD, FAAN
Marguerite J. Purnell, PhD, RN, AHN-BC

SPRINGER PUBLISHING COMPANY

NEW YORK

Springer Publishing Company, LLC
11 West 42nd Street
New York, NY 10036
www.springerpub.com

Acquisitions Editor: Allan Graubard
Cover Design: David Levy
Composition: Monotype, LLC

09 10 11 12 13 / 5 4 3 2 1
Ebook ISBN: **978-0-8261-2579-8**

Library of Congress Cataloging-in-Publication Data

A contemporary nursing process : the (un)bearable weight of knowing in nursing / [edited by] Rozzano C. Locsin, Marguerite J. Purnell.
   p. ; cm.
  Includes bibliographical references.
  ISBN 978-0-8261-2578-1
  1. Nurse and patient. 2. Nursing—Philosophy. I. Locsin, Rozzano C., 1954– II. Purnell, Marguerite J.
  [DNLM: 1. Nurse-Patient Relations. 2. Nursing Process. WY 87 C761 2009]
  RT86.3.C668 2009
  610.7306'99—dc22

                                             200900841

Printed in the United States of America by Hamilton Printing

DEDICATION

Rozzano Gregorio Ramon Agustin C. Locsin

This book is dedicated to my sisters, Lucilla Elizabeth Michaela and Maria Corazon Francisca; and my brother, Jose Maria Genaro. In memoriam.

The development of this book stemmed from the understanding that the focus of nursing practice is to know the other as person. Knowing is a dynamic process—the epitome of compassionate nursing practice.

Knowing and growing with my sisters and my brother was my nursing. They have gone before me. We will continue to know each other more and grow together in time.

Marguerite Josephine de la Hyde Purnell

The creativity and spirit for this book began several generations ago. The current is strong: My great-great-grandfather Charles Purnell; my great-grandfather Charles William Purnell; my grandfather Leslie Gordon Purnell; my uncle William Robert Purnell; and my father, John Leslie de la Hyde Purnell: all were adventurers, philanthropists, journalists, writers, poets, and artists who drank deeply of life.

This book is dedicated to them. They are ever-present reminders of my commitment to share and write about what is important. And so I walk in their footsteps in the creation of this book about my passion, nursing.

Contents

Section II: Processes of Knowing in Nursing: Practice Perspectives

Section III: Influences of Technology on Knowing in Nursing

Section IV: Knowing the Person Through Lenses of Culture and Community

Contributors

Anne Boykin, RN, PhD
Dean and Professor
Florida Atlantic University
Christine E. Lynn College of Nursing
Boca Raton, Florida

Savina O. Schoenhofer, RN, PhD
Professor of Nursing
Department of Graduate Nursing
Alcorn State University
Natchez, Mississippi

Lynne M. Dunphy, PhD, ARNP
Professor of Nursing and Routhier
Chair of Practice
At the College of Nursing University
of Rhode Island
Kingston, Rhode Island.

Pamela G. Reed, PhD, RN, FAAN
Professor
University of Arizona
College of Nursing
Tucson, Arizona

W. Richard Cowling III, RN, PhD, AP,
RN-BC, AHN-BC
Professor and Director, PhD Program
Editor, Journal of Holistic Nursing
School of Nursing
University of North Carolina Greensboro
Greensboro, North Carolina

Elizabeth Repede, PhD(c), FNP-BC,
CMH
School of Nursing
University of North Carolina
Greensboro
Greensboro, North Carolina

Gail J. Mitchell, RN, PhD
Associate Professor
School of Nursing, York University
Midland, Ontario, Canada

William K. Cody, RN, PhD, FAAN
Dean and Professor
Presbyterian School of Nursing at
Queens University
Charlotte, North Carolina

Marlaine C. Smith, RN, PhD, AHN-BC,
FAAN
Professor and Associate Dean for
Academic Programs
Helen Karpelenia Persson Eminent
Scholar
Christine E. Lynn College of Nursing
Florida Atlantic University
Boca Raton, Florida

Patricia L. Munhall, EdD, ARNP,
NCPsyA, FAAN
Founder and President, International
Institute for Human Understanding
Miami, Florida

Zane Robinson Wolf, PhD, RN, FAAN
Dean and Professor
School of Nursing and Health
Sciences
LaSalle University
Philadelphia, Pennsylvania

Christopher Johns, RN, PhD, PACT
Complementary Therapist and
Professor of Nursing
University of Bedfordshire
Bedfordshire, UK

Marian C. Turkel, RN, PhD
Director, Professional Nursing Practice
Albert Einstein Medical Center
Philadelphia, Pennsylvania

Marilyn A. Ray, RN, PhD, CTN
Professor Emeritus
Florida Atlantic University
Christine E. Lynn College of Nursing
Boca Raton, Florida

Susan K. Chase, EdD, ARNP, FNP-BC
Professor and Assistant Dean for
Graduate Programs
Christine E. Lynn College of Nursing
Florida Atlantic University
Boca Raton, Florida

Bernie Carter, PhD, PgC, PgC, BSc,
RSCN,
Professor of Children's Nursing
School of Nursing and Caring Sciences
University of Central Lancashire
Preston, United Kingdom

Marie Marshall, BSc (Hons), DipHE,
RSCN, RGN, EN
Children Community Specialist
Practitioner
Central Manchester and Manchester
Children's Hospitals, NHS
Stockport, United Kingdom

Caroline Sanders, RSCN, RN, BSc
(Hons), PgD Psychosexual Health
Consultant Nurse, Paediatric
Urology/Gynaecology
Royal Liverpool Children's Hospital
NHS Trust
Alder Hey, United Kingdom

Donna Carol Maheady, EdD, ARNP
Adjunct Assistant Professor
Christine E. Lynn College of Nursing
Florida Atlantic University
Boca Raton, Florida

Ruth McCaffrey, ARNP, DNP
Associate Professor of Nursing
Christine E. Lynn College of Nursing
Florida Atlantic University
Boca Raton, Florida

Alan Barnard, RN, BA, MA, PhD
Senior Lecturer
School of Nursing
Queensland University of Technology
Victoria Park Road, Kelvin Grove
Queensland, Australia

Marilyn Macdonald, RN, PhD
Assistant Professor
School of Nursing
Dalhousie University
Halifax, Nova Scotia, Canada

Charlotte D. Barry, RN, PhD, NCSN
Associate Professor
Christine E. Lynn College of Nursing
Florida Atlantic University
Boca Raton, Florida

Shirley C. Gordon, RN, PhD
Associate Professor
Christine E. Lynn College of Nursing
Florida Atlantic University
Port St. Lucie, Florida

Samantha M. C. Pang, PhD, RN
Professor and Head
School of Nursing
The Hong Kong Polytechnic
University
Hung Hom, Kowloon, Hong Kong
SAR, China

Michiko Yahiro, MSN, RN
PhD student
School of Nursing
The Hong Kong Polytechnic
University
Hung Hom, Kowloon, Hong Kong
SAR, China

Helen Y. L. Chan, BSN, RN
PhD student
School of Nursing
The Hong Kong Polytechnic
University
Hung Hom, Kowloon, Hong Kong
SAR, China

Yukie Takemura, RN, PhD
Vice Director of Nursing
The University of Tokyo Hospital
Bunkyo-ku, Tokyo, Japan

Katsuya Kanda, RN, PhD
Professor of Nursing Administration
Graduate School of Medicine
Department of Nursing
Administration
The University of Tokyo
Bunkyo-ku, Tokyo, Japan

Carolina Huerta, RN, EdD
Chair and Professor of Nursing
Department of Nursing
College of Health Science and Human
Services
University of Texas–Pan American
Edinburg, Texas

M. Sandra (Sandra) Sánchez, RN, PhD
Associate Professor of Nursing
Department of Nursing
College of Health Science and Human
Services
University of Texas–Pan American
Edinburg, Texas

Foreword

At the heart of a thoughtful practice process of nursing is coming to know persons. The realization that nursing cannot truly take place without the intentional and knowing engagement of the nurse with the one nursed is critical to advancing knowledgeable practice. Much has been written about knowing in nursing, initially stimulated by Carper's germinal study on fundamental patterns of knowing. Since then, scholars have identified and described other ways to come to know persons from a variety of perspectives. Nonetheless, these efforts to know are just beginnings—a place from where we might begin to reach higher, deeper, and broader. With this declaration, this book offers perspectives from contemporary nursing scholars for knowing persons—from the abstract reaches of philosophy to the realities of contemporary practice where the rules of convention may not fit, and where nurses are challenged to know themselves in order that they may truly know those nursed.

As a unity of scholarship, the book constitutes an active text for students to rise above the confines of the rudimentary traditional Nursing Process more popularly known as "APIE"—assessment, planning, intervention, and evaluation to a complex, creative, relational, and expert practice that extends across venues and specialties and is grounded in postmodernist/human science viewpoints. Indeed, the philosophical grounding of the traditional nursing process in positivism/empiricism is perpetuated by the notion that APIE is the scientific method, and therefore thinking by nurses outside of this linear process is discouraged, devalued, and contradictory to the established and popular health care practice process.

The goal of the book is to illuminate knowing of persons as a contemporary, human-centered, distinctive process of Nursing, in which knowing the person is the unfolding of the value of the nursed and nurse. The general theme of the book, transcending the confines of the traditional nursing process, is simply "knowing persons." It promotes the realization of ways of knowing other than those solely grounded in empiricist/objectivist viewpoints. The need to re-think the Traditional Nursing Process is emphasized, as is the need to re-envision and shift the focus of knowing the person as object, to knowing person as person. In this transformative and transcendent process of nursing with multiple dimensions for practice, both the nurse and the one nursed are honored as whole. The nurse is freed to nurse in a meaningful and creative way.

Locsin and Purnell believe that the postmodernist/human science views provide philosophical underpinnings that transform one's understanding of the traditional nursing process to a contemporary process of nursing that is of and with the person. Such a contemporary process of nursing is expressed uniquely in diverse ways. Maintained in this distinction is the understanding that the context for nursing is the nursing situation which Boykin and Schoenhofer (2001) describe as "those shared lived experiences in which the caring between the nurse and nursed enhances personhood" (p. 17). Fundamentally occurring in this nursing situation is continuous, moment-to-moment knowing of persons as caring. In knowing the person, the nurse intentionally focuses on coming to know person, on hearing the calls for nursing, and on creating unique and meaningful caring responses.

Today there are many challenges facing health care systems. I believe the most important of these is the call to create models of care which nurture, support, and celebrate nursing as a discipline and profession; Models of care which understand and appreciate that to nurse, the nurse must be fully engaged in the human situation... ...to nurse, the person(s) nursed must be known. In this compendium, Locsin and Purnell invite the reader to let go of the traditional nursing process as having served and outgrown its purpose, and to embrace a contemporary, substantive process of nursing grounded in knowing persons as participants in their care instead of being objects of our care.

Anne Boykin, RN, PhD
Dean and Professor
Florida Atlantic University
Christine E. Lynn College of Nursing
Boca Raton, Florida

Boykin, A., & Schoenhofer, S. O. (2001). Nursing as caring: A model for transforming practice. Sudbury, CT: Jones & Bartlett.

Prologue

The idea of this book evolved out of a decade or more of collaborative and pithy conversations over a steady ritual of afternoon tea, where we ruminated on subjects near and dear to us in nursing. The notion of the traditional nursing process as an impediment to reflective and thoughtful practice arose repeatedly. The institutionalization of the nursing process taught in most schools of nursing, along with its required use in hospital settings, was a focus of concern to us. In our discussions, we returned again and again to the idea that nurses appear to be programmed into a type of thinking that produces cyclical, prescriptive, and predictive practice with the use of the Traditional Nursing Process (assessment, planning, intervention, and evaluation) as the standard for nursing practice.

Indeed, the philosophy of the traditional nursing process is grounded in positivist and empiricist thoughts, and is perpetuated by the notion that the APIE is the scientific method and is therefore justified in its adoption as the practice norm. Persons are viewed as collections of parts, a process that begins when medical consultation is first sought. The process is perpetuated in health care institution systems where most nurses practice. Thinking outside the box, away from the linear process, is discouraged, devalued, and derided as contradictory to the scientific system.

In contrast, a transformative and transcendent process of nursing with multiple dimensions for practice honors both the nurse and the one nursed as whole. This transcendent process opens the way for co-creating mutual relationships and for affirming each other's hopes and dreams of health and well-being. This understanding advocates for, and indeed, demands the illumination of alternative views which advance contemporary nursing practice. The impetus for development of this book was borne out of this underlying moral stance.

As an overarching concept, knowing persons, the (un)bearable weight of practicing nursing encompasses the burden of reconciling two very different perspectives in nursing: the institutionalized processes for addressing problem-oriented nursing, and the processes of knowing persons that arise from a human science perspective. Can these views *ever* be reconciled? Is there a way to bring them together in a harmonious co-existence?

Currently, there exist various traditionally oriented processes of nursing, most of which are viewed from perspectives of humans that target wholeness as being made up of parts, and of nursing as making the person whole by completing the parts. However, in today's views of contemporary processes of nursing, we witness a different philosophical lens of human science that is becoming more acceptable and commonplace. Even with this growing appreciation, the popularized rote process of assessment, planning, intervention, and evaluation continues to maintain a highly recognized status as *the* nursing process, perpetuating its use primarily in clinical areas or in hospital nursing settings in which patient conditions of health are addressed by "disease and illness" care. Despite this pervasive institutionalization in protocols, software, and health care informatics, new and alternative processes of nursing are steadily being advanced, grounded in nursing philosophies and theories of nursing. These contemporary processes are framed in an appreciation of the fundamental valuing of knowing persons from a human science perspective. They are continually being realized, recognized, and appreciated by practicing professional nurses as valuable and integral to advancing thoughtful nursing practice.

It is the goal of this book to be instrumental to the discourse concerning contemporary nursing processes with selected topics found crucial to the articulation of a compassionate, informed practice process. With this goal, the book is designed to provoke advancing appreciation of various processes of Nursing grounded in multiple views of nursing practice. This book embraces the diverse philosophical and theoretical viewpoints of nurse scholars whose appreciation of persons as unitary beings underpins their understanding of professional nursing practice. The anthology of topics that comprise the essential substance of the book is directed toward the identification, description, clarification, and dissemination of leading-edge processes of nursing grounded in various perspectives within the realm of human science and human-centered care.

The book emphasizes the transformation of the process of nursing from a focus on the person as object of care to instead, the person as a knowledgeable participant in his or her care. In materializing the transcendent idea of nursing care, the significant thread encompassing these processes of nursing is the nursing practice concept of knowing the person. This concept is predicated upon the assumption that professional nursing practice is for the purpose of knowing persons as intimately involved in their own care.

Opportunities are provided in this collection of chapters for the practicing nurse to understand knowing the person through a lens that is responsive to what matters and is grounded in what matters: in knowing the person, the nurse accepts the "witness" role, bearing the weight of knowing the other as person. Each chapter author has created a perspective that fosters the description, explanation, and dissemination of a unique and celebratory process of professional nursing practice. We are indebted to their contribution to this growing horizon of practice processes that will serve as an inspiration and resource to others.

In each chapter, a view of nursing unfolds as the relationship among persons. As such, the focused trajectory is the clarification and illustration of the concept of persons, while "knowing persons" is articulated as a process that keeps evidence in synchrony with research data, illuminating nursing care as a deliberative acknowledgment of persons.

Each author has responded uniquely. To illuminate the writing styles and backgrounds of the contributing authors, a biographical sketch of each is included.

The contributors and coeditors are scholars and practitioners of nursing. They recognize that as a discipline of knowledge and practice profession, Nursing demands a legitimate understanding of its ontology and epistemology. How is nursing known, and what are the processes involved in this knowing? It is the vision of the editors and community of authors that the contents of this book will stimulate, motivate, and guide others toward knowing persons as participants in their care rather than as objects of our care. Knowing the experiences of the other and calling upon all in our knowing

in order to know the other as person is critical to the realization of a discipline of knowledge and a practice profession.
In "knowing person," Nursing lifts up its voice to advocate
and answer meaningfully to society; to those we nurse; and,
importantly, to ourselves.

Rozzano C. Locsin, RN, PhD, FAAN
Marguerite Purnell, RN, PhD, AHN-BC
Coeditors

Acknowledgements

In each journey, there comes an end, a time when the beginning is reconsidered and the journey is traveled again in spirit. We have both treasured and cherished each author and have understood their travails in trying to balance the myriad responsibilities of teaching, practice, research, and service while giving birth to a thoughtful, scholarly chapter for the benefit of Nursing. Additionally, our international colleagues struggled to meet challenges of time zones and technology. We have wondered, how could we have cared for them better during this process? How could we have helped alleviate the stress of meeting deadlines? We are proud of all the contributors to this book, of their consummate professionalism, and of their fine, creative works. Their lights shine.

The difficulty in naming names is that we may miss one who is important to us, and so we say that we would like to acknowledge *all*. In particular, we would like to thank Dr. Anne Boykin and Dr. Savina Schoenhofer, who have been colleagues of conscience in our efforts to stay true to our underlying beliefs and values centered in caring. Dr. Marilyn Parker's support has always been a steady stream, and Dr. Marilyn "Dee" Ray, Dr. Bernadette Lange, and Dr. Madeleine Leininger have always exhorted us to believe in ourselves and to seek the highest.

And finally, we thank Alan Graubard, our acquisitions editor at Springer, whose patience and witty rejoinders provided laughter and a sense of renewed energy. We are indeed grateful and offer our sincere thanks to all.

Rozzano C. Locsin and
Marguerite J. Purnell

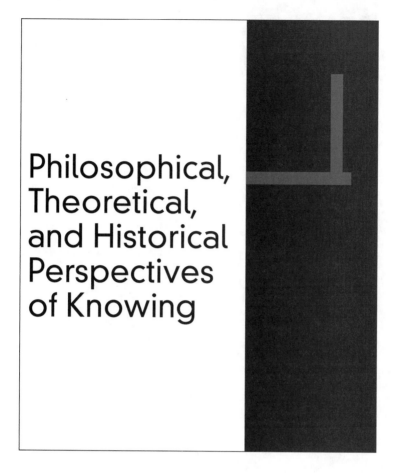

Philosophical, Theoretical, and Historical Perspectives of Knowing

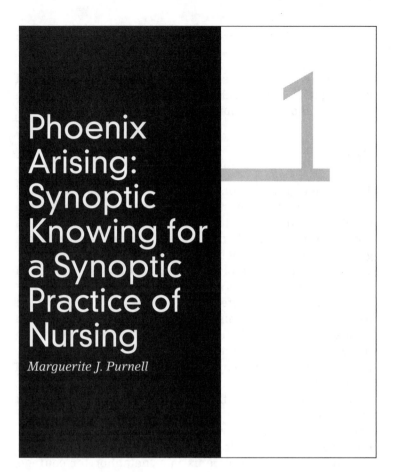

Phoenix Arising: Synoptic Knowing for a Synoptic Practice of Nursing

Marguerite J. Purnell

Chapter Overview

Since Carper's (1978) germinal research was published, nurse scholars have critiqued, extended, and sought to reconcile with practice the four fundamental patterns of knowing that she distinguished. This chapter retraces the provenance of Carper's (1976) research to its source to reveal two further patterns of knowing that may be similarly derived from Phenix's (1964) work: symbolic knowing and synoptic (integrative) knowing. Symbolic knowing is the fecund, undifferentiated pattern of tacit, unexpressed knowing, valuing, and meaning from which other patterns arise and are expressed. Synoptic knowing is the pattern in which all patterns are gathered together in unity and fullness. This is the pattern of knowing that answers to the complex, multidimensional knowing taking place within the caring relationship between the nurse and the one nursed.

Prelude

The mythological phoenix has captured the imagination and wonder of human beings for thousands of years. Chronicled in folklore of diverse and ancient peoples, this noble bird has appeared in the annals of civilizations flung far across the globe. The phoenix touches us with wonder. Its life is poignant. In Chinese mythology, the phoenix is a symbol of high virtue and gentle grace, sipping only upon drops of morning dew. Its venerable life spans 500 years. When the time of its death draws near, this noble bird collects branches and builds itself a large funeral pyre, finally settling sadly on the wood to draw its last breath and surrender life. As the phoenix bows its head low and slowly begins to die, the wood bursts into flames, consuming the bird until nothing is left. The world holds it breath, until suddenly, transformed out of the ashes, the phoenix arises triumphant, reborn stronger and more beautiful, to live again for another 500 years. It is no wonder that we are drawn to the story of this magnificent, unique creature. The phoenix is a metaphor for courage, transformation, and continuance. The old becomes the new, and knowledge is not lost in change, but becomes change. It is thus we turn our thoughts to nursing as a discipline, to the uniqueness of its knowledge, to our knowing and how we know what we know, and to informed courage in surrendering to necessary change.

Introduction

Since Carper's germinal research was published in 1978, nurse scholars have critiqued, extended, and sought to reconcile with practice the four fundamental patterns of knowing that she articulated. Commentary by more than one generation of scholars has ranged widely from unquestioning acceptance and integration to acerbic criticism. Formulaic recitation and description of Carper's four fundamental patterns of knowing—personal, empiric, ethical, and aesthetic—continues with singular predictability. These patterns tend to be applied in a linear, discrete fashion, rather than enlightening our knowing practice with a rich, multidimensional range of understandings as Carper intended.

While almost every work referring to knowing routinely pays homage in some way to Carper's unique understanding and contribution to nursing knowledge, other scholars have illuminated uncharted aspects of disciplinary knowing that simply did not fit well within the four fundamental patterns, or did not resonate with their knowing of what was meaningful in their practice. Additional ways of knowing such as unknowing (Munhall, 1993), sociopolitical knowing (White, 1995), and women's ways of knowing (Belenkey, Clinchy, Goldberg, & Tarule, 1986) are now cited routinely in tandem with Carper's original retinue of fundamental patterns. Carper rightfully declared then, and other nurse scholars continue to follow suit now, that other ways of knowing may exist. These disclaimers, however, point silently back to a lack of capacity or an inadequacy that is implicit in the original four fundamental patterns: The range and dimensions of their domains, in and of themselves, are insufficient to embrace other ways of knowing as they have been discovered and added to the knowledge base of nursing.

It is evident that Carper's four fundamental patterns of knowing, as they were originally presented in her 1978 landmark article, provide neither sufficiency nor capacity, given the struggles of nurse scholars to describe their knowing in nursing phenomena and processes of practice. Carper stressed that each pattern is necessary for achieving mastery in the discipline and that no pattern alone should be considered sufficient or mutually exclusive. The discussion, perhaps, should center on whether all patterns together should have the capacity not only for mutual inclusion, but also for being mutually inclusive—a somewhat different premise.

Carper's unique gift to nursing that explicated and illuminated the wide-ranging complexity of knowing and knowledge in practice may be better understood in light of the source of her inspiration for these patterns of knowing in Philip H. Phenix's (1964) *Realms of Meaning*. This chapter retraces the provenance of Carper's (1976) research to reveal two further realms of meaning that may similarly be found useful in Phenix's (1964) work: the symbolic and synoptic (integrative) realms. It is important, however, before embarking upon a retrospective journey, to examine the influence and conceptual significance of the language embedded in Carper's and Phenix's work.

Linguistic Interplay and Fuzzy Understanding

Knowing and Knowledge. In reflecting upon the multitude of articles referring to nurses' knowing, the rapid exchange in use between the words *knowing* and *knowledge* in the literature compromise clarity in communication of ideas. The two words *knowing* and *knowledge* are different parts of speech (gerund and noun, respectively) and have very distinct meanings and usages. Benoliel (1987) sees the need to illuminate the difference between knowing and knowledge:

> *Knowledge consists of concepts, theories, and ideas about an identified area of information, often presented in organized form in textbooks and monographs. Knowing can be viewed as an individual's perceptual awareness of the complexities of a particular situation and draws upon inner knowledge resources that have been garnered through experience in living. (p. 151)*

Jacobs-Kramer and Chinn (1988) define *personal knowledge* as expressing knowledge of self in experiencing, encountering, and focusing—all ongoing, subjective processes. Moch (1990) describes *personal knowing* as entailing a "shift in connectedness/transcendence" (p. 159) and defines components of personal knowing as experiential, interpersonal, and intuitive—all continuing as inner experiences.

Pattern and Way. As with the interchange of the words knowing and knowledge, the different words *pattern* and *way* undergo similar transfer and application. What is the difference between a pattern of knowing and a way of knowing? Each of Carper's patterns is customarily and interchangeably referred to using both descriptive words. However, the notion of *pattern* is specific and is a concept with dimensional implications. A way is more specific and relatively concrete, with limited horizons of use.

These other ways of knowing do not necessarily constitute new *patterns* of knowing commensurate with the complexity and scope of patterns introduced by Carper. This poses a problem in that all identified patterns are of value, but when ways that are context dependent or of a narrower focus are aligned among the four fundamental patterns, the dynamic relationship and unity among the original patterns lose balance and coherence. This alignment and difference in magnitude again point to and affirm the problem outlined earlier: There is a certain lack of capacity among Carper's four fundamental patterns of knowing.

Therefore, the scope of these later ways is better understood as a *sub-pattern, category,* or *aspect* that illustrates increasing complexity or specialization among larger patterns of knowing. From this narrower perspective, knowing as a way rather than a pattern becomes an appropriate fit.

The original problem remains, however, regardless of any taxonomy that one might propose at this point in the discussion: Nurse scholars are finding the fundamental patterns inadequate and are seeking meanings that answer their practice in ways of knowing beyond the perceived scope of the patterns.

Looking Beyond the Scope. In considering Carper's patterns of knowing, each appeals to cognition or psychological processes. Each also appears to be "thinned" in meaning or without a certain capacity when suited to the individual processes of knowing. The interchange between the words *knowing* and *knowledge* contributes to this thinning: Meaning from knowledge must be inferred and is somewhat removed from immediacy. Meaning in knowing is experienced in the moment. This is evidenced by the narrower conceptual level of the more recent idea of *embodied knowing* (Rischel, Larson, & Jackson, 2008) that resonates with the experience of so many nurses.

Carper states that understanding the four fundamental patterns "does not extend the range of knowledge, but rather involves critical attention to the question of what it means to know and what kinds of knowledge are held to be of most value in the discipline of nursing" (p. 13). This rather abstruse statement does not help our understanding in light of the frequent crossover in understanding of terms. The subtle distinction between *what it means to know,* as opposed to *what knowing means*, is taken up by Silva, Sorrell, and Sorrell (1995) in their description of an ontological philosophical shift in nursing. Silva et al. identify three major limitations of Carper's (1978) work.

They assert that first, the title of the article "Fundamental Patterns of Knowing in Nursing" suggests a process, but yet the patterns are shown as end products. How one comes to know the knowledge in these patterns is not adequately addressed. Second, they argue that each pattern is presented as a discrete entity, contributing to understanding, use, and research of the patterns discretely. That distinction results in the richness of Carper's work being lost or passed over in favor of a more linear, formulaic application. Third, and most important in this discussion, Silva, Sorrell, and Sorrell point out that two-dimensional aspects of knowing emerged instead of multidimensional aspects.

As a result of the dimensional paucity they perceived, Silva et al. (1995) coined the terms the *in-between* and *the beyond* (p. 3) to account for the ontological aspects they saw emerging from within Carper's epistemological focus. They observed the change in thinking spurred by cyberspace and virtual reality, and the trend of nurses toward raising ontological questions concerning the nature and meaning of reality. Thus, they found that when Carper's four patterns are used to address all types of epistemological and ontological knowing within nursing theory and research, the research questions become mixed and a certain dissonance ensues. Silva et al. (1995) state succinctly and poignantly 13 years later, "The issue is that often nurses do not recognize this dissonance and, even when appropriate, do not move beyond epistemological questions to ontological questions that address issues of reality, meaning, and being" (p. 4). Included among contemporary critics, however, are non-nurses with perspectives from other disciplines, who propose to further thin or limit the valuing and experience of nurses' knowing by relegating their experiences to the "supervisory and corrective function" (Paley, Cheyne, Dalgleish, Duncan, & Niven, 2007, p. 692) of rule-based, analytical forms of cognition in cognitive science. This interpolation of knowledge from other disciplines under the guise of "science" and "evidence" lends further impetus to the necessity of clarifying what is considered knowledge in the discipline of nursing, including its provenance and philosophical groundings within the relationship of the nurse and the one nursed. At this juncture, the separation in differences of meaning between knowledge and knowing is clear.

Turning to the Source. In turning to Phenix's (1964) work, *Realms of Meaning,* we are able to understand the foundational background to Carper's 1978 work, "Fundamental Patterns of Knowing in Nursing." The purpose in turning back to Phenix is to weigh ideas and search for answers that suggest how fundamental patterns of knowing might be drawn forward and re-visioned for a contemporary, meaningful practice of nursing. Carper's profound contribution has helped generations of nurses to distinguish their own practice as uniquely nursing, and to move away from non-nursing perspectives (Silva et al., 1995) and we thus honor her work.

In the introduction to his work, Phenix (1964) states, "General education is the process of engendering essential meanings" (p. 5). This is the prelude to his idea that meanings are found in realms and sub-realms of distinctive kinds of knowledge within the various disciplines. Six realms of meanings provide foundations for "all the meanings that enter the human experience" (p. 8). Each realm of meaning and its sub-realms has typical methods, leading ideas, and characteristic structures. In studying several disciplines held to be the most important at the time, Phenix examined the general logical character of the field, the distinctive subject matter of the discipline, the representative ideas, and the methods of inquiry. He found that various disciplines or *fields of knowledge* exhibit distinctive structures or patterns of meanings. Today these differences are apparent in the challenges of understanding often felt in interdisciplinary communications. The differences in focus, language, and meanings in disciplinary knowledge often arise from vastly different worldviews and types of endeavors.

These expressive realms of knowledge with their meanings are briefly described, with the *realms of meaning* from which Carper derived her *patterns of knowing.* Perhaps Carper's greatest and most frequently overlooked contribution to nursing is her understanding that whereas Phenix found distinctive realms of meaning and knowledge structures among clusters of similar disciplines, nursing uniquely engages in all realms simultaneously. The notion of matching one distinctive realm of meaning to one discipline correspondence fell far short in regard to nursing's complex practice. The following brief descriptions of Phenix's realms of meaning stem from foundational types of disciplinary knowledge.

Synnoetics or personal knowledge. Phenix states that synnoetics, or subjective knowledge, relates to the kind of personal knowledge such as that found in Martin Buber's close I-Thou relationship and reflects intersubjective understanding. Synnoetics implies relational direct awareness and refers to meanings in which a person has direct insight into other persons existing in relation. This kind of knowledge is concrete, direct, and existential, and it may apply to persons or objects. Most importantly for our consideration, personal knowledge is not developed through formal instruction, even though it refers to human association, beginning with the family and extending out to community, occupation, other cultures, and global associations. Phenix provides examples of four disciplines in this realm: religion, philosophy, psychology, and literature.

Empirics. Empirics (objective knowledge) includes the sciences of the physical world human beings, and other living things. Knowledge gained is based on observation and experimentation. Meanings are expressed as probable empirical truths using rules of evidence and verification. Disciplines whose knowledge structure is primarily empirical include physical sciences (matter), life sciences (life), psychology (mind), and social sciences (society).

Ethics. Ethics (objective knowledge) is the realm "that includes moral meanings that express obligation rather than fact, perceptual form, or awareness of relation" (p. 7). Ethics has to do with personal conduct based on free, responsible decision.

Esthetics. In this realm (objective), meanings take the form of contemplative perception of significant, particular things, such as are found in the various arts. These are expressions of subjective ideation or the creative mind, such as in music, visual arts, arts of movement, and literature.

The "Missing" Realms. Two other realms of meaning were proposed by Phenix: symbolic and synoptic. These realms are significant in that they are not addressed or included by Carper and their properties were not reconceptualized as fundamental patterns of knowing. In the discussion following, however, they shall be seen to be of significant and enduring value to nursing.

The Symbolic Realm and Pattern of Knowing. Phenix (1964) states that symbolic systems constitute the most fundamental of all realms because they must be used to express meanings of other realms. Symbolic knowing encompasses experience and history and relates to values, ideals, and purposes of existence. This realm of meaning is found in knowledge systems of ordinary language, nondiscursive, symbolic forms such as mathematics, rituals, gestures, and tacit understandings. Phenix holds that these "constitute the most fundamental of all of the realms of meaning and are foundational to expression of meanings in each of the other realms" (p. 6). This understanding is significant because it also encompasses and shares the inarticulate; the unexpressed or ineffable; the involuntary response; and abstraction, such as the idea of a round square. It also allows values to surface.

When the meaning extrapolated from this realm is transferred to the idea of knowing in a distinguishable pattern, the idea of symbolic knowing in nursing also becomes a fundamental pattern identified among Carper's original fundamental patterns. We can see that ideas are readily transferred to practice. For example, the image of a nurse's uniform invokes trust; a national flag calls forth meanings associated with birth and patriotism. Language is itself a symbol and is synonymous with culture. This is a pattern that is fundamental in its characteristics; however, it is here that the uniqueness and conceptual value of symbolic knowing changes how we might view the relationships among patterns of knowing in nursing. The symbolic realm, as Phenix noted, is foundational and gives rise to or informs all other realms.

From this perspective, although all patterns are of inherently "equal" value, a glimmer of a process is seen in this relationship. Symbolic knowing may be understood as undifferentiated potential with the capacity for giving rise—from itself—to other patterns of knowing that richly vary in combination, dimension, and form, according to the meanings called forth from the unique and complex disciplinary knowledge found in nursing practice.

It is this unique capacity on which we first focus our attention and offer explanation for the variety and scope of patterns of knowing extant in the nursing literature. In understanding the tacit nature of symbolic knowing, it becomes easy to understand, that this pattern of knowing is present always and answers to the meaning from nursing practice. The glimmer of a process can be seen further in the idea that symbolic knowing is active in the idea of call and response within the nursing situation. Other patterns are simultaneously being perceived tacitly and explicitly within the richness of nuanced practice. This capacity for expressing differentiation, then, is a distinctive and significant function of symbolic knowing in its role as a fundamental pattern, with the relationship between knowing and knowledge made clear. We now turn our attention to the realm that Phenix calls *synoptic,* which presents a paradox for consideration.

The Synoptic Realm and Pattern of Knowing. Phenix describes the synoptic realm as one in which meanings are "comprehensively integrative" (p. 7), and which includes history, religion, and philosophy. These disciplines combine empirical, esthetic, and synnoetic meanings into coherent wholes (Ibid), and their knowledge is described by Phenix as objective. Phenix states that synthesis of coordination with other realms through reflective interpretation of all other kinds of meaning *and* their relationships occurs in the synoptic realm. Of all the realms of meaning that Phenix illuminates, the synoptic realm is perhaps the most intriguing because it resonates with possibilities for the practice of nursing. Although Carper recognized that all patterns were inherent in nursing in the form of patterns of knowing, as previously noted, she did not include the idea of synoptic knowing itself as a pattern in which all other patterns were brought together and integrated as a whole. The necessary transference of the concept of the synoptic realm to patterns of knowing in nursing as synoptic or integrative knowing is as significant as the inclusion of symbolic knowing previously considered.

Synoptic knowing is the pattern that is at home within the nursing situation. Wholeness, caring, oneness, valuing, the "in between" and "the beyond" of Silva et al. (1995), transcendence, empathy, growth, intuition, and all such knowing that is perceived and informed are embraced and included within the nature of integration in this pattern. This is the role of synoptic or integrative knowing: to fuse or synopsize in a unitary whole. The idea of ultimate meanings and what Phenix terms "boundary concepts" (p. 7), such as the Whole, the Comprehensive, and the Transcendent where there are no boundaries, are included in synoptic knowing.

Creative characteristics of fundamental patterns of knowing are expressed through synoptic knowing in the nursing situation. Aesthetic knowing is inherently creative, and it is this aspect that is seen in the perception and understanding of new knowledge brought forth in the nursing situation; that is, nursing knowledge that might not yet be articulated. This is growth, an example of which may be understood as growing in caring, and includes both nurse and the one nursed. In nursing, synoptic knowing unites all knowledge and experience in the moment and creatively transforms them. This critical pattern of knowing enables an individual, or a discipline in the collective sense, to grow and transform with the integration of new knowledge and understandings.

The Unitary Nature of Symbolic and Synoptic Knowing

What has not been addressed at this juncture is the paradox alluded to in our discussion of synoptic knowing. We address this in a question. If symbolic knowing is the pattern from which all others arise, then it must include synoptic knowing; if synoptic knowing integrates all other patterns, then it must include symbolic knowing. Which is it? The answer is similarly puzzling: Neither and both.

Phenix provides the idea of a spectrum, at one end of which are the symbolic fields of knowledge, from which all meanings are expressed. At the other end of the spectrum are the synoptic fields, which gather up the entire range of meanings. In between these two realms are the four distinct but interdependent realms of empirics, esthetics, and synnoetics, which are "modes of significant human relatedness to the world and to existence" (p. 8). The symbolic and synoptic realms "serve as binding elements running throughout the various realms and welding them into a *single meaningful pattern*" (p. 9).

Patterns of symbolic knowing and synoptic knowing in nursing, therefore, are merely two different expressions of the same knowing, rather like a double helix, between which patterns of knowing such as personal, empiric, aesthetic, ethical, sociopolitical, and unknowing come into view and reveal their unique characteristics. The fusion of all the patterns of knowing into a single pattern, with meaning grounded in the disciplinary knowledge of nursing, is the pattern which we will now call *synoptic* or *integrative knowing* in nursing practice. The nursing literature reveals a growing number of integrative theories of nursing practice. The knowing addressed within these theories should also be reflective, and should reflect the whole, as does synoptic knowing.

At the beginning of this paper, we raised the idea of a perceived "thinness" of the four fundamental patterns of knowing. In Phenix's fundamental realms as discussed, meaning is drawn from the fields of knowledge that the realms typify and represent. When transferred as patterns of knowing in nursing, meaning is drawn from disciplinary nursing knowledge and infused into fundamental patterns of knowing. This gives *knowing* the life and fullness of *meaning* distinctive to nursing.

All patterns together are fluid and unbounded, and although they express different natures at different times, they are characteristic of the whole person within the nursing situation, yet remain connected with the universe. It is here that we see a new process of knowing and being that is integral to living in an unbounded universe—one that is increasingly supported by a bolder science and that turns conventional, Newtonian scientific thought on its head. If the focus of concern of the discipline of nursing is nursing in the human health experience, and if the essence of nursing is caring, the nurse grounds practice in an explicit conception of nursing grounded in caring (Boykin, Parker, & Schoenhofer, 1994; Boykin & Schoenhofer, 1993). This is where meaning resides. This is where synoptic or integrative knowing occurs. This is where there are no boundaries.

Phoenix Arising. This chapter began with the story of the mysterious phoenix as a metaphor for courage, change, and continuance. In telling the story of the epistemological roots of our knowing in nursing, we built our nest of wood and settled deep. The consuming of the old in the fire of insight and understanding has raised us up in a new form, more beautiful, and able to live on in wisdom and surety.

Both Barbara Carper, nursing scholar, and Philip Phenix, education scholar, whose opuses we have been considering, have provided the foundations for the re-visioning of this phoenix, or in true understanding of what the name means, metamorphosis or change. We are indebted to them.

Summary

We began this examination of fundamental patterns of knowing in nursing with the premise that something was missing from the patterns and was not explained or accounted for. We turned back the pages of our epistemology to seek to understand the realms of meaning whose sources were discovered in Phenix and expressed for nursing in Carper's work. Two realms of meaning—symbolic and synoptic—were not included in the envisioning of the four original fundamental patterns of knowing in nursing, but were found to answer uniquely to a contemporary process of knowing in nursing practice. Both newly termed as patterns of knowing in nursing, these were found to be two aspects of the same knowing that were differentiated by their functions. This knowing in nursing is called synoptic or integrative knowing.

Reflections

As a young discipline of knowledge with unique complexities in practice, we are only at the beginning of our journey. As human beings, our knowing and intentionality are more complex and wonderful than we have ever dreamed, yet we have hardly begun. Our unique nursing caring is the invitation for exquisite healing of those who are wounded, and the myriad ways this is being lived in practice have only begun to be chronicled. In a contemporary process of nursing, our unbounded knowing and being enables us to simultaneously be at the bedside and in the stars. Our search for knowledge is so that we can tell the story of our own humanity and the desire for goodness and kindness that thread their way through our lives. This we do through nursing.

Sullivan in Phenix (1964) states magnificently, "It is only when the world expands as a tissue of persons and interpersonal relations which are meaningful that knowledge becomes truly significant" (p. 200).

References

Belenky, M. F., Clinchey, B. M., Goldberg, N. R., & Tarule, J. M. (1986). *Women's ways of knowing: The development of self, voice, and mind.* NY: Basic Books.

Benoliel, J. Q. (1987). Response to "Toward holistic inquiry in nursing: A proposal for synthesis of patterns and methods". *Scholarly Inquiry for Nursing Practice: An International Journal, 1*(2), 147–152.

Boykin, A., & Parker, M. E., & Schoenhofer, S. O. (1994). Aesthetic knowing grounded in an explicit conception of nursing. *Nursing Science Quarterly, 7*(4), 158–161.

Boykin, A., & Schoenhofer, S. O. (1993). *Nursing as caring: A model for transforming practice.* New York: National League for Nursing Press.

Carper, B. A. (1976). *Fundamental patterns of knowing in nursing.* PhD Dissertation. Teachers College, Columbia University. UMI DAI-B 36/10, P. 4941

Carper, B. A. (1978). Fundamental patterns of knowing in nursing. *Advances in Nursing Science, 1*(1), 13–23.

Jacobs-Kramer, M. K., & Chinn, P. L. (1988). Perspectives on knowing: A model of nursing knowledge. *Scholarly Inquiry for Nursing Practice: An International Journal, 2*(2), 129–139.

Moch, S. D. (1990). Personal knowing: Evolving research and practice. *Scholarly Inquiry for Nursing Practice: An International Journal, 4*(2), 155–165.

Munhall, P. L. (1993). Unknowing: Toward another pattern of knowing. *Nursing Outlook, 41*, 125–128.

Paley, J., Cheyne, H., Dalgleish, L., Duncan, E., & Niven, C. (2007). Nursing's ways of knowing and dual process theories of cognition. *Journal of Advanced Nursing, 60*(6), 692–701.

Phenix, P. H. (1964). *Realms of meaning: A philosophy of the curriculum for general education.* New York: McGraw-Hill.

Rischel, V., Larsen, K., & Jackson, K. (2008). Embodied dispositions or experience? Identifying new patterns of professional competence. *Journal of Advanced Nursing, 61*(5), 512–521.

Silva, M. C., Sorrell, J. M., & Sorrell, C. D. (1995). From Carper's patterns of knowing to ways of being: An ontological philosophical shift in nursing. *Advances in Nursing Science, 18*(1), 1–13.

White, J. (1995). Patterns of knowing: Review, critique, and update. *Advances in Nursing Science, 17*(4), 73–86.

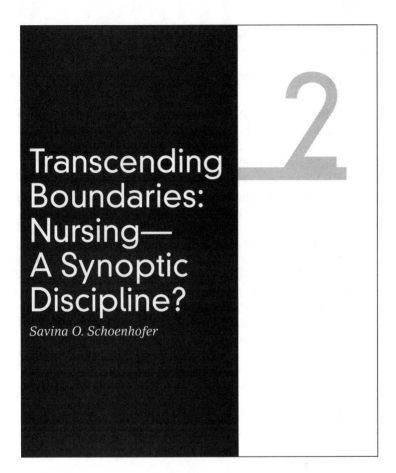

Transcending Boundaries: Nursing— A Synoptic Discipline?

Savina O. Schoenhofer

Chapter Overview

The guiding question explored in this chapter is this: What is nursing's characteristic pattern of meaning? I will use Phenix's (1964) classic *Realms of Meaning* as a framework for analyzing the discipline of nursing in terms of its characteristic meaning. The analysis will demonstrate how nursing's characteristic pattern of meaning encompasses and transcends the five initial realms of symbolics, empirics, aesthetics, synnoetics, and ethics, thus being best characterized as synoptic. The synoptic pattern of meaning integrates and unites the other patterns. Having argued the guiding question, I will then discuss the implications of scholarship, practice, and education in understanding nursing in the broadest sense of meaning.

Introduction

Philip Phenix, a philosopher of education, published in 1964 the book *Realms of Meaning*, written as a philosophy of curriculum for general education. Phenix's thesis was that meaning is the central element in the disciplines of knowledge. Thus, he took up the idea of characteristic patterns of meaning as a way to distinguish among groups of disciplines. While Phenix's purpose was to develop a philosophy of general education, I have found his "realms of meaning" useful for my own purposes, purposes having to do with understanding the meaning of nursing in the broadest possible sense, as a guide to practical work of nursing in the arenas of scholarship, policy, education, and practice.

Phenix posited six realms of meaning and illustrated the unique characteristics of each realm as a pattern. Those six realms of meaning, along with illustrative subjects, are the following:

1. Symbolics—subjects such as ordinary language; mathematics; and nondiscursive, symbolic forms
2. Empirics—subjects such as physical sciences, biology, psychology, and social sciences
3. Esthetics—such as music, visual arts, movement arts, and literature
4. Synnoetics—personal knowledge
5. Ethics—moral knowledge
6. Synoptics—such as history, religion, and philosophy; integrative, synopsizing disciplines that draw on the other realms of meaning

I will pursue the question of what nursing's characteristic pattern of meaning is by asking of each successive realm, "Is the meaning of nursing expressed in this realm?" I will also sketch out examples that demonstrate that nursing's meaning encompasses and transcends the boundaries of each of the first five realms (symbolics, empirics, esthetics, synnoetics, and ethics), and thus that nursing's meaning is best characterized by the realm of synoptics. And finally, I will attempt to respond to this question: Why is it meaningful to call nursing a synoptic discipline?

Before I begin that task, I think it is incumbent upon me to disclose my own perspectival orientation, the perspective of nursing that gave rise to the questions I want to explore with you. To quote our esteemed colleague June Kikuchi in her 1999 paper on clarifying the nature of conceptualizations about nursing, there can be no "presuppositionless" conceptions. My perspective on nursing is expressed well in the theory of Nursing As Caring—an integrated, comprehensive, systematized expression of nursing. Its central project is a system of value, language, and thought that offers an ontological grounding for epistemological, axiological, pedagogical, and praxeological concerns and activities. While I am not going to describe Nursing As Caring directly, I think it will be helpful to acknowledge up front that it does serve as my lens for viewing nursing. To reiterate, there can be no presuppositionless conceptions, so what I have to say necessarily emerges from my explicit and tacit Nursing As Caring perspective.

Now to return to the task of examining nursing's meaning in relation to Phenix's realms of meaning. I will begin with symbolics.

Symbolics

Symbolics refers to humanly constructed, symbolic formalisms, "formal expressive patterns created for the purpose of communication" (Phenix, 1964, p. 95). Knowledge in symbolics is of form and relations within a symbolic design (Ibid). Thus symbolic meaning is formal meaning, meaning pertaining to form. To what extent is nursing's meaning understood to be a language or system of symbols, a symbolic design of form and relations? It is not unusual to hear that the central project of nursing is communication—the act of becoming one with—whether in discursive or nondiscursive forms, verbal or nonverbal. Nursing scholars such as Hildegard Peplau, Ida Orlando, and Joyce Travelbee have proposed that communication in the form of relationship is what nursing is all about. In the theory of *Nursing as Caring* (2001), Boykin and I have modified Paterson and Zderad's (1988) concept of "the between." We have written that the living expression of nursing happens in the "caring between"—a phenomenal space, a loving relationship. We have even postulated that without the "caring between," there is no true nursing.

Since the mid-1970s in the United States, some nurses have viewed the meaning of nursing and its central project to be a symbolic system termed "the nursing process." In the

United Kingdom, Roper, Logan, and Tierney (1985) entered the fray with their nursing model called The Nursing Process. And although the centrality and even the value of the idea of nursing as a sequential process are widely disputed, I think we must acknowledge that our literature continues to proclaim nursing process as central to the meaning of nursing. Out of curiosity, I searched CINAHL for the term *nursing process*, restricted to the year 2002. I retrieved 48 titles from countries scattered literally all over the globe, from Australia, Brazil, and China to India, Nigeria, and Spain, to Sweden, Slovenia, South Africa, and Uruguay—powerful evidence that this symbolic system of nursing process has swept the nursing world and is giving a widely accepted voice to a view of nursing's meaning in symbolic form. I will have more to say about nursing process and nursing meaning in the final section of this chapter.

This brief excursion into symbolics as a realm of meaning for nursing recognizes that language, both verbal and nonverbal, makes an important contribution to nursing as a cultural enterprise. Let me now examine empirics as a possible pattern for nursing's meaning.

Empirics

In introducing empirics as a realm of meaning, Phenix (1964) acknowledges that although symbolics are employed to *express* empirical meaning, the symbols used do not *constitute* empirical knowledge per se. Empirics as a pattern of meaning is concerned with matters of fact, with fact understood as "particular data of observation" (Phenix, 1964, p. 99). The various sciences are the empirical disciplines, and they have as their collective project abstract descriptions "of different aspects of the experienced world" (p. 96), advancing theoretical understandings—that is, making meaning. Facts independent of a system of meaning are irrelevant; however, facts within a created system of meaning provide the stuff of further refinement of meaning expressions.

Nursing as a field of knowledge and practice was initially formalized largely through the leadership of Florence Nightingale. Empirics was crucial to the meaning nursing had for Nightingale. For example, her advocacy of light as an important element in a healing environment is based in part on her having noticed that patients tended to lie with their faces toward the sunlight (Todaro-Franceschi, 2001). Although Nightingale understood nursing practice as a calling, nursing knowledge was developed initially with an emphasis on the empirical—the deliberate gathering of facts for organization into a meaningful theoretical framework. The meaning of nursing as science was a major focal point of scholarly work in the decades of the 1970s through the 1990s. Carper's 1978 work on patterns of knowing fundamental to nursing clearly drew on Phenix's *Realms of Meaning* as a foundational text, and empirical knowing was one of the four patterns that Carper identified from her analysis of the nursing literature. It is widely accepted that nursing is an enterprise whose central meaning resides within the empirical realm. Nursing's meaning as science is debated today primarily in terms of which science—natural science or human science—with all kinds of labels thrown into the mix to try to get a firm, defensible fix on just what kind of science nursing is.

Although the late 1960s through the early 1990s was a time of active push-pull between nursing as science and nursing as ontology, the scientists have pretty well won out for the time being. The literature of the 1970s and even the 1980s was replete with fervent and fervid analyses of the question "Is nursing a science?" but thankfully we rarely hear that rhetorical plea today. In my scope of acquaintance and observation these days, even nurses in practice settings have begun to internalize the view that nursing is a science and that the practice of nursing is an applied science. In my own work, I have given some credence to the idea of nursing as science through the development of several approaches to nursing inquiry from the perspective of the theory of nursing as caring. However, while empirics is and always has been a characteristic meaning pattern of formal nursing, I submit that it is not the only pattern of meaning nor the most encompassing. Let's move on now to explore aesthetics as a potential realm of meaning for nursing.

Aesthetics

Phenix (1964) says that the chief distinction between esthetics as a meaning pattern and the meaning patterns of symbolics and empirics is that symbolics and science are both general, whereas esthetics is particular. In esthetics "The primary concern is not with types of things but with unique individual objects" (p. 142). "Meanings in the arts are ideal abstractions presented in particular created works" (p. 194). Phenix further asserts, "Esthetic meanings are gained by *acquaintance* and not by *description*" (p. 142). Esthetic understanding is immediate, directly perceived, rather than being mediated by concepts or propositions. Phenix tells us, "The successful artist is the one who *thinks well with the characteristic materials* of that field" (p. 154). Furthermore, cultivation of an immediate perception of the possibilities of the materials is best gained through actual practice. "Mastery in the arts grows out of prolonged imaginative experimentation with the material" (p. 155) as the materials are put together in patterned wholes (p. 156). "The meaning of a work of art consists in what its organized materials uniquely express" (p. 164).

How do all these ideas about esthetics comport with what we know of nursing? Although Nightingale emphasized the importance of empirics in nursing, she viewed nursing as an artful practice as well. Wiedenbach, in her 1964 book *Clinical Nursing: A Helping Art,* provided a formal conceptualization of nursing as art. A quote from that book graces the Web site dedicated to Wiedenbach's work. This quote reflects some of Phenix's thinking about art. Wiedenbach is quoted as saying "My thesis is that nursing art is not comprised of rational nor reactionary actions but rather of deliberative action" (*http:// healthsci.clayton.edu/eichelberger/wiedenbach.htm; retrieved September 16, 2008*). This quote from Wiedenbach connects with Phenix's exposition of esthetics as a realm of meaning in Wiedenbach's (1964) use of the term "deliberative action" and in Phenix's message of imaginative experimentation. It also connects with the idea of the successful artist as one who thinks well with the materials of his or her art.

Regardless of how we might evaluate Barbara Carper's (1978) work, initially in her doctoral dissertation and then published in the inaugural issue of *Advances in Nursing Science*, I think there is no question that her work, supported by Chinn and Kramer's (1999) book *Theory in Nursing,* launched a significant line of the development of aesthetics in nursing. On a personal note, I still have a very clear recollection of the moment over 20 years ago when I read Carper's *ANS* paper and experienced an "aha," a sense of liberation. The "aha," came primarily from the acknowledgement that aesthetic knowing was not only worthwhile but was actually an essential way of knowing in nursing.

In a critique of Carper's work, which I jointly authored with my colleagues Anne Boykin and Marilyn Parker, we expressed the view that, of Carper's four patterns of knowing (personal, empirical, ethical and aesthetic), it is the aesthetic pattern that encompasses the other three and permits an understanding that integrates and supersedes formerly competing claims of nursing as art/nursing as science (Boykin, Parker, & Schoenhofer, 1994). My involvement with practicing nurses has made it clear to me that the value of aesthetic understanding of nursing far supersedes that of the empirical at the grassroots level of the profession. To support this claim, I offer an early example and a recent example. The early example is *Nightingale Songs*, an "occasional paper" in which nurses share aesthetic expressions about their nursing. *Nightingale Songs* was conceived by my colleague Marilyn Parker and me and began publication on May 12, 1990. A more recent exposure to aesthetic expressions of the meaning of nursing to nurses is through the publication *The Heart and Hand of Nursing: A Collection of Poems*, published in 2003 by the University of Wisconsin-Madison Nurses' Alumni Organization. Although nursing's meaning is well characterized by the aesthetic pattern, other patterns apply as well.

Synnoetics

Phenix (1964) coined the term *synnoetics* to refer to "meanings in which a person has direct insight into other beings (or oneself) as concrete wholes existing in relation" (p. 193). At the time of Phenix's writing, synnoetics, along with ethics [to be addressed in a subsequent section], was not traditionally included in the subject areas with their own constituencies; however, Phenix considered synnoetics and ethics to be the most essential realms of meaning—most essential "because they deal with elemental human meanings that sustain all other knowledge....go[ing] most directly to the core of personhood and color[ing] every type of understanding" (p. 188). Synnoetics is distinct from the three preceding patterns of meaning (symbolics, empirics, aesthetics) in that knowledge development in the former requires detachment in the sense of subject-to-object relationship, whereas synnoetics requires engagement, subject-to-subject relationship, and intersubjectivity. Synnoetic meanings are concrete; they are not transformations of some other complete experience, but a "prototype of experience in its wholeness or concreteness" (p. 194). And Phenix, drawing on Michael Polyani, points out that tacit knowing is a personal act, not a formal operation. While symbolics, empirics, and aesthetics are concerned with essences, according to Phenix, synnoetics is existential, having to do with being itself, with concrete existence, with being in relation.

I would not be surprised if some consider synnoetics as just a special case of empirics; that view has its proponents. Even the research arm of the Institute of Noetic Sciences and nurse scientists working within the framework of the Science of Unitary Human Beings seem to be walking both sides of this street, with their efforts to demonstrate energy and energy fields as the operational construct in studies of intuition, therapeutic touch, and other occurrences—occurrences that some might consider as having a personal or tacit meaning, and therefore as unavailable for empirical knowing. Nursing conceptualizers like Parse (1981) and Roach (1987) draw on the work of Martin Buber, particularly the notion of "I-Thou" as an expression of personal relation as *the*, or at least *a*, seat of meaning for nursing. Subjectivity, and more accurately, intersubjectivity are important ideas associated with meaning that is synnoetic in character.

To make the claim that nursing meaning is most characteristically expressed in the synnoetic or personal realm may or may not be absurd, depending on one's presuppositions. While direct-practice nurses more and more refer to empirics as a primary pattern of nursing meaning, many acknowledge that personal insight and intuition are often final arbiters of their practice. There are many instances in the literature and in professional dialogue in which nurses refer to this insight and intuition as indispensable to their practice. As I mentioned earlier in this section, some may argue that insight and intuition are simply products of an as-yet-not-understood process that can eventually be recognized empirically. However, because I accept the "value added" contribution of personal knowing, I would not be one to make that argument. A growing emphasis on the inclusion of "experiential learning," "self-awareness," and personal relating in nursing education supports the view that nurse educators value this realm of meaning too. I will have more to say in relation to synnoetics and nursing education in the final section of this chapter. Let's now turn briefly to ethics as a realm of meaning.

Ethics

Phenix (1964) says that the essence of ethical meanings, or of moral knowledge, is "right deliberate action, or that which a person ought voluntarily to do" (p. 215). Ethics is concerned with value, rather than with fact: "The ethical realm of meaning is a realm of decision, commitment and engagement" (p. 220). Phenix holds that right action, although a personal, concrete, committed decision, refers ultimately to a general, universal principle of right. As Phenix puts it, morality is everybody's business and it enters into every department of life.

The American Nurses Association has long promulgated a code of ethics for nurses. A universal ethical code for Chinese nurses has recently been developed, led by the work of Professor Samantha Pang of Hong Kong Polytechnic University, and the Chinese Nurses Association. Professor Marilyn Parker of Florida Atlantic University is presently supporting Thai nurses in a similar enterprise. Although you may have strong criticisms of the nursing theories originated by Watson and by Boykin and me, I think you would agree that both of these theories explicitly ground the meaning of nursing practice in ethics. All in all, nurses recognize nursing as a moral enterprise and seek to craft significant expressions that portray ethics as a characteristic pattern of nursing meaning.

Synoptics

Thus far, I have briefly addressed Phenix's first five realms of meaning and have attempted in survey fashion to show that each realm has been considered a characteristic pattern of nursing's meaning. I would now like to begin to construct the argument that nursing's meaning can be considered synoptic in pattern and then to explain why I think that is a useful perspective to hold.

Phenix (1964) writes that synoptic meanings have an "*integrative* function, uniting meanings from all the realms into a unified perspective, that is, providing a single vision or synopsis of meanings" (p. 235). Phenix associates certain disciplines or subjects with each of the realms to illustrate characteristic meaning patterns. The disciplines he uses to explicate the synoptic realm are history, religion, and philosophy. However, he does clearly state that the disciplines he mentions are not meant to be an exhaustive list. Therefore, I think that I am not misusing his work as I talk about the synoptic character of nursing's meaning.

It is time now to return to my explicit perspective of nursing, that which is expressed in the theory of nursing as caring. From that perspective, nursing is not exclusively or even predominantly about sickness, nor is it about brokenness, nor suffering; nursing is not understood to have a "fix-it" focus or purpose. Neither is nursing about health or wellness. In my 31-year career in nursing, which began in the late 1960s and early 1970s, at a time when the concept of wellness was sweeping the world, I have time and again seen that when health and/or wellness are used as concepts to transcend a focus on illness and disease, the explications always get back, one way or another, to the reciprocal: illness and disease. As I have experienced and conceptualized nursing through a career that has taken me to many practice settings as practitioner, teacher, and researcher, I have come to understand that nursing is about living human life—not *about* human life, in the general, abstract sense, but about *living* human life— the day-to-day, personal and interpersonal valuing, deciding, and acting that is living. Nursing, in the form of interest, knowledge development, and participation, ranges over the whole course of human living. I think it was this realization of the scope of nursing that opened the way to my attraction to the idea of caring as the core of what it means to be human, and thus as the central project of nursing. At any moment, for any purpose, nurses in any field of nursing (practical or conceptual) can focus on meaning patterns from any one or several patterns of nursing meaning. When nurses function too inflexibly from within a single pattern or a partial grouping of patterns, critique arises as the pendulum swings: too much focus on science to the detriment of personal relationship, too much emphasis on intangibles like intuition and value to the detriment of empirical systematization, and so forth.

Ascribing to the synoptic realm of meaning can help to promote creative discourse within various emphases in nursing. Taking a synoptic view of the meaning of nursing could mean that differing positions and competing areas of focus could be welcomed as belonging rather than rejected as erroneous or irrelevant. Scholars, thinkers, and philosophers of nursing, giving the broadest possible latitude in describing the meaning of nursing, could perhaps surmount apparent incongruities and discover or create new, more integrative truths. Knowledge workers are attempting to transcend currently dichotomous philosophies of nursing science, and although the call for triangulation and blending is not working well, its failure is demonstrating that transcendent thinking is needed. Complexity theory has shown some promise in this regard.

From my perspective, the synoptic value of articulated conceptualizations of nursing, what Kikuchi (1999) calls philosophic nursing theories (and what others have called nursing models), has not yet been widely realized in nursing. To some extent, the literature has been bogged down in what became largely technical arguments about denotations and connotations, and then arguments against the labeled materials. By the same token, what some have declared to be fraudulent self-aggrandizement on the part of individual theoreticians has led to what seems to be unexamined rejection of the ideas themselves. Meanwhile, the value of articulated synoptic visions of nursing has not been sufficiently explored in nursing scholarship, practice, and education. Just as there is yet unmined value in addressing the relevance of Phenix's realms of meaning, there are two particular works I want to mention that have not been sufficiently understood and incorporated into nursing as a structure for meaning. The first of these works is the classic text *Concept Formalization in Nursing: Process and Product*, written by the Orem study group in 1979. Granted, some technical ideas espoused therein are passé; however, there is significant value there that has not yet been grasped in nursing. The second work that could help us realize the synoptic value of the philosophical nursing theories was written by Pamela Reed in *ANS* in 1995, the work entitled "A Treatise on Nursing Knowledge Development for the 21st Century: Beyond Postmodernism." One of the services that Reed provides in this work is suggesting *how* nursing theories might be useful as philosophical orientation and grounding. The large cadre of nursing-knowledge workers today have specialization in their experience, specialization in one or more of the realms of meaning, even specialization in one or more *branches* of a single realm. Some of the works I have commended to you have been around for three decades, and

I do commend them because I think that perhaps the time is ripe now for a swing of the pendulum toward an interest in integration, in synoptics. The specialists have so much to bring to a new synoptic understanding of nursing, and a synoptic understanding can extend context and meaning for the work of the specialists. Part of what I have tried to suggest is that structures for integration are already available, in the philosophic theories of nursing. Not all of the philosophic theories of nursing will survive, and new, superseding ones will emerge. But each of the so-called extant theories of nursing offers an integrating statement of the meaning of nursing that is valued by a significant cadre of nursing, and a structure for elaborating on that meaning.

How might the synoptic perspective of the meaning of nursing be useful in nursing education enterprises? The most important contribution, of course, would be to a broad generosity of thought, facilitating the energizing tension of freedom and anchor—freedom to explore in novel directions and anchoring orientation to dynamic, meaningful purpose.

Let me just touch on a couple of vulnerable and rather ubiquitous sacred cows of nursing education.

- Basing nursing education programs on a symbolic system such as nursing process rather than on synoptic meaning leaves the student nurse without orientation to a central organizing purpose for operating the process.
- Overemphasis on critical thinking as *a set of procedures* is a limiting-empirics approach, without a synoptic-meaning frame that would give purpose to the critical thinking.
- Teaching nursing as a set of highly skilled and systematized operations rather than as a discipline of valuing, knowing, and living leaves nurses in a diaspora. There *is* no home to come home to, no common ground of meaning, no synoptic grasp of nursing's meaning.
- An overemphasis on empirics as the most valued realm of nursing meaning is accompanied by downplaying other patterns of meaning that are necessary to an understanding of the fullness of nursing. Meaning patterns like intuition and aesthetics in particular are

downplayed or completely passed over; approaches taken to ethical meaning are, by and large, leaden and mechanical. A synoptic commitment from educators would assist nurses in exploring all of nursing and in creating novel meaning. And perhaps that possibility of creating novel meaning is, in itself, a threat?

Concluding Statements

I would like to end this chapter by suggesting some ways in which taking the perspective of nursing as synoptic in meaning may bring a welcome transformation to practice.

Mature nurses in practice and administrative positions frequently complain about the loss of critical thinking in the nursing profession. That complaint often translates to an explanation that although nurses who were educated more recently have a great depth of knowledge about technical issues related to nursing care, they frequently do not see the forest for the trees and cannot make good decisions. This complaint seems to be a plea for the synoptic perspective of the meaning of nursing.

Practice environments tend to emphasize piecework and attention to technology, leading to considerable demoralization. A synoptic perspective of nursing as a life-affirming enterprise could help provide nurses with the grounding necessary to effectively advocate for increased freedom and true responsibility in the practice setting. I have seen this happen.

I have attempted to explore the fit of Phenix's various realms of meaning with the meaning of nursing, and then to sketch out a beginning argument for the adoption of a synoptic perspective for nursing. I have made the claim that the various philosophical nursing theories offer synoptic statements about nursing's meaning. It is my hope that this presentation will stimulate a reawakening of discourse about the scope of nursing—discourse that can be taken to a new level through the enriching experience of the last 30 years of specialization. Discourse can then be taken toward a new and renewed commitment to the creation of satisfying and useful synoptic expressions of the meaning of nursing.

References

Boykin, A., Parker, M., & Schoenhofer, S. O. (1994). Aesthetic knowing grounded in an explicit conception of nursing. *Nursing Science Quarterly, 7,* 158–161.

Boykin, A., & Schoenhofer, S. O. (2001). *Nursing as caring: A model for transforming practice.* Sudbury, CT: Jones & Bartlett.

Carper, B. A. (1978). Fundamental patterns of knowing in nursing. *Advances in Nursing Science, 1*(1), 13–24.

Chinn, P. A., & Kramer, M. K. (1999). *Theory and nursing: Integrated knowledge development* (5th ed.). St. Louis: Mosby.

Kikuchi, J. F. (1999). The nature of conceptualizations about nursing. *Canadian Journal of Nursing Research, 30*(4), 115–128.

Orem, D. E. (Ed.). (1979). *Concept formalization in nursing: Process and product.* Boston: Little, Brown.

Parse, R. R. (1981). *Man—living—health: A theory of nursing.* New York: Wiley.

Paterson, J. G., & Zderad, L. T. (1988). *Humanistic nursing.* New York: NLN Press.

Phenix, P. H. (1964). *Realms of meaning.* New York: McGraw-Hill.

Reed, P. G. (1995). A treatise on nursing knowledge development for the 21st century: Beyond postmodernism. *Advances in Nursing Science, 17*(3), 70–84.

Roach, M. S. (1987). *The human act of caring.* Ottawa, ONT: Canadian Hospital Association.

Roper, N., Logan, W., & Tierney, A. (1985). *Elements of nursing.* Edinburgh: Churchill Livingstone.

Todaro-Franceschi, V. (2001). Energy: A bridging concept for nursing science. *Nursing Science Quarterly, 14,* 132–140.

University of Wisconsin-Madison Nurses' Alumni Organization, Eds. (2003). *The heart and hands of nursing: A collection of poems.* Madison, WI: University of Wisconsin-Madison Nurses' Alumni Organization.

Weidenbach, E. (1964). *Clinical nursing: A helping art.* NY: Springer.

"With the Very Best of Intentions": The Development of Nursing Process as a Way of Knowing

3

Lynne M. Dunphy

Chapter Overview

This chapter approaches the emergence of the concept of nursing diagnosis, the use of the nursing process for decision-making in nursing, and the justifications for the development of nursing classification systems structured around the nursing process in their historical context. Because these developments occurred during the latter half of the 20th century, they are examined within the context of the medical thought of the time, and their influence on changing ideas in education, especially concerning curriculum. Here, nursing knowledge is contextually situated and explained as such. This chapter portrays some of the foundations that motivated the concepts mentioned above—concepts often obscured over time as they became institutionalized. The author makes the case that nursing is a discipline of knowledge with a history and that this history is an important link to interpretations of subsequent knowledge development.

Introduction

In preparing this chapter, I reflected on my own nursing education in a hospital-based diploma program in the late 1960s and early 1970s. Nothing about the "nursing process" surfaced in my memories. Nor could I recall doing "nursing care plans," although once I began teaching nursing in the mid-1980s my teaching life, as prescribed by the curriculum, became rapidly consumed with these care plans, lengthy things that students labored over for hours. I do distinctly recall a series of staff in-service education sessions when I was a staff RN in the late 1970s explaining this process but can recall little else. Thus, I was amazed to discover, as I began to search the literature, articles as early as 1953 on nursing diagnosis (Hornung, 1953; Fry, 1953). The purpose of this chapter is to situate the development and emergence of nursing process as a way of knowing in nursing practice and education in its sociohistorical context. The case is made that the development and formalization of "the nursing process" and its attendant strategy of "nursing diagnosis" have been a response/reaction to certain broader societal mandates. Concerns of other professional disciplines that have long influenced nursing, medicine, and education come into play. Awareness of the context of knowledge development and structure is critical to a full understanding and evaluation of that knowledge. This chapter assumes nursing diagnosis as a key component of the nursing process.

The term *nursing process* has become a broad rubric, with many and various meanings and usages. Murray and Atkinson's (2000) book *Understanding the Nursing Process in a Changing Care Environment* defines the nursing process as the "way one thinks like a nurse" and identifies the nursing process as "the foundation, the essential, enduring skill that has characterized nursing from the beginning of the profession" (p. 2).

According to these authors, the nursing process is divided into six steps: assessment, diagnosis, outcome identification, planning, implementation, and evaluation. They relate these steps to a form of "scientific problem solving" (p. 3) and see the nurse as using these steps in every interaction with a patient, no matter how brief. It is speculated that the nurse has so internalized the process that he or she is unaware of using separate steps. These authors also identify the emergence of managed care and the emphasis on quality as two other forces that underpin the need for nursing process, calling it a "tool for nurses in all settings to use to continually evaluate and improve the quality of nursing care" (p. 5).

According to Lynda Carpenito-Moyet (2006), the term *nursing diagnosis* was introduced in a 1953 article by Vera Fry, published in the *American Journal of Nursing*, entitled "The Creative Approach to Nursing" to describe a step necessary in developing a nursing care plan (p. 4). Carpenito-Moyet (2006) makes the point that before the development of a taxonomy of nursing diagnoses, nurses used "whatever word they wanted to describe client problems" (p. 4). She also makes the case that a taxonomy of diagnoses for nursing defines the body of knowledge for which nursing is held accountable. She references the American Nurses Association's (ANA) 1973 *Standards of Nursing Practice* and ANA's *Social Policy Statement* (1980) as establishing nursing as "the diagnosis and treatment of human responses to actual or potential health problems" (p. 4). The revised Social Policy Statement (ANA, 1995) identified four essential aspects of nursing practice that include the following:

1. Nursing includes attention to the full range of human experiences and responses to health and illness, without restriction to a problem-focused orientation.
2. Nursing integrates objective data with the knowledge gained from an understanding of the patient's subjective experience.
3. Nursing includes the application of scientific knowledge to the processes of diagnosis and treatment.
4. Nursing provides a caring relationship that facilitates health and healing.

The 1995 revised Social Policy Statement reaffirms the 1980 statement that "nursing is the diagnosis and treatment of human responses to actual or potential health problems" (ANA, 1995, p. 9) and further elaborates, "Diagnoses facilitate communication among health care providers and the recipients of care and provide for initial direction in choice of treatments and subsequent evaluation of the outcomes of care (Ibid). The ANA's 1998 *Standards of Clinical Nursing Practice*, which define the responsibilities of all registered nurses engaged in clinical practice, are structured around the categories of assessment, diagnosis, outcome identification, planning, implementation, and evaluation. ANA and more than 15 specialty organizations jointly developed these standards. Many state-implemented nurse practice acts describe nursing legally as in accordance with these definitions. The 1999 Joint Commission on Accreditation of Healthcare Organizations (JCAHO) standards also build on aspects of the nursing process, specifically assessment, reassessment, and periodic evaluation.

The ninth conference of the North American Nursing Diagnosis Association (NANDA) approved an official definition of nursing diagnosis (NANDA, 1992): "Nursing diagnosis is a clinical judgment about individual, family, or community responses to actual or potential health problems/life processes. Nursing diagnosis provides the basis for selection of nursing interventions to achieve outcomes for which the nurse is held accountable" (p. 10).

Background

The first conference on nursing diagnosis was held in 1973 to create the groundwork for a classification system of nursing knowledge that would be amenable to computerization. As a result of this conference, the National Group for the Classification of Nursing Diagnosis was formed, composed of nurses from different regions of the United States and Canada, and representing practice, education, and research. This group took the lead in developing a standardized language, or classification system, for the human responses that nurses treat. This group continued to meet through a series of invitational conferences and, by 1982, produced an alphabetical list of 50 nursing diagnoses accepted for clinical testing. The third national conference saw the creation of an initial theorist group concerned with the development of a conceptual framework for the emerging diagnostic classification system.

In 1985, a formal taxonomy committee was appointed to draft a conceptual framework that would provide a classification schema for the diagnoses, or taxonomy, based on human-response patterns. The work of the committee resulted in Taxonomy I, which comprised nine categories of human responses. This work was presented and approved, along with 21 new nursing diagnoses, at the next national conference (McLane, 1987). Taxonomy I was submitted to the World Health Organization (WHO) for inclusion in the 10th version of the International Classification of Diseases in 1989. It was not accepted (Fitzpatrick et al., 1989). A Taxonomy II was proposed at the 1990 conference, but no consensus was reached on its acceptance. Indeed the 10th, 11th, and 12th conferences were scenes of continued debate about the proposed structure for the taxonomy. The research team of Gloria M. Bulechek and Joanne C. McClosky of the University of Iowa College of Nursing formed a collaborative agreement for a joint venture with NANDA to continue to extend the work of NANDA, with the stated goal of improving the comprehensiveness, scope, and clinical usefulness of the NANDA taxonomy (Craft-Rosenberg & Delaney, 1997).

Two important works were published concurrently in 1985: *Nursing Interventions: Treatments* (Bulechek & McCloskey, 1985) and *Independent Nursing Interventions* (Snyder, 1985). Both texts proposed "nursing interventions"—essentially, nurse-initiated treatments—as symbolic concepts that required a series of actions for implementation in response to a nursing diagnosis. These works paved the way for the publication in 1992 of the *Nursing Interventions Classification* (*NIC*), the first volume of 336 nursing interventions made up of a nursing label (diagnosis), a definition, and a set of activities for implementation, with appropriate references. This standardized, comprehensive language to describe nursing treatments or interventions was developed by the research team of Bulechek and McCloskey as part of the Center for Nursing Classification at the University of Iowa College of Nursing and was funded by the National Institutes of Health, National Institute for Nursing Research. As described in Bulechek and McCloskey (1999), this research, which originally began in 1987, went through three phases: Phase I, construction of the classification; Phase II, construction of the taxonomy; and Phase III, clinical testing and refinement using multiple research methods. The first phase used a more inductive approach to develop the classification, with Phase II, Construction of the Taxonomy, relying on more quantitative methods such as similarity analysis, hierarchical clustering, and multidimensional scaling (Bulechek & McCloskey, 1999, p. 11). Phase III involved clinical field testing.

Closely tied to the nursing intervention classification system (NIC) has been the development of nursing outcomes classification (NOC). Using a research process similar to that used in the development of NIC, a second research team at the University of Iowa, headed by Marion Johnson and Meridean Maas and funded by Sigma Theta Tau International and NINR, developed a classification of patient-care outcomes sensitive to nursing care. Outcomes are defined as "behaviors, responses and feelings of the patient in response to the care provided" and serve as the criteria against which to judge the success of a nursing intervention (Bulechek & McCloskey, 1999, p. 13).

In 2000, NANDA approved a new Taxonomy II, which encompassed 13 domains, 106 classes, and 155 diagnoses (NANDA, 2001). The domains include the following:

- Health promotion
- Nutrition
- Elimination
- Activity/rest
- Perception/cognition
- Self-perception
- Role relationships
- Sexuality
- Coping/stress tolerance
- Life principles
- Safety/protection
- Comfort
- Growth/development

The second level, classes, is considered useful for assessment criteria, and the third level, diagnostic concepts, considered the most useful for clinicians, is the nursing diagnosis labels (Carpenito-Moyet, 2006, p. 6).

Issues

Confusion arises over the nature of nursing diagnosis. Is it a process or outcome? For example, a nursing diagnosis may be the second step in the nursing process, in which the nurse analyzes data collected during assessment and evaluation of the client's health status. However, not all the data that a professional nurse collects during the assessment phase, or the concerns identified, lead to a "nursing" diagnosis; identified problems may require treatment by professionals from a number of different disciplines, such as medicine. Carpenito-Moyet (2006) recommends using the term *diagnosis* when discussing the second step of the nursing process, and using the terms *diagnostic label* or *nursing diagnosis* when describing health states that nurses legally diagnose and treat (p. 5).

When moving into the area of treatment or the nursing intervention, a primary consideration is to identify one that will help the patient move toward one or more desired outcomes. When discussing the selection of a nursing intervention, Bulechek and McCloskey (1999) suggest that a variety of factors come into play, although they do cite the desired patient outcome as the most important (p. 14). The nature of the nursing diagnosis itself is also seen as critically important, the intent being to direct the intervention toward altering the related factors (the etiology) of the diagnosis. If the underlying cause (etiology) is correctly identified during the nursing-assessment phase of the nursing process, and if the intervention is successful in altering the cause, the patient's status should improve and/or change. This improvement, ideally, can be measured by a change in the outcome criteria associated with the diagnosis. The feasibility of successfully implementing the intervention, the acceptability of the intervention to the patient, and the capability of the nurse are also all considered important in successfully implementing nursing interventions. Psychomotor and/or interpersonal skills are necessary in implementing many interventions, as well as the ability of the professional nurse to effectively use health care resources. The patient's values, beliefs, and culture must be considered in selecting the appropriate nursing intervention.

There has been continuing controversy about the use of physiological diagnoses in the taxonomy, given that this type of diagnosis is usually more impacted by medical care. Also, given the philosophical claim of health promotion as a basis for nursing practice, how can this wellness perspective be factored into what is essentially a problem-identification and problem-solving approach? In addition, given the fluctuating nature of human responses, the associated diagnostic categories are much more fluid and changeable than, for example, medical diagnostic categories.

A Confluence of Factors and Compelling Reasons

Sources from the 1970s to the 2000s were relatively consistent on the need for a "nursing classification system." Such a development was seen as essential in documenting and clearly defining an explicit base of nursing practice. A consensus of forces within organized nursing, including the ANA and the International Council of Nurses (ICN), endorsed the need for a standardized language in the areas of diagnoses, interventions, and outcomes. It was thought that as nursing's ability to link diagnoses, interventions, and outcomes grew, middle-range theories for nursing practice would evolve (Blegen & Tripp-Reimer, 1997). A number of compelling reasons lay behind these arguments, including the theory that standardized databases would provide ongoing evaluation and documentation of nursing's effectiveness in achieving patient-care outcomes.

Nursing documentation, however, had not been systematically organized to advance nursing knowledge or to develop nursing practice. R. D. Zielstroff (1984) identified deficiencies in nursing's knowledge base as the major stumbling block to the development of computerized nursing information systems. Subsequently, a 1988 Conference on Research Priorities in Nursing Science sponsored by the National Center for Nursing Research (now the National Institute for Nursing Research [NINR]) identified the development of nursing information systems as a high priority (Hinshaw, 1988). This identification helped lay the groundwork for the subsequent funding of NIC and NOC at the University of Iowa College of Nursing.

The emergence of guidelines for patient management based on scientific evidence and expert opinion was another impetus to the development of a nursing classification system, or at least a more systematized approach to nursing knowledge. In 1990, an ad hoc advisory panel of nurses to the Agency for Health Care Policy and Research (AHCPR—now the Agency for Healthcare Quality and Research [AHQR]) concluded that the purpose of guidelines "is to guide practice by providing linkages among diagnoses, treatments, and outcomes" (AHCPR, 1990).

Another widely cited use of nursing classification systems was to facilitate the teaching of decision making to nursing students. Clinical judgment and critical thinking in nursing began to be widely used terms and the need was emphasized for students to have electronic access to information systems and databases from actual clinical practice situations in order to enhance clinical judgment abilities. Physician reimbursement was driven by the American Medical Association's codification of physician services in the form of the manual *Physician's Current Procedural Terminology* (CPT) as well as the *International Classification of Diseases* (ICD). In reality, nurses often performed some of the procedures for which physicians are paid (Griffith, Thomas, & Griffith, 1991). There was consensus that nursing needed an accepted "coding" system that would capture nursing treatments for reimbursement to nurses by third-party payers (Bulechek & McCloskey, 1999). Several critical health data sets were developed in the 1990s under the auspices of the National Committee on Vital and Health Statistics, notably, the Uniform Hospital Discharge Data Set (UHDDS), the Ambulatory Medical Care Minimum Data Set, and the Long-Term Health Care Minimum Data Set, none of which are representative of nursing practice.

Existing data sets and classification systems that are instrumental in defining United States health care policies did not reflect nursing data. Thus the reasons for the development of nursing classification systems, rooted in nursing diagnoses, interventions (NIC), and outcomes (NOC), all of which were arrived at or determined through some manifestations of the nursing process, were clearly compelling. These developments, however, must be viewed in context.

The Context of 20th-Century Medicine

Medical diagnosis and treatment seem to have always been with us. It is difficult to recall sometimes how recent these developments really are. In addition, far from being written in stone, medical diagnostic categories and therapeutics frequently morph or change into new modes of being. The Diagnostic and Statistical Manual of Mental Disorders, 4th edition (DSM-IV), originally published in 1994, underwent a text revision in 2000 but has failed to have a whole new edition published, as debates regarding "spectrums" of disorders and "dual-diagnosis" rage. In reality, medical "science" as we know it is a recent phenomenon, and medical taxonomies did not really begin in any real way until the late 18th and early 19th centuries.

John Pickstone (2000), historian of science, technology, and medicine, discusses "ways of knowing" that are interconnected and nonlinear, although one mode may dominate in certain periods over another. He sees these "ways of knowing" as transcending specific disciplines, but nonetheless, they have significance when tracing the development of knowledge in medicine. Pickstone (2000) identifies these ways of knowing as "world-readings (hermeneutics), natural history, analysis, experimentation, and technoscience" (p. xi). World-readings are akin to natural philosophy but include human creations and refer to "'de-coding' of the world and to the systems of meaning found there" (p. 8). Natural history, for example, is about the describing and classification of phenomena, a phase that medicine pursued when it began to describe signs and symptoms clusters and naming pathological states, or diseases. Analyzing is about breaking things into various elements, such as germ layers, cells, and chemical elements, in the case of medicine, organs, and tissues. Experimenting is where we control phenomena, such as in randomized, controlled, blinded studies. Pickstone is especially interested in demonstrating how ways of knowing are linked to ways of production—to ways of making things. He elaborates, "Or to ways of tending and mending (in agriculture and medicine), or of defending or destroying (military science and technologies)" (p. 3), with particular emphasis on the ways in which knowledge is built into commodities or other products, such as pharmaceuticals.

Edmund D. Pellegrino (1980) states, "Nothing more clearly sets contemporary medicine apart from its antecedents than its remarkable therapeutic effectiveness," noting that physicians now intervene, "specifically and radically," in the natural history of previously fatal diseases: "No disorder, however complex or intractable, is beyond the possibility of conquest" (p. 245). In reviewing a history of medicine in general, one is struck by the transition from the 19th-century notion of health as balance, which had grounded medicine since Greek times, to the emerging idea of diseases as discrete clinical entities. An early challenge to the idea of illness as a whole-body phenomenon came from Thomas Sydenham's (1724–1689) insistence on a nosology of disease based on observation and reason rather than on all-embracing systems of ultimate causes (Lourdon, 1997). Although his writing was reminiscent of Hippocrates' in its insistence on observation, he sought to group cases with similar symptoms into classes, creating identifiable clinical entities. He also believed that therapy could be improved by careful observation of the patient's responses to treatment, thus leading to validation of specific remedies.

Almost a century after Sydenham, the great anatomist G. B. Morgagni (1682–1771) provided tangible evidence that clinical illness could be anatomically localized—in other words, that external signs and symptoms of diseases might be correlated with internal lesions on specific organs. The trend toward etiological discreteness in medicine was extended by Xavier Bichat (1771–1802), founder of the "Paris School," to specific tissues, and extended still further by Rudolf Virchow (1821–1902) to the cellular level, and by Linus Pauling (1901–1994) to the molecular level (Lourdon, 1997). It has now been extended even further to the genome. According to Pellegrino (1980), "The modern concepts of molecular, subcellular, and biochemical pathology are extensions of this search for morphological substrata for the symptomatic manifestations and natural history of disease" (p. 251). Shades of Pickstone categorizations of knowing are heard throughout (Pickstone, 2000).

At the end of the 19th century, many physicians were still loath to give up old understandings in favor of the new conception of a type of therapeutics specifically tailored to particular disease entities. Advancements in anesthesia, surgery, chemistry, and pharmaceuticals, however, tipped the balance in favor "of the discrete and radical in therapeutics" (Pellegrino, 1980, p. 247). The 21st century promises to continue this trend toward ever-greater specificity in medicine, with the potential capability of effecting cures at the genetic loci of diseases, as well as the identification of medicine with its technical armamentarium This movement toward ever-greater specificity is consistent with Pickstone's description of technoscience. It is clear that the successes of modern medicine—indeed, 20th-century progress in general—were rooted in positivism and reductionism. Ultimate causes for diseases were sought in the basic sciences such as chemistry and physics, and now are sought in genetics. To quote Pellegrino (1980), "The success of these efforts has revived the dreams of seventeenth-century Cartesians—the iatrochemists and iatrophysicists—who first sought ulti-mate explanations for disease in mathematical and scientific terms" (p. 257). It is not hard to see the jump to classification systems of diseases: the ICD and CPT codes for billing and reimbursement. In addition, given the stunning successes of the scientific model as lived out in 20th-century medicine, as well as the cultural dominance of medicine as a profession in seizing and using the scientific model, it is hard to see how nursing could not have attempted to follow suit.

Additionally, the 1970s saw the emergence in medicine of the development of the problem-oriented medical record (POMR) by physician Lawrence Weed. Originally designed as a teaching tool for medical students and influenced by the emergence of behaviorist concepts in the discipline of education (discussed in our next section), it also provided a means of enhancing quality care. Its principles and tech-niques were widely adapted to many different health care educational and practice settings, including nursing. Also called the Problem/Need-Oriented System, the POMR took the problem-solving techniques used in everyday life and applied them to health care settings. The steps mimic what we as nurses understand as nursing process: collect data, define problems/needs, forecast outcomes, formulate care plan, implement plan, and evaluate progress (Goldberg, Benoit, Docken, Hoagberg, & Wesselman, 1978). The use of this system in a variety of health care settings speeded its adaptation and entrenchment in nursing.

The Intertwining of Medical and Nursing Knowledge

An overview of nursing content since the founding of the first formal nursing programs (under Florence Nightingale's influ-ence in Great Britain in 1860, and in this country in 1873) illustrates the intertwining of the disciplines of medicine and nursing. An analysis of planned curriculum content in nurs-ing, authored by Ina Madge Longway in 1972, divides the approach to content in nursing into six different periods: the folklore era, prior to Nightingale; the Nightingale era; the era of "local pathology"; the patient-care areas approach;

the body-system approach; and the person-centered curriculum that Longway saw as the emerging model in 1972 (pp. 116–121). These periods often mirrored changes in medicine. Nursing instruction during the folklore era was dominated by word of mouth from one nurse to another and by watching others who were deemed successful in caring for the sick. The specifics of care varied with the underlying medical theories of the day. Nightingale, however, carried out a job analysis of nursing based on current practices and the requirements of employers of potential future "professional" nurses. She identified the skills and procedures necessary for delivery of nursing care (Stewart, 1943, pp. 61–62). Despite the fact that Nightingale wrote extensively about health promotion, disease prevention, and sanitary reform, the emergence of hospitals both as the setting to increasingly provide care for ill persons and as the site to "educate" nurses led to curriculum structures that from the beginning prioritized the care of the acutely ill.

According to Longway (1972), Nightingale systematized nursing content around three major areas: (1) a body of technical skills and procedures, (2) rules and precepts related to hygiene and sanitation, and (3) a philosophy of nursing and a code of ethics (p. 117). These three major categorizations still have relevance today. The content making up each of these areas has varied considerably and was often linked to the medical knowledge of the time. Educational theory, as described later in this chapter, often dictated the process by which the students received this content.

The "local pathology" era occurred around 1900 and was tied to the increasingly specific identification of causes of illness and their specific associated treatments, such as salvarsan for syphilis. The organization of content around disease had a great deal of validity at that time: Because nursing content at that time was sparse, it was borrowed from medicine and usually taught by physicians. Emphasis was on how things were done in one institution or locality. Students checked off on a card how many patients they had cared for in each disease category. Emphasis on the disease often led to neglect of the patient as a person by both physicians and nurses. In addition, as knowledge increased about all diseases and new treatments were constantly under development, the disease approach became insufficient. The patient-care and body-system approaches occurred simultaneously, not sequentially, and overlapped from setting to setting.

Hospital patients were frequently grouped for the convenience of the physician admitting them, such as surgical patients on one floor for the surgeons, and medical patients in a different area for the internists. Nursing students rotating through the different patient-care areas would study content related to each area. Nursing instructors tended to remain in their specialized spheres, leading to compartmentalization and lack of communication between courses, and often, overlap in content. The body-system organization of content was a logical extension and is still with us today. Again, nursing knowledge being taught was dominated by medical knowledge, with knowledge of the person being divided into various body systems such as muscular, nervous, gastrointestinal, and the like. Tissues from each system were consistent from one person to another, and diseases from particular systems, whatever the disease-producing agent, tended to have similar manifestations requiring similar therapies and associated nursing care. This approach made student learning easier by allowing nursing educators to group many diseases together. This approach, however, was clearly rooted in the biological and medical sciences and tended to obscure the person as a whole.

The Context of 20th-Century Education and Its Impact on Nursing Education

Education was not immune to the lure of quantification. Indeed, many of the changes in educational thought that permeated the 20th century led to preparing the soil of nursing education for the development of nursing diagnoses and nursing process. Review of a classic text in nursing education, *Teaching and Learning in Schools of Nursing* (1965), by Loretta Heidgerken, reveal similar processes to those already discussed when talking about definitions of learning. She refers to learning as a "series of operations," which include observation; description; analysis; validation of the learning products; and evaluation, or testing the learning products through usage (p. 21). In addition, one sees the influence of educational psychology with the introduction of "objectives on a psychological basis," described as follows.

According to Em Olivia Bevis and Jean Watson, noted nurse educators and experts in curriculum design, "No other nursing activity or enterprise has so affected nursing's

3.1 Objectives on a Psychological Basis.

Mental Functions	Learning Outcomes	
	In General	In Detail
Cognition (knowing)	Knowledge	Facts, meaning, principles, laws, and other concepts of relationships. Primary objective is understanding and ability to interpret and apply concepts.
Affection (feeling)	Attitudes	Ideals, interests, and appreciations. Primary objective is to build right habits of conduct.
Conation (doing)	Abilities	Skills, including specific motor and general adaptive abilities and mental skills. Primary objective is concerned with mastery of skills, the acquisition of facility in the use of these abilities.

Heidgerken, L. (1965). Teaching and learning in schools of nursing (3rd ed.), Table 5, p. 101. © J. B. Lippincott.

historical course and its practice than the curriculum-development paradigm used for the last 40 years" (Bevis & Watson, 1989, p. 11). Bevis and Watson were referring to the Tylerian curriculum-development model that placed nursing curriculum into a behaviorist framework, reinforcing the pre-existing training mentality that had governed nursing education since its 19th-century emergence in hospital training schools. Bevis and Watson (1989) placed the blame on behavioral objectives and behaviorist evaluation for perpetuation of "the stylized, rule-driven, problem-solving format called the *nursing process*" (p. 11). They decry "competency-based education and evaluation as well as the dedication of nurses to nursing diagnosis" (Ibid), although they do give credit to these trends for some improvement in quality. They fault primarily the institutionalization of these processes.

There was a time in early nursing's professional development that fostered a need for standardization of curriculum. The rise of hospitals as a setting in which the ill received medical care was also to have a profound influence on nursing's development. As quickly as hospitals sprang up at the turn of the 20th century, so did schools of nursing within them. As noted earlier, care was often defined locally and idiosyncratically. Most early nursing schools in America used a curriculum based on a list of bedside functions to be mastered, copied from the one developed and used in the Nightingale schools. Aside from this, there was little uniformity. Indeed, neither pedagogy nor curriculum had yet emerged as specialized fields of study. The prevailing approach to instruction relied upon the assumptions inherent in the classical tradition, "a process of disciplining the mind through a series of exercises, just as muscles are developed through use" (National League for Nursing, 1951). Memorization and recitation were expected.

This apprentice system that did not rely on formal education was still considered an acceptable preparation for entry to practice in both medicine and law. Both the normal schools established for the training of teachers and the proprietary medical schools of the period had created precedent for the development of single-purpose institutions to prepare for professional practice (Murdock, 1986). Ward experience constituted learning with little thought or attention paid to either the sequence or the relative proportion of each of the experiences within the total curriculum. Classroom instruction was limited to lectures by physicians.

Economic realities of the late 19th century had forced nursing educational programs to surrender operational control to their respective hospital boards. Financial independence for nursing schools from the hospitals that housed them had been a sacred underpinning (seldom realized) of the Nightingale model. The education of the students had become secondary to the needs of the institution. This reality generated concern among the nursing leadership. Reform was on the mind of these leaders during their first meeting in 1893 at the International Congress of Charities held in association with the Chicago World's Fair.

The meeting led to the founding of the American Society of Superintendents of Training Schools for Nurses. One aim was the improved education of those in charge of training schools, a goal realized with the establishment of a postgraduate course for nurses at Teachers College, Columbia University in New York City. Another major effort of the society was establishing an improved, standardized curriculum for the rapidly burgeoning schools of nursing. This goal saw fruition with the publication of the *Standard Curriculum* in 1917. This book was the product of the Education Committee of the Society for Superintendents (which had by then become the National League for Nursing Education) and was begun in 1914, taking 3 years to prepare and publish. In 1927 the work was revised and the word *standard* was dropped from the title. A third edition, entitled *A Curriculum Guide for Schools of Nursing*, was published in 1937.

The 1917 edition was divided into two major sections, the first dealing with admission requirements for students, qualifications for teaching, specific guidelines for the physical facilities, financial resources, and administrative control of the schools. The second section provided a curriculum plan with objectives, content, methods, resources, and operational schedules. A plan of practical instruction was also included that outlined the time and sequencing of recommended experiences. This was a relatively sophisticated text. Most members of the Education Committee were graduates of the Teachers College program and had contact with such prominent figures in education and psychology as Edward Thorndike, John Dewey, and Frank McMurray, mainstream thinkers in the movement for overall educational reform. Dewey's scientific orientation predominated. Frank McMurray's perspective was rooted in the philosophy of Johann Herbart, who preached that the mind actively creates a unity out of the raw materials of ideas presented to it. This led to methods of instruction and techniques of curriculum development that would support the assimilation of knowledge and foster the correlation of the subject matter to the curriculum (Seguel, 1966).

The decades between the publication of the first and second editions saw a societal emphasis on efficiency, an outgrowth of industrialization, and the development of mass manufacturing. Concurrently, the study of curriculum came into existence as a specialized field of study and as a process rather than a focus on specific content or structure. Educational theorist J. Franklin Bobbit used industry as his controlling metaphor, comparing schools to "factories" and the child to "the raw materials" (Seguel, 1966, p. 80). W. W. Charters, another educator of this era, emphasized the development and testing of curriculum construction, with teachers actively participating in this curriculum-development process through an organized committee structure, engaging in an orderly sequence (Caswell, 1966; Kliebard, 1968). Any current nursing educator in the United States can see this process is still alive today in nursing schools and colleges.

A concurrent trend was the establishment in 1926 of the Committee of the Grading of Nursing Schools, also an outgrowth of the work of the National League for Nursing Education. This committee recommended that the league develop an accreditation system for schools of nursing, a project held up during the years of the Great Depression in the 1930s. What did move forward were plans for a new curriculum guide. The 1937 curriculum guide reflected a more philosophical approach to curriculum than the mechanistic methods employed in the 1927 edition. This was reflective of the educational and curriculum theorists of that particular era, such as Hollis Caswell (1966), who saw the philosopher as contributing a body of principles and the researcher as developing techniques helpful in meeting commonly recurring problems in curriculum situations. Caswell viewed curriculum development as a matter of judgment rather than technique, and he felt that maximum participation was necessary by what today would be referred to as "stakeholders." Caswell's (1966) methodology served as the guide for the construction of this revision of curriculum. Additionally, and also reflective of an era still governed by ideas from industry and efficiency, the 1937 third edition of *A Curriculum Guide for Schools of Nursing* was based on an activity analysis in nursing conducted by 22 subcommittees of the Education Committee of the National League for Nursing Education. Each subcommittee was composed of nurses representing all parts of the country and all areas of practice. The concept of adjustment was accepted as the overall aim of nursing education. According to Murdock (1986), "With the selection of the concept of adjustment as its guiding framework, nursing moved away from its traditional aims of discipline, service, practical utility, and technical efficiency, and closer to the democratic ideals expressed by the progressive educators of the period" (p. 23).

It might also be speculated that with the construction of nursing content still revolving heavily around medical content, and with significant numbers of early nurse educators as products of Teachers College, the creativity and intellect of nurse educators of the day were thrown into the structuring of nursing knowledge through curriculum development, at the expense of ideas about the practice of nursing itself. The driving force behind the 1937 edition of the curriculum guide was Isabel Stewart of Teachers College. As an educator rather than a clinician, and as one in charge of a school of education, her view of science was broad. In a 1929 article entitled "The Science and Art of Nursing," she called for an end to "empiric" nursing, arguing for a "scientific inquiry" into nursing procedures. She meant, "Not only bacteriological and physiological and chemical tests... but economic and psychological and sociological measurements also" (cited in Reverby, 1987, p. 143).

By the mid-1940s, Dewey's influence on educational theory was waning, giving way to behaviorism, a school of thought rooted in Thorndike's famous assertion that "Whatever exists, exists in some amount" (Thorndike, 1940, p. 19) and therefore can be measured. Because Thorndike was an educational psychologist at Teachers College, it was inevitable that the quantification afoot in all social sciences would seep further into education. Bloom's works on mastery (1968) and, with colleagues, on the educational domains (1956) were outgrowths of this worldview. According to Bevis (1989), "All—or most all—curriculum-evaluation paradigms arise from the empiricist-behaviorist tradition" (p. 26). A prime mover of this movement was Ralph Tyler. Bevis (1989) identified the work of Tyler and its institutionalization by the approval and accrediting bodies of nursing in the 1950s and '60s as the next major impact on nursing curriculum structures (p. 22). Tyler's guide, originally a syllabus for a curriculum course he taught at the University of Chicago, was first published as *Syllabus for Education 360* and was reprinted in 1950 as *Basic Principles of Curriculum and Instruction.* Tyler then became a consultant on a 3-year action research project conducted at the University of Washington School of Nursing and published in 1955. Reports from this study were published in three volumes (Sand, 1955; Sand & Belcher, 1958; Tschudin, Belcher, & Nedelsky, 1958) and "substantiated the practicality of using the Tyler Rationale to develop nursing curriculum" (Bevis, 1989, p. 22). Bevis's own (1972) book on curriculum development translated primary and secondary school-curriculum-development behaviorist theory into a useful handbook for the practice field of nursing and became a classic reference. Mager's book *Preparing*

Instructional Objectives (1962) clinched the deal. Measurable behavioral objectives were the order of the day. Most significant was the growth in nursing programs within schools of higher education, including the community college movement spawned by the work of Mildred Montag in the early 1950s. These programs all embraced the Tylerian approach to curriculum development. It was Tyler who suggested using major content threads—concepts, values, and skills—as organizing elements. Evaluation completed the cycle, providing data for measuring achievement of the program objectives (Murdock, 1986, p. 28).

Additionally, most nurse educators of the time seeking higher education were still studying in schools of education, where behaviorism reigned supreme. In addition, behaviorism was another reflection of the dominance of traditional science as the predominant discourse of the 20th century. It was difficult for nursing, surrounded by medicine's staggering successes and education's quest for scientific validity, not to throw its lot in the same direction. This focus provided fertile soil for the subsequent development of nursing process as a problem-solving method, and for the classification of nursing knowledge.

Bevis herself authored the 1989 classic *Toward a Caring Curriculum* with Jean Watson in which she made a clean break with her Tylerian past. The introduction affirms the book's ambitious aims: nothing less than a new curriculum-development paradigm for nursing education, "liberating both student and faculty from the authoritarian restraints of empiricist/behaviorist models as represented by specified behavioral objectives" (p. 1). The goals were to enable nursing graduates to be more responsive to societal needs and the needs of their patients, to humanize the increasingly technical world of health care, to foster creativity, and generate more insight into ethical and moral problems. However, was this really new?

Origins of the Problem-Based Approach to Patient Care

Although nursing was influenced by the respective disciplines of medicine and education, which in turn built on other trends and ideas, there were nurses who attempted to separate nursing practice unto itself. Nursing practice and education in the 1950s were facing major problems because of increasing technology, continued advances in medical science, and social change in general. Methods of education and nursing practice based on body systems and medical services were inadequate to meet the demands of rapid change. Longway (1972) noted when discussing the curriculum developments of the 1960s, "When a new organization of content for nursing became imperative, the *person* emerged as a logical focal point. It seems self-evident that nurses are in existence to nurse *persons*, not diseases, organs, or body systems" (p. 120).

Faye Abdellah and colleagues called for "patient-centered approaches to nursing," stating, "Disease and procedure approach to nursing [are] no longer adequate" (Abdellah, Beland, Martin, & Matheney, 1960, p. v). Abdellah's research, funded in 1953 by the Division of Nursing Resources of the U.S. Public Health Service, was carried out in a sample of 30 general hospitals with and without schools of nursing. It was the first direct attempt to develop a classification of common nursing problems presented by patients. Abdellah and her coinvestigator, Eugene Levine, classified the medical diagnoses of more than 1,700 patients into 58 categories thought to represent common nursing problems (Abdellah & Levine, 1954). This was the first direct attempt to develop a typology of nursing problems presented by patients and a concomitant typology of nursing treatments. A nursing problem presented by a patient was defined as a condition or situation faced by the patient or his or her family in which the nurse can assist through the performance of professional functions. Abdellah et al. state the injunction "Learn to know the patient" as the first step in any problem identification in Chapter 1 of the book *Patient-Centered Approaches to Nursing* (Abdellah et al., 1960, p. 13). Abdellah's (1955) dissertation work, *Methods of Determining Covert Aspects of Nursing Problems as a Basis for Improved Clinical Teaching,* was designed to identify which interview techniques provided the most complete list of patients' problems. What this study revealed was that a free-answer method elicited more covert—or emotional-social—problems than a pictorial-interview technique or direct-questioning approach (Abdellah, 1957).

In 1955 the National League for Nursing (NLN) Committee on Records formed a subcommittee to develop a meaningful clinical evaluation tool, a topic of great fascination to nurse educators newly infatuated with the curriculum work of Tyler. With feedback from more than 40 NLN-accredited collegiate schools of nursing, the 58 patient categories identified by Abdellah and Levine (1954) were compressed into 21 common nursing problems as representative of all. This work was reported in the 1960 book *Patient-centered Approaches to Nursing*. Abdellah et al. (1960) identified nursing diagnosis as a sub concept of the problem-solving focus, defining it as the "determination of the nature" (p. 9) and extent of nursing problems identified by individual patients or families receiving care.

The problem-solving process identified and presented by Abdellah used words that underpinned what later became known as the nursing process. Even then it was "outcome driven," with Abdellah (1960) stating, "Her [the nurse's] professional competence would be based on her ability to solve key nursing problems presented by patients not on the number of beds that she made, the number of major operations, or the number of days on a particular service caring for a number of diagnoses" (pp. 12–13).

Virginia Henderson, prominent nurse author and educator, enjoyed a lengthy career in nursing. In a course for advanced students in medical-surgical nursing that Henderson taught at Teachers College in the 1940s, she developed an approach that was "unique because it was patient-centered and organized around major nursing problems rather than medical diagnoses and diseases of body systems" (Henderson, 1966, p. 14). It was the beginning of teaching nurses to care for a whole patient, not just to perform a series of tasks, and Henderson was one of the first to use the phrase "Nursing is both a unique science and an art" (cited in Thorson & Halloran, 2005, p. 70).

Prior conceptualizations drew on nursing as an art, and science built on the tasks of the nurse as the art, as Henderson carried out the science of medicine. Drawing on her commitment to and understanding of physiologic concepts, "Henderson began to see the possibility of, in her metaphor, a 'complete marriage between nursing and science' and spent the rest of her career negotiating the terms of this 'nuptial contract'" (Reverby, 1989, p. 147). Reverby (1989) also noted that Henderson sent her students to the library to investigate the underlying theories of particular nursing problems. She then had her students "list the unanswered questions needing further research" when no scientific theory was found to frame a given nursing situation (Ibid). Henderson was also influenced by Thorndike's teachings on psychology at Teachers College, focusing on social and cultural environments as much as on individuals.

Henderson did present nursing as a systematic process involving analytical thinking and evaluation of patient needs; in this sense, her thinking was pivotal to the evolution of the nursing process (Fulton, 1987). However, she did *not* subscribe to nursing being a process, and she said that there is no such thing as *the* nursing process or even *a* nursing process because the word constrains the word *nursing* (Thorson & Halloran, 2005, p. 78). In a 1982 article entitled "The Nursing Process—Is the Title Right?" Henderson observes that the nursing process as it existed then was weighted so heavily on the scientific side that it seemed "to belittle the intuitive artistic side of nursing" (cited in Halloran, 1995, p. 208). She goes on to state, "The process depends to a large extent on the knowledge that the nurse has acquired, but the intuitive intervention of the nurse depends on the kind of person he or she is. To use an old-fashioned term, upon character" (Ibid).

The 6th edition of Henderson and Nite's widely used text *Principles and Practice of Nursing* (1978) does contain what might be considered nursing diagnoses. Henderson refers to them as "symptoms," although nursing diagnoses as defined by NANDA do appear in certain portions of the text. Of greater interest is the fact that the nursing interventions found in this text, in substance if not in the schema and organization used in NIC (McCloskey & Bulechek, 2000), are still in use today. The text does not use the specific term *patient-care outcomes* but rather, more in keeping with Henderson's times, the word *evaluation*. According to Thorson and Halloran (2005), "Henderson believed that professionals in health care should avoid the use of jargon and speak in plain language" Citing some of the commonly observed critiques of nursing classification systems, as well as formalized nursing process, they go on say, "Some of the terms used in both NIC and NOC are clearly nursing jargon, and classification schemas that separate nurses from all other health and illness management will isolate nurses from patient needs that they can reasonably manage" (pp. 78–79). However, viewed in the light of history, it is clear that these classifications and problem-solving approaches rooted in the literature and presaging evidence-based practice emerged with the very best of intentions: keeping the patient first, knowing the patient, and establishing a clearly articulated base for nursing practice. It is the subsequent institutionalization and codifications that, although they may be necessary in the 21st century, have come to obscure the true aims and intent. Nursing, emerging from medical dominance, was compelled to develop some of its initial language in opposition to what existed.

Origins of Nursing Process

Another clear example of this initial languaging is the work of Ida Jean Orlando, noted developer of "Nursing Process Theory" (Fischer, Marriner-Tomey, Mills, & Sauter, 1994; Schmieding, 1993). Her overall goal was to find an organizing principle for professional nursing; that is, a distinct function (Orlando, 1961, p. viii). This goal obsessed the thinking of nurses in the 1950s and '60s. Emerging from medicalized cocoons and repressive curriculum models, these early nurses struggled to make sense of, and to articulate, what it was they "did" as nurses. Doctoral study for nurses was just beginning to emerge, and concurrently, the beginnings of formal theory development in nursing, a trajectory that continues to the present day. However, what did nurses do that was uniquely nursing?

Orlando was a psychiatric nurse, a field that proved fertile for nurses of that era, and a field that grounded much of nurse theorizing in the interpersonal relationship. Orlando's 1958 book, *The Dynamic Nurse-Patient Relationship: Function, Process and Principles,* not published until 1961, offered a conceptualization of nursing that was built around the reciprocal relationship between patient and nurse. Grounded in the psychodynamic thinking of the time, Orlando's approach to nursing process was composed of the following elements: (1) the behavior of the patient, (2) the reaction of the nurse, and (3) the nursing actions that are designed for the patient's benefit. The interaction of these elements with each other is the nursing process.

Orlando viewed the nurse as providing direct assistance to the patient in whatever setting for the purpose of "avoiding, relieving, diminishing, or curing the person's sense of helplessness" (Forchuk, 1991, p. 41). Nursing actions with positive results were called a "deliberative nursing process," whereas nurse actions that produced negative patient outcomes were called "automatic personal reactions" (Schmieding, 1993, p. 23). It was Orlando who founded the learning tool of the "process recording" as a way for the professional nurse to reflect on his or her practice (Fischer et al., 1994). It is clear that the interpersonal process elements identified by influential nurse leaders and visionaries of the 1950s and 1960s were some of the basic building blocks to the subsequent development of the more conventional nursing process as a problem-solving method. It was always assumed, although perhaps not always made explicit, that there was a relational grounding.

Throwing out the Baby With the Bathwater: Art or Science—or Both?

There is no doubt that science has been the dominant discourse of the 20th century. Professions staking their claims on the rock of science prospered; it was inevitable that nursing would attempt to do the same, as the endeavor toward classification systems of nursing knowledge has attempted to do. However, as an emerging profession composed primarily of women, nursing has had an unusual set of issues with which to deal. Heavily influenced by both medical science and educational theories rooted in behaviorist approaches, the struggle for the birth of a science of nursing has been difficult.

From the very beginning, aspects of nursing, and many individual nurses, were at odds with scientific approaches to the nursing of patients. Nightingale, for example, was opposed to the registration of nurses, feeling that as a "moral art," nursing could not be so regulated (Reverby, 1986). Susan Reverby in *Ordered to Care* (1986) quotes a nurse named Annette Fiske, who spent her career in the 1920s arguing against increasing educational standards for nurses. Rather, according to Reverby (1987), "She called for a reinfusion into nursing of spirituality and service, assuming that this would result in nursing's receiving greater 'love, respect, and admiration'" (p. 9). And despite the fact that women have gained greater social, economic, legal, and even political power in the late 20th and early 21st centuries, many in nursing continue to rely on this virtue script and a view of nursing as rooted in a repackaging of "nursing's traditional stereotype of women born to be good, kind, and self-sacrificing—not educated, to provide care based on science and practical skill" (Gordon & Nelson, 2005, p. 63).

There are no simple answers. The problem-solving approach of the nursing process, the work involved in the attempted classification of nursing-based knowledge through the labeling of nursing diagnosis, and nursing interventions measured by patient-care outcomes, are all historical developments of work not to be thrown away or discarded. Henderson points out, "The nursing process has served a useful purpose in reminding nurses that they should practice the habit of inquiry throughout their lives in nursing practice" (Halloran, 1995, p. 210). Clearly this habit of inquiry has served as an underpinning of the current evidence-based-practice craze. But the nursing process must be examined and understood in context, in the context of the times in which it developed, and in the richness of other ideas and understandings whose humanistic underpinnings must not be forgotten. It seems fitting in any work on nursing to end with some thoughts by nursing's founder, Florence Nightingale. I quote Nightingale from a work by noted nurse educator Isabel Stewart: "No system can endure that does not march. Are we walking to the future or the past? Don't let us stereotype mediocrity" (Stewart, 1943, p. 138). However, the work of nursing diagnosis and nursing process must be seen as just a recent part of a lengthy trajectory of valued nursing knowledge, rooted in knowing the person.

In 2004, nurse-historian Sioban Nelson and journalist Suzanne Gordon published an article entitled "The Rhetoric of Rupture: Nursing as a Practice With a History?" in *Nursing Outlook*. Their goal, they state, in paraphrasing the British social historian E. P. Thompson, was to "rescue" nursing from the "enormous condescension of posterity" (Thompson, cited in Nelson & Gordon, 2004, p. 255). This chapter attempts to document the work of nursing educators and thinkers in the context of their times, as they have struggled to align the valuable practice of nursing rooted in a knowing of the patient, and as Henderson said so succinctly, rested upon the character of the nurse (Halloran, 1995, p. 208) and linked to the prevailing social discourse and mores of those times. Nelson and Gordon (2004) conclude with the statement, "Arguments for advancement of the profession have to be based on this understanding and respect for nursing as a practice with a history" (p. 260). I would expand that argument to include an understanding and respect for nursing as a discipline of ideas with a history. Only then can we achieve a true integration of theory and practice.

References

Abdellah, F. G. (1955). *Methods of determining covert aspects of nursing problems as a Basis for improved clinical teaching.* Unpublished doctoral dissertation, Teachers College, Columbia University.

Abdellah, F. G. (1957). Methods of identifying covert aspects of nursing problems. *Nursing Research, 6*(4), 118–124.

Abdellah, F. G., Beland, I., Martin, A., & Matheney, R. V. (1960). *Patient-centered approaches to patient care.* New York: Macmillan.

Abdellah, F. G., & Levine, E. (1954). *Appraising the clinical resources in small hospitals.* Washington, DC: Public Health Service Monograph No. 24. Department of Health, Education, & Welfare.

Agency for Health Care Policy & Research [AHCPR]. (1990, September). *Nursing advisory panel for guideline development: Summary* (program note). Washington, DC: U.S. Department of Health & Human Services, Public Health Service, AHCPR.

American Nurses Association. (1973). *Standards of nursing practice.* Kansas City: Author.

American Nurses Association. (1980). *Nursing: A social policy statement.* Kansas City: Author.

American Nurses Association. (1995). *Nursing: A social policy statement.* Washington, DC: Author.

American Psychiatric Association. (2000). Diagnostic and statistical manual of mental disorders (4th ed.). TR. Author.

Bevis, E. O. (1972). *Curriculum building in nursing: A process.* St. Louis: Mosby.

Bevis, E. O., & Watson, J. (1989). *Toward a caring curriculum.* New York: National League for Nursing, Pub. No. 15-2278.

Blegen, M. A., & Tripp-Reimer, T. (1997). Implications of nursing taxonomies for middle-range theory development. *Advances in Nursing Science, 19(3),* 37–49.

Bloom, B. S. (1968, May). Learning for mastery. *Evaluation Comment,* 1–11.

Bloom, B. S., Englehart, M. D., Furst, E. J., Hill, W. H., & Drathwohl, D. R. (Eds.). (1956). *Taxonomy of educational objectives.* New York: Longmans, Green.

Bulechek, G. M., & McCloskey, J. C. (Eds.). (1985). *Nursing interventions: Treatments for nursing diagnoses.* Philadelphia: W. B. Saunders.

Bulechek, G. M., & McCloskey, J. C. (Eds.). (1999). *Nursing interventions: Effective nursing treatments.* Philadelphia: W. B. Saunders.

Carpenito-Moyet, L. (2006). *Nursing diagnosis: Application to clinical practice.* Philadelphia: Lippincott Williams & Wilkins.

Caswell, H. L. (1966). Emergence of the curriculum as a field of study. In H. Robison (Ed.), *Precedents and promise in the curriculum field.* New York: Teachers College Press.

Craft-Rosenberg, M., & Delaney, C. (1997). Nursing diagnosis extension and classification (NDEC). In M. Rantz & P. LeMone (Eds.), *Classification of nursing diagnoses: Proceeding of the twelfth conference* (26–31). Glendale, CA: Cumulative Index to Nursing & Allied Health Literature.

Fischer, S., Marriner-Tomey, A., Mills, D. I., & Sauter, M. K. (1994). Ida Jean Orlando (Pelletier): Nursing process theory. In A. Marriner-Tomey (Ed.), *Nursing theorists and their work* (3rd ed.). St. Louis: Mosby.

Fitzpatrick, J. J., Kerr, M. E., Saba, V. K., Hoskins, L. M., Hurley, M. E., Rottkamp, B. C., et al. (1989). Translating nursing diagnosis into ICD code. *American Journal of Nursing, 89*(12), 493–495.

Forchuk, C. (1991). A comparison of the works of Peplau and Orlando. *Archives of Psychiatric Nursing, 5*(1), 38–45.

Fry, V. S. (1953). The creative approach to nursing. *American Journal of Nursing, 53,* 301–302.

Fulton, J. S. (1987). Virginia Henderson: Theorist, prophet, poet. *Advances in Nursing Science, 10*(1), 1–9.

Goldberg, L., Benoit, C., Docken, T. R. S., Hoagberg, E. & Wesselman, J. (1978). *The problem/need-oriented approach to planning and evaluation of patient care.* Minneapolis: Medallion Communications.

Gordon, S. & Nelson, S. (2005). An end to angels. *American Journal of Nursing, 105* (5), 62–69.

Griffith, H. M., Thomas, N., & Griffith, L. (1991). MDs bill for these routine nursing tasks. *American Journal of Nursing, 91*(1), 22–27.

Halloran, E. J. (Ed). (1995). *A Virginia Henderson reader.* New York: Springer.

Heidgerken, L. E. (1965). *Teaching and learning in schools of nursing: Principles and methods* (3rd ed.). Philadelphia: J. B. Lippincott.

Henderson, V. (1995). The nursing process—is the title right? In E. J. Halloran (Ed.), *A Virginia Henderson reader: Excellence in nursing.* New York: Springer.

Henderson, V. (1966). *The nature of nursing.* New York: Macmillan.

Henderson, V., & Nite, G. (1978). *Principles and practice of nursing* (6th ed.). New York: Macmillan.

Hinshaw, A. S. (1988). The new national center for nursing research: Patient care research programs. *Applied Nursing Research, 1*(1), 2–4.

Hornung, B. A. (1953). The nursing diagnosis: An exercise in judgment. *Nursing Outlook, 4,* 29–30.

Joint Commission on the Accreditation of Healthcare Organizations (1999). *Hospital Accreditation Standards.* Chicago: Author.

Kliebard, H. (1968). The curriculum field in retrospect. In P. W. F. Witt (Ed)., *Technology & the curriculum.* New York: Teachers College Press.

Longway, I. M. (1972). Curriculum concepts: An historical analysis. *Nursing Outlook, 20*(2), 116–120.

Lourdon, I. (1997). *Western Medicine: An illustrated history.* New York: Oxford University Press.

Mager, R. (1962). *Preparing instructional objectives.* Belmont, CA: Feron Publishers.

McCloskey, J. C., & Bulechek, G. M. (2000). *Nursing interventions classification* (NIC) (3rd ed.). St. Louis: Mosby.

McLane, A. M. (Ed.). (1987). *Classification of nursing diagnoses: Proceeding of the seventh national conference.* St. Louis: Mosby.

Murdock, J. E. (1986). Evolution of the nursing curriculum. *Journal of Nursing History, 2*(1), 16–35.

Murray, M. E., & Atkinson, L. D. (2000). *Understanding the nursing process in a changing care environment.* New York: McGraw-Hill.

National League for Nursing. (1951). Department of services to schools. *In Joint Nursing Curriculum Conference, Curriculum Bulletin,* No. 2. New York: Author.

Nelson, S. & Gordon, S. (2004). The rhetoric of rupture: Nursing as a practice with a history? *Nursing Outlook, 52,* 255–261.

North American Nursing Diagnosis Association. (1992). *Taxonomy of nursing diagnoses.* Philadelphia: Author.

North American Nursing Diagnosis Association. (2001). *Nursing diagnoses: Definitions & classification, 2000–2001.* Philadelphia: Author.

North American Nursing Diagnosis Association. (2002). Nursing diagnoses: Definitions & classification, 2001–2002. Philadelphia: Author.

Orlando, I. J. (1961). *The dynamic nurse-patient relationship: Function, process and principles.* New York: G. P. Putnam's Sons.

Pellegrino, E. (1980). The sociocultural impact of twentieth-century therapeutics. In C. E. Rosenberg & J. Golden (Eds.),*Framing disease: Studies in cultural history* (pp. 245–267). Rutgers University Press.

Pickstone, J. (2000). *Ways of knowing.* Chicago: University of Chicago Press.

Reverby, S. (1986). *Ordered to care.* Cambridge, MA: Harvard University Press.

Reverby, S. (1987). A caring dilemma: Womanhood and nursing in historical perspective. *Nursing Research, 36*(1), 5–11.

Reverby, S. (1989). A legitimate relationship: Nursing, hospitals, and science in the twentieth century. In D. Long & J. Golden (Eds.), *The American general hospital: Communities and social context* (pp. 135–156). Ithaca, NY: Cornell University Press.

Sand, O. (1955). *Curriculum study in basic nursing education.* New York: G. P. Putnam's Sons.

Sand, O. & Belcher, H. C. (1958).*An experience in basic nursing education.* New York: G. P. Putnam's Sons.

Schmieding, N. J. (1993). *Ida Jean Orlando: A nursing process theory.* Newbury Park, CA: Sage.

Seguel, M. L. (1966). *The curriculum field: Its formative years.* New York: Teachers College Press.

Snyder, M. (1985). *Independent nursing interventions.* New York: Wiley.

Stewart, I. M. (1943). *Education of nurses.* New York: Macmillan.

Thorndike, E. L. (1940). *Selected writings from a connectionist's psychology.* New York: Appleton-Century-Crofts.

Thorson, M. J., & Halloran, E. J. (2005). Henderson's conceptualization of nursing. In J. J. Fitzpatrick & A. L. Whall (Eds.), *Conceptual models of nursing: Analysis and application* (pp. 68–82). Upper Saddle River, NJ: Pearson Prentice Hall.

Tschudin, M. S., Belcher, H. C., & Nedelsky, L. (1958). *Evaluation in basic nursing Education.* New York: G. P. Putnam's Sons.

Zielstroff, R. D. (1984). Why aren't there more significant automated nursing information systems? *Journal of Nursing Administration, 14*(1), 7–10.

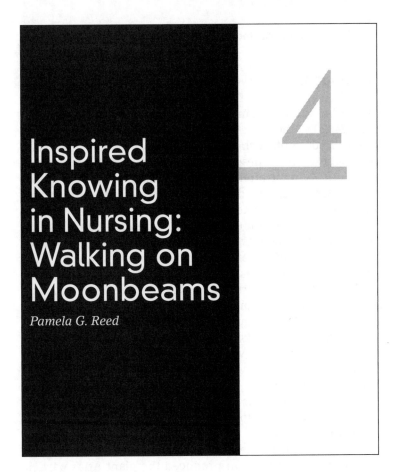

Inspired Knowing in Nursing: Walking on Moonbeams

Pamela G. Reed

Chapter Overview

This chapter focuses on *inspired knowing* as a practice-based approach to knowledge development in nursing. Historical perspectives on the philosophy of science are presented as background to a new philosophical perspective for knowing: neomodernism. In addition, *nursing process* is radically redefined in a way that provides a substantive focus for knowing and practice in nursing. Strategies that facilitate *inspired knowing* and its accompanying theory development are discussed.

Introduction

It traveled 422 million miles from Earth for 10 months. Then on May 24, 2008, the three-legged Phoenix Lander slowed down from 12,500 mph with help from a parachute, the Martian atmosphere, and 12 descent thrusters for a safe touchdown on Mars at 4:38 in the afternoon (Mountain Standard Time). The vehicle landed during the Martian summer, when the weather is like that in Canada's Northwest Territories where the sun never sets this time of year. The scientists had a window of time about 3 months long to complete their data collection on soil composition before winter, when the sun would disappear and the coldness would encase the Lander spacecraft in dry ice. The project required a team of 160 scientists, engineers, and other personnel and $420 million. After six failed missions to Mars, scientists from the University of Arizona and NASA's Jet Propulsion Lab were ecstatic. As one reporter described, they were "walking on moonbeams." Their major goal for scientific knowledge was to find evidence of water and elements of life by analyzing soil and ice samples scooped from an arctic plain of Mars. A broader question on the minds of all who followed the story was whether we are alone in the universe.

Back on earth, the work of 2,200 researchers from 37 countries and $10 billion produced the giant Atlas particle detector at the European particle physics lab CERN. In August 2008, scientists would start up the Large Hadron Collider machine, housed in a 17-mile-long tunnel 300 feet below farmland in eastern France. Superconducting magnets in the Collider would be used to steer the beams of protons around the tunnel at a speed of 11,000 circuits per second, smashing protons together with as much force as occurred when the universe burst into existence and exploded into an inferno of particles. The theory-driven goal was that the energy would materialize into new heavy particles; these particles could give evidence of other dimensions in the universe and reveal more about the mysterious dark form of matter that composes 80% of the universe. A broader goal was to better understand the laws of nature and human existence.

In this chapter, we will explore an idea about a new pattern of knowing that may open new horizons for your nursing practice and research. If crisis is "the reaching of our limits of knowing" (Carlsen, 1988, p. 234), then the vast scope of the scientific projects described above minimizes any possibility of that kind of crisis. The summer of 2008 provided two dramatic examples of how scientists go about knowing. Scientists' knowing begins with their disciplinary focus, followed by accepted practices of science in their discipline. Approaches to knowing are pulled by their particular disciplinary focuses.

In terms of a disciplinary focus, for example, geologists study geological matter and processes of a solid body such as Earth, Earth's moon, and Mars. Chemists study chemical processes in organic and inorganic matter. Psychologists study psychological processes of humans and other animals. Physicists study the processes and phenomena of a physical system. Medical doctors focus on pathology and the medical approaches to disease. And nurses, at a fundamental level, focus on nursing processes of human beings and nursing approaches to health, healing, and well-being (Reed, 1997).

From Mars to Human Beings

The focuses on the geologic aspects of Martian rock and on the chemical elements in Martian soil and ice required certain approaches to knowing, ranging from microscopy and mass spectrometry to baking ovens and an 8-ft robotic arm to dig into the soil. Scientists had to shift their sleep cycles to match the day-night cycle on Mars. The questions physicists asked of their phenomena required that they build a 17-mile tunnel and instruments for observing protons and analyzing the data. Nurses' research and practice require distinct approaches to knowing as well.

Nursing phenomena of interest, human healing processes in the context of health events, are no less complex than Martian soil or colliding protons. Each discipline presents its own unique challenges in building knowledge. Architecture, for example, has its "burdens of linearity" (Ingraham, 1998). Nursing, because its unit of care is the whole (not parts) of human beings in process with their environment, has its burden of holism. To students who want the challenge of a discipline that has access to human beings and their holistic processes of healing and well-being, nursing offers diverse patterns of knowing. These patterns include but also extend beyond the traditional approaches to knowledge.

Historical Views on Knowing

In the mid-20th century, sociologists and historians of science, of which Thomas Kuhn (1970) was one of the most revolutionary, challenged basic assumptions from Western theory of scientific knowing that had taken root in the 16th and 17th centuries. These assumptions, described by the terms *objectivism,* and *positivism* or *post-positivism*, were based upon values of objectivity, disinterestedness, and rationality in the observer. The assumptions included these ideas: there is an independent truth about the order of nature, there is one best scientific method for knowing, this method can be used to eventually produce mirror-like representations of reality, and scientific knowledge accumulates and progresses over time. An alternative theory about knowledge, described as *constructivism* or *co-constructivism*, is that nature's order is constructed by societies rather than discovered universally, and that cultures and societies may develop their own approaches to knowledge and its verification.

A third framework in science studies about knowing is *postcolonialism*. Postcolonial theory originated in the 1960s in the aftermath of formal European colonialism. It is critical of colonizers' oppression and hegemony over indigenous groups at institutional, societal, or cultural levels. Often, colonizers extract local knowledge and technology at the expense of the indigenes' economic, social, and physical well-being. This critique also acknowledges that all cultures beyond those in the Western and Northern hemispheres have been producing knowledge since recorded history.

Ways of knowing within this view do not privilege the Eurocentric, rational "man" and disinterested observer. Instead, postcolonial views about knowledge value the perspective of the *other*, which originally referred to non-European cultures and the economically and politically vulnerable people who lived in them (Harding, 1998). Harding's overall argument is that modern science is fundamentally multicultural; knowledge and technology have been borrowed—Connor (2005) called it "knowledge robbery"—across many cultures, albeit without recognizing those cultures as playing a vital role in knowledge production. She points out that traditional scientific approaches to knowing can also promote "systematic ignorance" (p. 55).

From a postcolonial perspective on knowing in health care, one could say that the colonization of nursing by other health care professionals and management systems has limited development and expression of nursing knowledge. Nurses who are recruited to tend to physician orders (in all their ramifications, including transcribing, verifying, and implementing) and to conduct medical and pharmaceutical research, deplete the workforce of creative knowledge builders who have access, unlike any other professional caregiver, to ways of knowing patients.

In the desire to be recognized as a science-based discipline, nursing historically has traded away some of its science of caregiving to adopt the science focus and ways of knowing of the dominant health care provider. Medical discourse is still prevalent in some nursing curricula, research, publications, and marketing strategies in a way that can confuse development of nursing students' identity and knowledge. However, despite economic and social forces that have limited development of nursing knowledge, nursing has epistemological potential to survive and even thrive in a postcolonial era of health care. Doctoral-level education of practitioners and researchers, along with other trends, is stimulating (if not demanding) innovations in knowledge production that can emancipate nurses and nursing knowledge.

Innovations in Knowing

One innovation for knowing proposed here derives from a movement toward practice-based knowledge production (Reed, 2006b; Reed & Lawrence, 2008; Rolfe, 2006). This approach challenges the traditional hierarchy whereby knowledge is produced by the researcher and then handed down—for application, utilization, translation or evaluation—to the practicing nurse. In contrast, within a paradigm of practice-based knowledge production, the nurse in practice is regarded as a discoverer or originator of theory-based knowledge, as well as a user of knowledge (Ellis, 1969). Practice is the place where general knowledge is transformed into nursing knowledge (Reed, 1996; Peplau, 1988). Yet practitioners have been marginalized in the knowledge-production enterprise. For example, American Association of Colleges of Nursing (2004) guidelines on curricular content for educating the Doctor of Nursing Practice (DNP) student stipulates that DNP nurses are to be knowledge users, not knowledge producers.

During the mid-19th century, Louis Pasteur generated knowledge about microbes, fermentation, pasteurization, and other significant biochemical processes by combining his imagination with logic, linking data with theoretical concepts, and hypothesizing situations for empirical testing. What Nightingale had initially dismissed as mystical (germs) Pasteur transformed into theory (as in the germ theory) to create life-changing and life-saving scientific knowledge. Latour (1988), a sociologist of science studies, explained, however, that Pasteur had to turn physicians into scientists to enable physicians to understand his development of scientific knowledge.

As nursing moves deeper into the 21st century, we may want to consider inverting Pasteur's approach and instead focus on turning scientists into practitioners. The intent would be to situate nursing knowledge development closer to the source of inspiration for building nursing knowledge — patients and their processes of healing and well-being. Post-colonial theory recognizes the experiences of the vulnerable other as an important resource for the growth of knowledge (Harding, 1998). Therefore, one particular strategy of practice-based knowledge production is centered on the nurse-patient caregiving relationship.

Caregiving as a Source of Inspiration in Knowing

Caring and knowing have been linked in the educational and nursing literature in previous decades with the idea that sufficient knowledge is needed first before one can adequately care for someone (Benner & Wrubel, 1989; Noddings, 1992). Knowing and caring were two separate events. However, new thinking has suggested the possibility of an inspired knowing where caring and knowing are a mutual process; the relational, technical, and moral context of caregiving informs knowing. Caregiving, itself a nursing process, is regarded as a path to knowing the patient and learning about other nursing processes of healing and well-being. Knowing is fueled by nursing practice, particularly by the interpersonal relationships between nurses and patients and their families.

Inspired knowing emerged from a new philosophical stance toward nursing knowledge and practice—a stance that reaches beyond modern and postmodern perspectives to embrace a post-postmodern or *neomodern* view (Reed, 2006a). For one, it entails new thinking about nursing process, now an anachronism that originated during mid-20th century positivist science. In accord with neomodern thought, the nursing process can be reformulated to be something other than an elementary problem-solving approach external to the patient: a process of healing and well-being that resides within and among human systems (individuals, groups, and communities) (Reed, 1997). This process defines a substantive focus of nursing that distinguishes advanced practice nursing from other practice disciplines (Arslanian-Engoren, Hicks, Whall, & Algase, 2005; Whall & Hicks, 2002). It also entails a belief in the patient's ability to participate at some level in facilitating this inner process of healing and well-being. Within neomodernism there is also a critical realist view acknowledging the person's capacity for self-organization, spirituality, innovative change, agency, and empowerment.

The tenets of neomodernism propose bringing science and practice together more deliberately and extending the nursing epistemology put forth in Carper's (1978) seminal philosophical inquiry. For example, the neomodernist view posits a nursing practice that embraces the patient's knowing participation in the caregiving process beyond that depicted in Carper's (1978) aesthetic pattern of knowing. Her aesthetic pattern emphasized only the *nurse's* knowing, skill, empathy, and artistry in interactions with the patient. Within neomodern epistemology, nurses and patients partner their skill and artistry to develop nursing knowledge based on abstracted particulars in caregiving.

In addition, original descriptions of the empiricist pattern of knowing (Carper, 1978; Chinn & Kramer, 2008) have been extended to value the *patient's* participation in knowledge production where patient and nurse engage in a "collaborative empiricism" (Carlsen, 1988, p. 96), identifying the problem, gathering data, interpreting findings, making connections between concepts, and refining and building nursing theory together.

The clinical setting is not only a place of knowledge application; it is also a place where nurse-patient encounters produce important data for building knowledge. It is a knowing context that includes but extends beyond the scientific method to transform scientific knowledge into nursing knowledge.

Inspired Knowing and Theory Generation

Inspired knowing is a mutual process of meaning making that can generate nursing theories about a person's inner processes of well-being. The adult developmental psychologist Kegan (1982) explained that the most fundamental things we do with what happens to us are organizing the experiences and composing meaning out of them. Meaning making can be done for scientific purposes to generate theories, or for existential reasons to facilitate personal healing and well-being. Some theories may apply only to a specific, local context (Rolfe, 2006), whereas others apply to a broader context; the theory-development strategies used by the nurse and patient influence the scope of a theory.

There are several strategies for knowledge production in practice that may be used with patients to generate nursing theory for either scientific or therapeutic purposes. These strategies include the following methods of clinical inquiry: Glaser's (1978) grounded theory (methodology), Pesut and Herman's (1999) clinical reasoning model, Rolfe and Gardner's (2005) reflexive model of evidence-based practice, Schön's (1983) reflection-in-action and single-case experimentation, and development of clinical conceptual frameworks for practice (Reed and Lawrence, 2008). Less conventional approaches for developing theory-based knowledge are abductive reasoning (Montgomery, 2006) and guerrilla theorizing (Reed, 2008).

At the heart of these theory-building strategies is a wild and passionate component of inspired knowing, where knowledge is produced in context, in touch with others, in the messiness of practice; where practice and knowing are one and ongoing; and yet where knowledge is partial and always under construction (Reed, 2008). Characteristics of persons who practice inspired knowing are also characteristics of emotional and cognitive maturity and are found in a therapeutic relationship. Some examples are as follows:

- Sense of trust
- Openness and flexibility
- Appreciation of contradiction and conflict
- Comfort with or tolerance of ambiguity
- Honoring of others' wisdom or experience
- Nonjudgmental attitude
- Creative construction of patterns
- Validation of observed patterns with another
- Reflective thinking
- Self-transcendence
- Spiritual and emotional intelligence

Inspired knowing is a sophisticated ability, and its development is facilitated by personal reflection, educational preparation, and engagement in a process of interaction with others.

Inspired knowing recognizes and values the nursing processes that reside within and among individuals, families, and communities; the patient's inner capacity for organization and well-being; and the knowledge-building synergy that exists in encounters between nurse and patient, science and practice. Inspired knowing delights in discerning patterns in persons' lives (Boyd, 2008) and in helping others recognize those patterns to facilitate positive change. Inspired knowing dissolves destructive distinctions between self and other and generates a sense of compassion and connection. And in revealing the patterns and resources for healing and well-being, inspired knowing facilitates knowledge-based health care practices and hope.

The popular and greatly revered American pragmatist philosopher Richard Rorty (1931–2007) challenged the modernist push toward foundational knowledge, methods that strove to discover truth, and frameworks that claimed to represent objective reality. Most relevant here, however, is an article in which he wrote about the necessity of inspired reading (Rorty, 1996). In the article, Rorty warned against a desire for knowingness that sacrificed inspiration for analysis, enthusiasm for professionalism, hope for understanding, and self-transformation for knowledge. He instructed that the path to inspiration is one where we take a balanced approach to knowing, and where we do not strive to know it all but instead allow the situation to recontextualize us; that is, to transform what we know and how we perceive the world.

And so it is with our quest for knowing in nursing: it seems desirable to make room for both the spiritual and the scientific, to be wild as well as systematic in our theorizing. May we embrace patterns of knowing that sustain us and our patients in practice, and make us feel as though we are walking on moonbeams.

References

American Association of College of Nursing. (2004). *Position statement on the practice doctorate in nursing.* Washington, DC: Author.

Arslanian-Engoren, C., Hicks, F. D., Whall, A. L., & Algase, D. L. (2005). An ontological view of advanced practice nursing. *Research and Theory for Nursing Practice, 19*(4), 315–322.

Benner, P., & Wrubel, J. (1989). *The primacy of caring: Stress and coping in health and illness.* Menlo Park, CA: Addison-Wesley.

Boyd, B. (2008). The art of literature and the science of literature: The delight we get from detecting patterns in books, and in life, can be measured and understood. *American Scholar, 77*(2), 118–127.

Carlsen, M. B. (1988). *Meaning-making: Therapeutic processes in adult development.* New York: Norton.

Carper, B. A. (1978). Fundamental patterns of knowing in nursing. *Advances in Nursing Science, 1*(1), 13–23.

Chinn, P. L., & Kramer, M. K. (2008). *Integrated theory and knowledge development in nursing* (7th ed.). St. Louis: Mosby.

Connor, D. (2005). *A people's history of science: Miners, midwives, and "low mechanics."* New York: Nation Books.

Ellis, R. (1969). Practitioner as theorist. *American Journal of Nursing, 69,* 1434–1438.

Glaser, B. G. (1978). *Theoretical sensitivity.* Mill Valley, CA: The Sociology Press.

Harding, S. (1998). *Is science multicultural? Postcolonialisms, feminisms, and epistemologies.* Indianapolis: Indiana University Press.

Ingraham, C. (1998). *Architecture and the burdens of linearity.* New Haven, CT: Yale University Press.

Kegan, R. G. (1982). *The evolving self: Problem and process in human development.* Cambridge, MA: Harvard University Press.

Kuhn, T. S. (1970). *The structure of scientific revolutions* (2nd ed.). Chicago: University of Chicago Press. Latour, B. (1988). *The pasteurization of France.* (Trans. as *Microbes* by A. Sheridan & J. Law). Cambridge: Harvard University Press.

Montgomery, K. (2006). *How doctors think: Clinical judgment and the practice of medicine.* New York: Oxford University Press.

Noddings, N. (1992). *The challenge to care in schools: An alternative approach to education.* New York: Teachers College Press.

Peplau, H. E. (1988). The art and science of nursing: Similarities, differences, and relations. *Nursing Science Quarterly, 1*, 8–15.

Pesut, D. J., & Herman, J. (1999). *Clinical reasoning: The art and science of critical and creative thinking.* Albany, NY: Delmar Publishers.

Reed, P. G. (1996). Transforming practice knowledge into nursing knowledge: A revisionist analysis of Peplau. *Journal of Nursing Scholarship, 28*, 29–33.

Reed, P. G. (1997). Nursing: The ontology of the discipline. *Nursing Science Quarterly, 10*(2), 76–79.

Reed, P. G. (2006a). Neomodernism and evidence based nursing: Implications for the production of nursing knowledge. *Nursing Outlook, 54*(1), 36–38.

Reed, P. G. (2006b). The practice turn in nursing epistemology. *Nursing Science Quarterly, 19*(1), 36–38.

Reed, P. G. (2008). Practitioner as theorist: A reprise. *Nursing Science Quarterly, 21*(4), 315–322.

Reed, P. G., & Lawrence, L. A. (2008). A paradigm for the production of practice-based knowledge. *Journal of Nursing Management, 16*, 422–432.

Rolfe, G. (2006). Nursing praxis and the science of the unique. *Nursing Science Quarterly, 19*(1), 39–43.

Rolfe, G., & Gardner, L. (2005). Towards a nursing science of the unique: Evidence, reflexivity and the study of persons. *Journal of Research in Nursing, 10*, 297–310.

Rorty, R. (1996). The necessity of inspired reading. *The Chronicle of Higher Education, 43*(1), 48.

Schön, D. A. (1983). *The reflective practitioner: How professionals think in action.* New York: Basic Books.

Whall, A. L., & Hicks, F. D. (2002). The unrecognized paradigm shift in nursing: Implications, problems, and possibilities. *Nursing Outlook, 50*, 72–76.

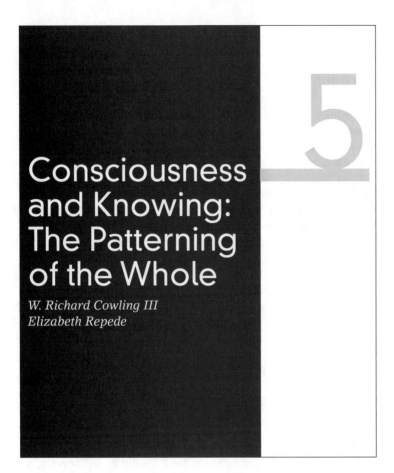

Consciousness and Knowing: The Patterning of the Whole

W. Richard Cowling III
Elizabeth Repede

Chapter Overview

This chapter focuses on knowing the person through the lens of a unitary perspective based upon the wholeness and the uniqueness of each life as expressed through patterning. The relationship of consciousness to ways of knowing and how they shape nursing practice and human betterment is addressed. A unitary theory of healing is presented, offering a reconceptualization of nursing practice responding to the wholeness of human life. Nursing from a unitary theoretical perspective is guided by appreciative and participatory processes aimed at the fullest involvement of people in their own emancipation in health care.

Introduction

The major premise of this chapter is that consciousness and knowing are practical tools to be used to capture the patterning of the whole of human life—a distinctive concern of nursing practice and science. There has been a great deal written about consciousness across a variety of disciplines. Consciousness has been explored as a psychological construct in general and as a cognitive construct in particular. Research has suggested that the source of consciousness can be traced to areas of the brain and understood as a neurophysiological phenomenon (Bekinschtein & Manes, 2008; Feinberg & Keenan, 2005). Consciousness has been described, delineated, and explained conceptually and theoretically across a variety of scientific and spiritual disciplines. Forms of consciousness, such as unitive consciousness (associated with holism and spirituality), have been explicated and correlated with modes of thinking and processing information.

Consciousness and Knowing as Patterning of the Whole

Nursing science has reached a crossroads. Two predominating and conflicting epistemological paths have been converging toward a common point. The empirical models of nursing have provided the primary philosophical underpinnings of nursing science for almost a century. The postmodern discourse that has had a steadily increasing influence on nursing as science and art since 1970 is bringing us full circle to our historical roots as an embodied discipline. The dissonance between these philosophies is moving the profession toward a necessary synthesis of these two divergent paradigms. Since the introduction of health and human beings as unitary concepts by Martha Rogers (1970), nursing theorists have sought ways to understand health and humans both empirically and humanistically. The philosophy of a discipline necessarily drives research, practice, and education. To date, much of this triumvirate has been grounded in the positivist model. When we expand our philosophical orientation to an inclusive stance encompassing both positivist and postmodernist philosophies, the boundaries of knowledge and compassion are limitless (Newman, 2002, 2003).

In a recent description of the state of nursing knowledge development and science, consciousness was delineated as one of the concepts central to the discipline along with health, caring, mutual process, patterning, presence, and meaning (Newman, Smith, Pharris, & Jones, 2008). Putting these in theoretical context, health is viewed as the intent of the relationship, caring as the nature of the relationship, consciousness as the informational pattern of the relationship, mutual process as the way in which the relationship unfolds, patterning as the evolving configuration of the relationship, presence as the resonance of the relationship, and meaning as the importance of the relationship. When consciousness is conceived as a patterning of information, information can facilitate turning points in which patterning is transformed and new insights develop. This is an outgrowth of Newman's (1979) conceptualization of health as expanding consciousness, including the idea of consciousness as incorporating the total information of the field (nurse-patient-environment). Newman and her colleagues (2008) advocated for a "consensus in the collective consciousness of the nursing profession" (p. E25) that supports relationship-centered practice that expresses our shared values and the depth of our purpose and meaning to current health care.

Rogers defined nursing as a unitary, transformative science based upon scientific and theoretical understandings of the universe as an energy field which is simultaneously unique and universal, is constantly changing, and is a unified whole (Rogers, 1970). The scientific and theoretical postulates that were the basis of Rogers' work developed concurrently across disciplines such as quantum physics, transpersonal psychology, philosophy, and energy medicine (Watson, 2005). We are on the threshold of an emerging collective consciousness that is changing the way we view our universe (Curtis & Hurtak, 2004; Sarath, 2006). This consciousness is creating waves of transformation and emancipation from reductionist and separatist worldviews, and it may well be the key to an ecology of health and healing (Watson, 2005).

Elliot Dacher (2005) has proposed four elements that characterize and frame a postmodern concept of an integral health care system: expanded consciousness, holism, intentionality, and a larger self. Expanded consciousness is the foundation that transforms our vision to an inclusive landscape by embracing what has gone before while transcending older perspectives: "Through the exploration and full development of consciousness we will at first rediscover the profound and denied inner aspects of healing—wholeness, peace, love, joy, and wisdom—and then seamlessly interweave the two traditional aspects of healing—outer and inner—into a new medicine" (Dacher, 2005, p. 10).

Holism from a unitary perspective would require an understanding of the cosmos and everything in it as a seamless whole. Subjective and objective and inner and outer ways of knowing are all part of the same pattern. Intentionality is the cornerstone of our ability to self-regulate and to consciously create changes in health and well-being. Growing into a mature awareness of authentic self-discovery and self-actualization within the context of our interconnectedness with all of nature will move us beyond the egocentric and self-serving individualism that has contributed to environmental and global chaos. These elements of a postmodern shift require the ability to consciously hold the paradox of both individual uniqueness and universal interconnectivity simultaneously.

The basis of consciousness and knowing in nursing arises from a common ground of caring, wholeness, and healing within an expanded epistemological framework (Cowling, Smith, & Watson, 2008). The concepts of wholeness, pattern, mutual process, consciousness, transcendence, and transformation are unifying themes pulled from several nursing theories and presented as a "transcendent unity of the theories of nursing" by Margaret Newman (2003, p. 243). Newman went on to define praxis as a "melding of theory, research, and practice" (Ibid), which reflects a unitary nursing science. Within a unitary, transformative perspective, the boundaries between science and art, stories and numbers, and sense and soul; and between research, theory, and practice disappear (Cowling, 2007; Newman, 2003). This perspective allows for the appreciation of wholeness to emerge, while retaining an empirical framework that is grounded in extended ways of knowing.

The Consciousness of Wholeness

Ingrained in Western ideologies, consciousness is often conceptualized as simply awareness of one's surroundings and is narrowly defined as being awake. Consciousness from this perspective originates solely in the mind. Thought is the structural foundation for knowing, and understanding comes through an empirical, logico-reductionist, and sensory-based model.

In contrast, a unitary perspective of consciousness extends beyond thoughts to encompass both logic and analogic, body and mind, and spirit and form in a unified wholeness which is inherent in and contiguous with the universe. Ways of knowing arise from personal discovery, intuition, cognition, sensation, empathy, emotion, participation, and creative expression, to name a few. A unitary paradigm is boundaryless, ever changing, and relational (Cowling, 2001). Health is viewed as a dynamic process, and life patterning can be appreciated and understood within this context of wholeness through a synoptic lens. Synopsis is a way of perceiving the universe through the intentional viewing together of human aspects that are normally understood as separate (Cowling, 2001).

In a unitary worldview, the entire cosmos is understood as an integral whole. Instead of isolated planets drifting in a vacuum of space, the entire fabric of the universe is a beautiful, interconnected web, in which waves of energy speed up and slow down to create matter and space. The underlying foundation of the universe is information, embedded in the energetic matrix, and consciousness is one aspect of this energy (Newman, 2002). The universe is not breakable into separate parts which comprise a whole. Rather, it is unitary and indivisible. Because it is interconnected, any thought, action, or emotion is experienced by the whole. Both separatist ways of being in which aggressive individualism based upon a drive for power, egocentrism, and material accumulation (Dacher, 2005); and unitary ways of being based upon sharing, peace, and caring ripple around the world. A conscious awareness of these ways of being allows us to choose how we use and direct these ripples through our thoughts and actions. Albert Einstein, in his reflections on the quantum nature of human consciousness, described his perception of the human being as existing within the wholeness of the universe:

> He experiences himself, his thoughts and feelings as something separated from the rest—a kind of optical delusion of his consciousness. This delusion is a kind of prison for us, restricting us to our personal desires and to affection

*for a few persons nearest to us. Our task must be to free
ourselves from this prison by widening our circle of compassion to embrace all living creatures and the whole of
nature in its beauty. Nobody is able to achieve this completely, but the striving for such achievement is in itself a
part of the liberation, and a foundation for inner security.
The true value of a human being is determined primarily
by the measure in which he has attained liberation from the
self. (as cited in Nagler, 1982, p. 11)*

In a humanistic discipline such as nursing, unitary consciousness can provide the space for a caring perspective that
is participatory, transformative, and creative. Ways of knowing
that are synoptic, holographic, relational, ecological, and holar-
chical (wholes within wholes) are needed for a unitary science
of nursing, which seeks to understand and appreciate humans
in their wholeness (Cowling, 2001). As individuals attune to a
unity consciousness, infinite possibilities are born, and the sta-
sis of a finite consciousness disappears in the beauty of movement and flow, revealing a kaleidoscope of patterns that are
ever-changing (Ibid).

Knowing and Consciousness

Knowing has been given particular attention in the field of
nursing, most notably as spelled out by Chinn and Kramer
(2007) in their text *Integrated Theory and Knowledge Development in Nursing*, which is used widely in schools of nursing across the United States and world. Chinn and Kramer
described five ways of knowing central to nursing: empirical,
personal, ethical, and aesthetic, with all of these culminating
in emancipatory knowing. White (1995) described another
way of knowing central to nursing as sociopolitical knowing. The specific process, products, and criteria for evaluation associated with each of these ways of knowing were
described in detail to assist nurses in understanding how
they are used. Chinn and Kramer (2007) depicted nursing
science and art as an integration of all these ways of knowing. The integration culminates in the practice of nursing
with and for people.

In addition to the nursing literature, there are a variety
of perspectives on knowing and ways or forms of knowing
addressed in other disciplinary writings. A classical text on

feminist perspective and ways of knowing (Belenky, Clinchy, Goldberger, & Tarule, 1986) portrays how women form and use knowledge distinctive to their gender. One important aspect of their work that has relevance for nursing is bringing an understanding of how women's ways of knowing have been dismissed in favor of more masculine models of knowledge. Nursing has always embraced and valued a variety of ways of knowing that provide understandings beyond more empirical models of knowing. These alternative and complementary ways of knowing have brought understandings to patient situations that have been useful in promoting health and well-being beyond the biomedical perspective.

The variety of perspectives on consciousness and knowing may illuminate *and* confuse understandings about the nature of these phenomena and their practical value to nursing. It is critical to explore the context of a perspective on consciousness and knowing as presented by the proponents of that perspective in their writings and work. For instance, there are quite different meanings, understandings, and potentials for application of consciousness, depending on whether it is conceptualized as a psychological or spiritual or biomedical phenomenon. Knowing may be conceptualized as specific to a particular need or grounded in a particular worldview that would have implications for how one would develop, use, and evaluate that knowledge. For instance, there are those who advocate for evidence-based practice and have a very specific set of criteria about which forms of evidence should be given primacy and even what actually counts as evidence for practice. These advocates have a distinct view of knowledge with certain assumptions. When someone in practice adheres to one of these perspectives, he or she may screen out certain information as useful or not useful knowledge even though there are a variety of forms of knowledge available.

This chapter advocates for a model of consciousness and knowing that is grounded in a unitary view of human life and is designed to assist those nurses who seek to know and understand human life in its wholeness in order to help clients realize their greatest possibilities for health and well-being through this knowing and understanding. The model is based on the premise stated previously, that consciousness and knowing can serve nurses in very practical ways when providing care based on the inherent wholeness of human life. It seeks to more fully address significant questions that dominate much of the nursing disciplinary discourse: What does it mean to have a nursing perspective that accepts and embraces human wholeness from the vantage points of nurses and those who are engaged in their care? How do nurses use this perspective in active ways in their practices? What differences can be made in the health and well-being of humans and humankind by using such a perspective?

A Unitary Perspective on Consciousness and Knowing

A unitary perspective on consciousness and knowing is derived from the broad conceptual model known as the science of unitary human beings. This model was proposed and developed by Martha E. Rogers (1970, 1992, a noted nurse theorist. This conceptual model has led to the development and testing of a number of theories, and has served to orient the development of the theoretical frameworks of health as expanding consciousness (Newman, 1994) and human becoming (Parse, 1981, 1999). Central ideas from the science of unitary human beings that are used to guide a unitary perspective of consciousness and knowing are these:

1. Humans are essentially and inherently whole, unified beings (energy fields).
2. Human life coexists and emerges through its relationship and participation with the environment (mutual process).
3. Human life expresses itself in patterning that can be known through its manifestations, some directly and some indirectly sensed (pattern).
4. Human life has infinite potentials for health and well-being (pandimensionality and unpredictability).

What does this mean for conceptualizing consciousness and knowing as unitary? From a unitary perspective, consciousness is not a cognitive or psychological phenomenon or process. Rather, consciousness is a process that integrates all of the senses, creating an awareness of life as whole. This consciousness is multisensory and goes beyond cognition and cognitive processing of information. Unitary consciousness takes into account a wide variety of information from an array of sources. It is a bridge to knowing that rests upon the assumption that it is possible to be consciously aware of wholeness—that it is a matter of appreciating fully all the information with which we are provided, both within ourselves and from others and the environment.

From a unitary perspective, knowing arises within the context of unitary consciousness. Consciousness provides the orientation and the openness to seek to know human life as a whole. Rogers did not refer to consciousness in her writings and presentations because she believed that there was confusion about conceptualizations of consciousness and a tendency for many to regard consciousness as a cognitive or mental phenomenon. Unitary consciousness provides a conceptualization that is consistent with key tenets of unitary science. In this conceptualization that is meant to provide a context for both practice and research, knowing occurs through choosing to understand information that is available through the senses and through our sensitivity to the person and environment. Knowing through unitary consciousness opens the doors of perception to appreciate the wholeness of human life and the patterning that is underlying what the client or research participant perceives to be important or of concern.

This requires developing sensitivity and sensibility of what counts as information by embracing a new approach to understanding the information as it is made available to the practitioner or researcher. In the last few decades, nursing has used a predominantly systems-based approach to knowledge in the assessment of patients, in the creation of plans of care that reflect nursing diagnoses about health and illness, and in the research of human health conditions (Cowling, 1993). Koplowitz (1984) described unitary thinking as a cognitive stage beyond systems thinking, and his description of this stage is for the most part in concert with unitary science. Based upon a systems thinking approach (Ibid), there are four major perceptions that shape our understanding of the human-environment-health-nurse metaparadigm. These are (1) the cause and effect of different actions, perceptions, and environmental factors that affect health and illness; (2) the variables, which are objects or forces that affect human health and their relationship to each other; (3) the boundaries that separate each part of the human system and subsystems from the other parts; and (4) the awareness of the human about his or her health in the context of the internal and external environment of the person or community.

In a general systems model, the focus of practice or inquiry is on the parts as they relate and how they make sense of the whole (Cowling, 1993). Cause and effect occur as cycles of actions and reactions in a general systems view of the world. The nurse would study patterns of interactions in an effort to understand how different variables relate to each other in a cause-and-effect model of health or illness. For example, a diet high in carbohydrates, refined sugars, and fats combined with a genetic predisposition and sedentary lifestyle would predispose an individual to illnesses such as diabetes or heart disease. In general systems theory, these variables are considered interdependent. Changing any one variable (diet, exercise) in the system will have an effect on all of the other elements of the system, potentially offsetting the genetics.

Boundaries are considered bidirectional in a general systems theory. Boundaries allow for the exchange of information and energy between the system and its environment. Boundaries are considered open in general systems theory because they do not clearly separate the internal from the external environments. For example, the boundaries within the human body are fluid, allowing exchange of energy and information across cell membranes. The boundaries between the environment and the human reflect a fluid exchange of nutrients, gases, and energy. These boundaries may appear as more visible and are evidenced by patterns of eating, breathing, and moving through the world of objects and energy. Variables which are phenomena or energy affect the entire system. Eating a candy bar or a peach are variables that will have different effects upon the human at all levels of the system, from perception and meaning to physiological responses at the cellular level.

The concept of permanent objects in general systems is that the object is known as an independent reality apart from the knower, but with personal meanings specific to the person, constructed through an array of experiences unique to the individual. For example, the candy bar is separate from the person eating it, but the meaning of the candy may represent more than something to eat—it may represent a reward or be more tasteful to the individual than the peach, affecting the choice and thus affecting the whole system (Bertalanaffy, 1968; Cowling, 1993).

All of these concepts can be viewed from the smallest subsystems at the microscopic and cellular levels to ever-increasing levels of complexity of the universe. Systems thinking has broadened the scope of nursing so that the focus of nursing care is no longer the patient as a discrete unit, but the patient within the context of the family, the health care system, and the community in ever-increasing levels of rela-tionship and reflexivity (Cowling, 1993). However, advanc-ing knowledge in sciences such as quantum physics, chaos theory, string theory, and fractal geometry has opened our conception of systems to a subtle level of understanding in which the boundaries of time, space, and consciousness no longer exist even as discrete entities. Unitary thinking has arisen in a conceptual system that expands the concepts of the original systems theory and thinking. Energy theories have demonstrated that we live in a vast quantum pattern of energetic information. What was perceived as solid atomic particles is now understood to be simply energetic waves or vibrations oscillating at different speeds or frequencies, which are slowed way down and experienced by human senses as form. These energy fields are contiguous between the field and the object. Objects occur in the field as a slower, denser vibrational frequency of energy, which *is* information itself, or as a matrix of energy and information moving in waves. These waves occur in patterns that are continuously changing. These patterns are pandimensional rather than multidimensional. Multidimensional implies multiple sepa-rate forces or factors occurring over time. Pandimensional is all-encompassing, like the ripples in a pond after a stone is thrown into the water. The ripples move in increasing pat-terns of diversity and complexity simultaneously. Those rip-ples are the reflection of patterns of energy moving through the water that cannot be appreciated directly. But by becom-ing aware of the patterns as they are reflected in the ripples, we can gain an awareness of the whole movement as a field of flowing water that is inclusive of the energy, the water, the stone, and our perception of it. So the perceiver is not sepa-rate from the events or the forms.

In unitary thinking, systems thinking is embraced yet expanded and explicated according to Koplowitz (1984). Time and space are not separate. In this perspective, all things are connected in a unitary reality that is unable to be broken into parts. The ripples, the water, the stone, and the energy with which the stone was thrown into the water are appreciated as a whole rather than as elements of the whole. Variables of objects and forces and their characteristics are complex field phenomena in unitary thinking, rather than a constellation of interdependent constructs as they are in general systems theory. Because these are moving waves of energy and perception, there are no definable boundaries. So we have extended the systems concept of open boundaries to a unitary conception of systems which is boundaryless, and therefore open to infinite possibilities (Cowling, 2001).

This moves our perception in nursing from a dichotomous health-illness continuum to a dynamic perceptual field of shifting realities (Cowling, 1993). Figure 5.1 shows the conceptual schema for how we would use information and observations from a systems perspective in nursing practice.

Figure 5.2 shows a conceptual schema that might guide a unitary nurse to see all information and observations as integral to the patterning of the person.

5.1

Systems perspective on gathering and using information and observations

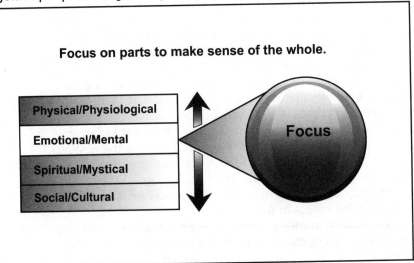

5.2

Unitary perspective on gathering and using information and observations

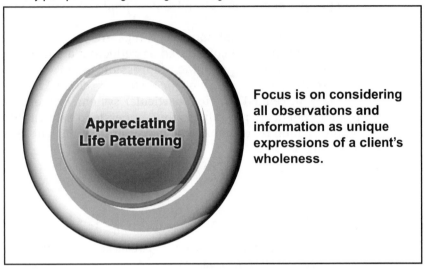

Appreciating Life Patterning

Focus is on considering all observations and information as unique expressions of a client's wholeness.

This diagram is intended to convey the process of using the unitary lens to configure information and observations as expressions of an underlying patterning of wholeness. Nursing assessment from a traditional systems model is based upon the subsystem analysis of physical/physiological, emotional/mental, spiritual/mystical, and social/cultural subsystems of the client. Diagnosis is the result of a synthesis of large amounts of existing information about the patient into a pattern that has meaning for the caregiver and care receiver. In a unitary perspective, nursing practice is aimed at appreciating each area of information and observations as an expression of wholeness—not as an expression of subsystems or parts. This appreciation requires a greater emphasis on synopsis and synthesis rather than analysis and diagnosis. In addition, this appreciation suggests that the unitary nurse would develop creative ways of organizing information and observations to be able to see the patterning beyond the parts. The nurse is engaged in moving and focusing the unitary lens in order to see the clearest picture or kaleidoscope of patterning that best represents what is happening with the client.

Figure 5.3 compares how information and observations are considered and contextualized from a systems perspective and from a unitary perspective within nursing practice. This figure is demonstrates in table format how a nurse with each perspective might look at and understand the phenomena available to them.

From a systems perspective, things are placed in categories and then are considered as reflecting a particular single category. For example, depression as an emotion representing a neurophysiological state is reduced to one category; or related only to a particular system. Depression from a systems perspective is thus understood as a variety of information that combines to make sense of the whole in a summative way.

5.3

Comparison of unitary and systems perspectives regarding how information and observations are considered and contextualized.

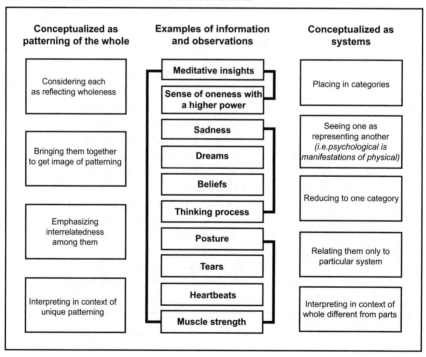

The unitary perspective guides a more synoptic approach, in which each phenomenon is considered as reflecting the whole. Bringing them together provides a deeper and wider appreciation of the patterning through emphasizing the interrelatedness of the phenomena. They are contextualized as providing an image or picture of the unique patterning of the individual.

Unitary Healing: Consciousness and Knowing in Action

Unitary healing, a new conceptual and theoretical perspective, creates a context for the practice of nursing integrating a variety of modalities. It is grounded in the science of unitary human beings (Rogers, 1992) and builds upon a decade of practice and research on women that focused on abuse, despair, and healing (Cowling, 2008). However, unitary healing can be used as an orientation for many forms of nursing practice across a variety of settings. Unitary healing is viewed as appreciating human wholeness through participating knowingly in emancipatory change and transformation. In this model, nurses seek to appreciate the wholeness of their clients and their clients' lives by engaging and involving them in a mutual process, using consciousness and knowing in unitary ways. As the engagement and involvement with clients unfolds with wholeness being appreciated and understood, change and transformation occur. The change and transformation is targeted at freeing the client (person, family, group, or community) from perceived limitations in his or her health and well-being.

The concept and theory of unitary healing can be contrasted with current conceptualizations of healing that suggest that healing is aimed at creating or facilitating wholeness. In the unitary healing view, wholeness already exists; it is consciousness and knowledge of the patterning of that wholeness that guides practice. This does not mean that a client's perception of feeling fragmented or limited is not valid or real, rather that this perception is one of the ways that the client might be expressing his or her patterning. The current patterning reflects a sensation of being fragmented or limited. Nurses work with clients to come to know and appreciate the patterning of wholeness associated with this sensation and to explore possibilities of using this knowledge and appreciation to create wanted change and transformation. The unitary healing perspective is also informed by the theory of power as knowing participation in change (Barrett, Caroselli, Smith, & Smith, 1997) and by the broader participatory worldview (Reason & Bradbury, 2001).

The term *pattern* was originally used by Dr. Rogers in her conceptual framework of unitary science (1992) to describe the unique identifying feature of each human being. She defined each person as being a field of energy, with pattern as the distinguishing feature of the particular human being. The view was that each person is distinguishable from others, although they might share similar characteristics. This led to a prior practice model that articulated a view of a "pattern-focused practice" for nursing (Cowling, 1993). More recently, Alligood and Fawcett (2004) did a historical conceptual analysis of *pattern* and suggested that the word *patterning* reflects a more dynamic perspective of the evolving nature of the human field pattern. The word *pattern* as a noun implies a static phenomenon, whereas *patterning* is a gerund that implies movement and process and is therefore more consistent with a unitary framework. The authors concluded that patterning of the client's life is an observable reflection of the person-environment process and that *patterning* (as described by Martha Rogers) is more useful than *pattern* in nursing practice as a reflection of the nurse-client encounter as process. This may in fact be distinct from the current movement in nursing toward outcome evaluation.

More recently, Newman et al. (2008) have conceptualized patterning as the evolving configuration of the relationship of the nurse and patient. This builds upon Newman's (1994) conceptualization of pattern as a characteristic of wholeness: "Pattern is information that depicts the whole, understanding the meaning of all the relationships at once" (Newman, 1994, p. 71); "Patterning reveals the evolving nature of the whole" (Newman et al., 2008, E22).

Conceptual and Theoretical Structure

Six focal and process aspects form the conceptual and theoretical structure of unitary healing. These aspects reflect a possible structure and process that could be used as grounds for a unitary healing practice. These are:

- Wholeness
- Appreciation
- Participation
- Knowledge
- Emancipation
- Change/transformation

Wholeness. A core dimension of unitary healing is a notion of inherent wholeness in human life. This compares with other healing perspectives that suggest that healing is associated with promoting, facilitating, and developing wholeness. The goal of unitary nursing is not aimed at helping persons create wholeness in their lives, but rather to help them appreciate and understand the patterning in their lives that reflects the wholeness that already exists. What is crucial in the unitary nursing process is helping the client see how all the various aspects of their experiences are interrelated. The patterning of wholeness for each individual is unique in that no client has the same patterning as other clients.

It is important to note that this patterning expresses itself in a variety of ways across the spectrum of human experience—physically, emotionally/mentally, spiritually, culturally. The real challenge for the unitary nurse is to use the information and observations from these domains of experiences in a way that puts them in the context of wholeness and patterning rather than to resort to using them separately as data about that single domain. In other words, physical information is really information about wholeness and patterning, mental/emotional information is really information about wholeness and patterning, spiritual information is really information about wholeness and patterning, and cultural information is really information about wholeness and patterning. The process of understanding all of these in a unified context rather than a system-specific context is called *synopsis*.

Appreciation. The core process dimension of unitary healing is appreciation of wholeness. This appreciation requires a conceptual orientation that is consistent with wholeness as inherent and with learning to develop oneself as an instrument to see and understand wholeness. This orientation is applied to a person's life. The appreciating process involves grasping the wholeness of human life from a synoptic perspective. What appears as separate, fragmented, or disparate is brought together to see a "patterning within wholeness." This involves nurses attempting to go beyond processes that only see human experience in terms of diagnoses, symptoms, and diseases. In a unitary healing frame of reference, all of these are important but are understood through consciousness and knowing as expressions of the patterning of the client's wholeness. When appreciated in this context, diagnoses, symptoms, and diseases become more deeply and widely useful in assisting the client to create needed change and transformation. In addition, unitary appreciation suggests that these experiences cannot be generalized in the same way to all clients, but they have peculiar or specific meaning for each person experiencing the diagnosis, disease, and symptom.

Appreciation is intended to replace the general notion of problem solving in nursing practice. In problem solving, there is an assumption that something is not whole but rather fragmented or broken and in need of fixing. According to Cooperrider and Srivastva (1987), "The function of problem solving is to integrate, stabilize, and help raise to full potential" (p. 153). Implied is that "through analysis, diagnosis, treatment, and follow-up evaluation" (p. 157), the person can be kept on a steady course of productivity and health. The function of appreciation is to seek to grasp the patterning that underlies the human life, and in that act of seeking, to discover hidden possibilities for change and transformation. Appreciation does not seek to stabilize because it assumes the person is in a constant state of flux and flow that can be mobilized into desired change. It does not seek to integrate because it assumes the person is already fully whole or integrated. It does not seek to raise the person to a full potential because it assumes that the person has unimaginable possibilities for change and transformation. Rather than aiming for a steady course of productivity and health, it aims to assist people in freeing themselves from constraints and limitations on reaching their desired futures.

Participation. Participation is an approach and way of being that accommodates appreciating wholeness. This flows from the unitary perspective of a world that is in continuous, mutual process. In a sense, the nurse is capitalizing on this mutual process to mobilize strengths and possibilities available to the client for change and transformation. The nurse chooses to participate in particular ways with the client so that they together deepen and broaden their understanding and appreciation of the client's patterning of wholeness. Through this participatory process, the client and nurse cooperate to bring about desired changes, considering what is learned in the context of the wholeness of human life and the patterning of the individual.

From this process of participation, a distinctive way of knowing emerges that is different from other forms of knowing. The nurse develops his or her own consciousness to be aware of participatory knowing. For instance, when working with clients, there is a heavy emphasis on what is happening from the client's perspective. The perspective of the client is highly regarded and valued and used to guide unitary nursing practice. The nurse contributes to this knowing by actively including her observations and perceptions based on her general knowledge and the unique knowledge she is gaining from involvement with the client. The nurse shares these actively with the client to ascertain whether the nurse's synopsis of knowledge represents what is going on with the client from the client's perspective. The nurse is cautious that the voice of the client is given precedence in the construction of what the nurse sees as the patterning of the whole.

Knowledge. Unitary healing involves practitioners considering a variety of forms and processes of knowing and knowledge. The focal point of knowledge is the patterning of wholeness of the client's life and experience; that is, the nurse seeks to grasp the knowledge that helps the nurse appreciate the wholeness of the client's life. This knowledge becomes available to the nurse through the participatory process that is guided by the intent of appreciating wholeness and by a high regard for inclusion of the client's perspective. Giving attention to appreciating wholeness leads to a variety of forms of knowledge that culminate in practical emancipatory change and transformation. These types and forms are not fully distinct from one another. They create a patterning of knowing and knowledge that is consistent with the patterning of wholeness of the individual or group; in other words, participation creates knowing in line with appreciating wholeness.

Examples of knowing that are participatory in nature and reflect an appreciation of wholeness are experiential, presentational, propositional, and, culminating from these three, practical (Heron & Reason, 2001). Experiential knowing refers to what happens in the direct encounters with clients—described as knowing through empathy and resonance that is almost impossible to put into words. Presentational knowing arises from experiential knowing and is conveyed through expressions such as "story, picture, sculpture, movement, dance, drawing on aesthetic imagery" (Heron & Reason, 2001, p. 9). Propositional knowing is the form of knowing that draws on concepts, ideas, and theories concerning what is happening—in this case related to the patterning of the client. Finally, "practical knowing consummates the other forms" (Ibid) through the development of competencies and skills that clients can use to better their lives. Other types of knowing and forms of knowledge that may be associated with unitary healing are relational, feminine, holistic, and systemic (Cowling, 2007).

Emancipation. Unitary healing is characterized by emancipation in a variety of forms and expressions. Unitary healing is associated with a sense of freedom across all dimensions of a person's life. The freedom that is experienced in unitary healing arises from the participatory process of discovering and appreciating the person's patterning of wholeness. As the person and nurse participate in uncovering this patterning, they become aware of possibilities for change and transformation that free the person from perceived limitations. The limitations may involve many aspects of human life and the human experience. An example of this comes from our work with women who were abused as children. Many of the women became aware of the larger and deeper association of these abusive experiences to their relationships, their health, and their sense of self. Through the participatory and appreciative process involved in unitary healing, new understandings and realizations emerged. For instance, a woman realized that what had happened to her and what had seemed benign when she was a child, was extremely traumatic and pervasive in her life. She moved from anger to feeling the power that knowing this could free her from self-doubt and blame. She decided to employ this personal power to help herself and others. The sense of emancipation pervaded her life and spilled over into her well-being and encouraged community action.

The varieties of understanding that come forth with unitary consciousness and knowing suggest to clients what may work differently in their lives to free them from constraints across all aspects of their health and well-being. There is an insightful awareness that leads to envisioning greater possibilities for change and transformation. Appreciation and participation make possible enlightened awareness and action, providing the means for creating desired changes and potential transformation in one's life. A primary ideal of unitary nursing is to enhance the fullest expression of human freedom in the lives of those who seek these services. The unitary healing theory guides nurses to creatively use the processes of appreciation and participation to actualize this ideal.

It is important to note that through a unitary lens of perception, people are viewed as unlimited, with infinite potential. Therefore one could question the ideal of a unitary healing theory that seeks to help people be freed from limits and constraints. This is similar to the conundrums that people are whole but feel fragmented and that people are connected yet experience life as separate. The sense of constraints and limitations is similar in that people experience these in spite of the infinite nature of human potential. In a subtle way, unitary healing implies that the appreciation of wholeness also involves an appreciation of infinite possibilities, which in itself frees people to explore a wider range of options for desired change. Unitary consciousness and knowing are integral to discovering a deepening sense of freedom that is essential to moving beyond previously limiting choices.

The unitary healing perspective on emancipation, freedom, and liberation in no way implies that there are not substantive constraints placed on people through others, including relationships, families, communities, and governments. These constraints are imposed in such forms as discriminatory practices and policies; stereotypes of individuals and groups, governmental and legal regulations; social conditions of poverty; imbalances in resource allocations; and the phenomena of racism, sexism, homophobia, ageism, and ethnic hatred.

One goal of nursing from a unitary healing perspective is to help people develop their fullest capabilities at moderating, if not overcoming, these constraints. It is hoped that by using appreciative and participatory approaches, individuals as well as groups will see the possibilities for community and societal change and transformation while developing competencies and skills to facilitate social action. As part of these unitary healing processes, people can not only discover the connection between their personal power and these constraints but also uncover the subtle ways in which many of these constraints are used and allowed to limit personal freedom and health.

Change/transformation. According to the unitary worldview (Rogers, 1992), change is constant, inevitable, and unpredictable. This includes change in human life, given that the universe is always fluctuating and flowing, not stagnant and static. However, change can be facilitated and guided by persons using a process called "knowing participation in change." The unitary healing interpretation of this principle of knowing participation in change is to use nursing practice to mobilize the possibilities for emancipatory change through the participatory and appreciative processes described previously.

For over 25 years, Dr. Elizabeth Barrett has been developing and using the theory of power as knowing participation in change to guide her work and others' in both the research and practice arenas (Caroselli & Barrett, 1998). She described the potential of this power also in terms of freedom: "Power is being aware of what one is choosing to do, feeling free to do it, and doing it intentionally. Awareness and freedom to act intentionally guide participation in choices and involvement in creating changes" (Caroselli & Barrett, 1998, p. 9). Having power—including the power of choices—is directly related to feeling free to act as one wishes. Likewise, how one participates in changes, and the nature of one's involvement, relates to both the type and potency of choices: "Awareness permeates the entirety of the power process" (Ibid). It is clear from this power theory that people share actively in creating their reality.

The theory of unitary healing embraces fully the notion and nature of power as described by Barrett and her colleagues (1997), which places freedom in a primary role in the process of emerging power. In addition, unitary healing suggests that through consciously appreciating the patterning of wholeness using a participatory process of knowing, people become more aware of possibilities for emancipation of themselves and others. In a sense, this inherent sense of freedom is enhanced and expressed throughout their lives and is integral to unitary healing. As noted in Barrett's theory, people actively participate in creating their own reality—a reality that can be characterized by perceptions of constraints and limitations as well as by possibilities for being and feeling free.

In the unitary healing perspective, transformation is viewed as a particular form of change. This is consistent with the unitary-transformative paradigm of nursing (Newman, Sime, & Corcoran-Perry, 1991). Newman (2003) described the recognition of pattern as spurring transformation that happens through the relationship of theory and action. In unitary healing terms, transformation occurs as appreciative and participatory processes unfold through consciousness into new forms of knowing that guide emancipatory changes in the client's life patterning. Newman describes transformation in a way that implies a changing of form in a literal sense leading to a new view or orientation, an entirely different angle. In unitary healing, transformation may occur in the form of a person seeing for the first time within his or her patterning of wholeness, many new possibilities and approaches that might support desires and aspirations for creating changes.

Change and transformation are expressed in manifestations that emerge from the appreciative and participatory processes used in unitary healing. They are closely associated with innovative and creative consciousness and knowing that suggest possibilities for fulfilling the dreams and visions of those engaged in these processes. Both the nurse and client benefit from this engagement. The participatory nature of human life, coupled with the appreciative orientation, are principle source of change and transformation. Through using an appreciative stance toward the wholeness of life, encouraging knowing participation in change, and using awareness and action aimed at emancipation, change and transformation are shaped by the individuals who seek the assistance of nursing.

Summary

How we understand, perceive, and act in our world reflects our consciousness and defines our ways of knowing. The ultimate question for the nurse is, How do I conceive of the universe, and what is my relationship to it? If the perception is one of a unitary synthesis in which everything and everyone is integral and exists in a unitary wholeness, then everything I think, do, or say is associated with each and every other aspect of the universe. The patient and nurse are not separate fields, but rather integral to one another. If, on the other hand, the perception is of a universe with separate parts that are distinct from each other, the locus of consciousness will reside predominantly in the self, thereby narrowing the choices, possibilities, and impact of relating to others.

Unitary healing is consciousness and knowing in action. Through an appreciation of our own wholeness, knowledge, and knowing participation in change, we consciously begin to create new patterning by envisioning infinite possibilities that can transform our lives and bring freedom from perceived limitations. By actively seeking to expand our conceptions of who we in the broader context of what it means to be human in a participatory universe, we can collectively and consciously guide nursing science and practice into a unitary field of knowledge without predefined boundaries on healing.

References

Alligood, M. R. & Fawcett, J. (2004). An interpretive study of Martha Rogers' conception of pattern. *Visions: The Journal of Rogerian Nursing Science, 12*(1), 8–13.

Barrett, E. A. M., Caroselli, C., Smith, A. S., & Smith, D. W. (1997). Power as knowing participation in change: Theoretical, practice, and methodological issues, insights, and ideas. In M. Madrid (Ed.), *Rogerian patterns of knowing* (pp. 31–46). New York: National League for Nursing.

Bekinschtein, T. A. & Manes, F. F. (2008). Neurobiology of consciousness. *Vertex, 19*(78), 35–44.

Belenky, M., Clinchy, B., Goldberger, N., & Tarule, J. (1986). *Womens' ways of knowing: the development of self, voice, and mind*. New York: Basic Books.

Bertalanaffy, L. von. (1968). *General system theory*. New York: Braziller.

Caroselli, C., & Barrett, E. A. M. (1998). A review of the power as knowing participation in change literature. *Nursing Science Quarterly, 11*(1), 9–16.

Chinn, P. L. & Kramer, M. K. (2007). *Integrated theory and knowledge development in nursing* (7th ed.). St Louis: Elsevier.

Cooperrider, D. L., & Srivastva, S. (1987). Appreciative inquiry and organizational life. *Research in Organizational Change and Development, 1*, 129–169.

Cowling, W. R. (1993). Unitary knowing in nursing practice. *Nursing Science Quarterly, 6*(4), 201–207.

Cowling, W. R. (2001). Unitary appreciative inquiry. *Advances in Nursing Science, 23*(4), 32–48.

Cowling, W. R. (2007). A unitary participatory vision of nursing knowledge. *Advances in Nursing Science, 30*(1), 61–70.

Cowling, W. R. (2008). An essay on women, despair, and healing: A personal narrative. *Advances in Nursing Science, 31*(3), 249–258.

Cowling, W. R., Smith, M. C., & Watson, J. (2008). The power of wholeness, consciousness, and caring: A dialogue on nursing science, art, and healing. *Advances in Nursing Science, 31*(1), E41–E51.

Curtis, B. D. & Hurtak, J. J. (2004). Consciousness and quantum information processing: uncovering the foundation for a medicine of light. *Journal of Alternative and Complementary Therapies, 10*(1), 27–39.

Dacher, E. S. (2005). Towards a postmodern integral medicine. In M. Schlitz, T. Amorak, & M. Micozzi (Eds.), *Consciousness and healing: Integral approaches to mind-body medicine*, (pp. 8–16). Philadelphia: Churchill Livingstone.

Feinberg, T. E., & Keenan, J. P. (2005). Where in the brain is the self? *Consciousness and Cognition, 14*, 661–678.

Heron, J. & Reason, P. (2001). The practice of cooperative inquiry: Research with rather than on people. In P. Reason & H. Bradbury (Eds.) *Handbook of action research: Participative inquiry and practice* (pp. 179–188). Thousand Oaks, CA: Sage.

Koplowitz, H. (1984). A projection beyond Piaget's formal operations stage: A general systems stage and a unitary stage. In M. L. Commons, F. A. Richards, & C. Armon (Eds.), *Beyond formal operations: Late adolescent and adult cognitive development* (pp. 272–295). New York: Macmillan.

Nagler, M. (1982). *America without violence: Why violence persists and how you can stop it.* Covelo, CA: Island Press.

Newman, M.A. (1979). *Theory Development in Nursing.* Philadelphia: F.A. Davis.

Newman, M. A. (1994). *Health as expanding consciousness* (2nd ed.). New York: National League of Nursing.

Newman, M. A. (2002). The pattern that connects. *Advances in Nursing Science, 24*(3), 1–7.

Newman, M. A. (2003). A world of no boundaries. *Advances in Nursing Science, 26*(4), 240–245.

Newman, M. A., Sime, A. M., & Corcoran-Perry, S. A. (1991). The focus of the discipline of nursing. *Advances in Nursing Science, 14*(1), 1–6.

Newman, M. A., Smith, M. C., Pharris, M. D., & Jones, D. (2008). The focus of the discipline revisited. *Advances in Nursing Science, 31*(1), E16–E27.

Parse, R. R. (1981). *Man—living—health: A theory of nursing.* New York: Wiley.

Parse, R. R. (1999). *Hope: An international human becoming perspective.* Sudbury, MA; Jones and Bartlett.

Reason, P., & Bradbury, H. (2001). Inquiry and participation in search of a world worthy of human aspiration. In P. Reason & H. Bradbury (Eds.) *Handbook of action research: Participative inquiry and practice* (pp. 1–14). Thousand Oaks, CA: Sage.

Rogers, M. E. (1970). An introduction to the theoretical basis of nursing. Philadelphia: Davis.

Rogers, M. E. (1992). Nursing and the space age. *Nursing Science Quarterly, 5*, 27–33.

Sarath, E. (2006). Meditation, creativity, and consciousness: charting future terrain within higher education. *Teachers College Record, 108*(9), 1816–1841.

Watson, J. (2005). *Caring science as sacred science.* Philadelphia: F. A. Davis.

White, J. (1995). Patterns of knowing. *Advances in Nursing Science, 17*(4), 73–86.

Evidence, Knowledge, and Wisdom: Nursing Practice in a Universe of Complexity and Mystery

6

Gail J. Mitchell

Chapter Overview

This chapter explores concepts of evidence, knowledge, and wisdom in light of philosophy, human science, complexity science, and nursing theory. Five kinds of activities are identified as being familiar and present in the nursing care of persons and families: simple, complicated, complex, unspeakable, and unknowable. Evidence is shown to be relevant in the simple and complicated activities that nurses participate in; it is less relevant in activities that are complex, unspeakable, and unknowable. Nursing actions are considered in light of thinking and doing, and wisdom is described as a quality that calls nurses to be open, present, and reverent to the unfolding possibilities in the nurse-person process.

Introduction

Over the years, particular concepts, theories, and processes have been developed and promoted with the intent of helping nurses enhance quality of care and service. The nursing process, theory-based practice, relational nursing, client-centered care, and evidence-based practice are several of the more common initiatives that nurses have developed and promoted. I have grown, benefited, and struggled with these initiatives and others during my years as a practicing nurse and as a nurse leader/educator trying to support and enable nurses in their work. Recently, insights from authors of complexity science, knowledge development, and nursing theory/philosophy have clarified and opened space for new thinking about the nature of nursing practice, in particular the relevance of evidence in a universe of connectedness.

Evidence: Contextualizing Applications. There is a kind of paradox about evidence that is intriguing. On the one hand, evidence has been presented as a need of nurses and other professionals—in order for them to be informed and competent (Boswell & Cannon, 2007). Some authors have presented evidence-based practice (EVP) as if there are no questions as to its relevance and fit for nursing. And yet, in numerous disciplines there have been both calls for EVP and cautions against or denunciations of it (see Davies, 2003; Pope, 2003; Rogers, 2004; Saarni & Gylling, 2004; Van Zelm, 2006). Nurses have also expressed diverging views and perspectives about the nature of evidence and its place, if any, in the care of persons and families who are complex, mysterious, and open to possibilities (Cody, 2006; Holmes, Perron, & O'Byrne, 2006; Kirkham, Baumbusch, Schultz, & Anderson, 2007; Milton, 2007; Mitchell, 1991, 1995, 1999; Parse, 2008; Reeder, 2007). As claims and counterclaims have pushed boundaries of understanding, some new insights of connectedness and divergence have surfaced.

Evidence is typically understood to be the product of studies that investigate what was in order to predict what might be. Evidence is based on laws of probability and is vulnerable to the next discovery that may confirm or derail the assumptions and theory accompanying the current line of reasoning. Evidence is constructed from research that studies proximal physical causes; it is typically presented and understood in terms of *this* causes *that* or *this* increases risk of *that*. Despite understanding many texts and articles on evidence-based practice, I found myself struggling with the ideas and joined others who were asking these questions: What counts as evidence? What is the place of evidence in nursing practice? How does it fit? Or, where does it fit? When is it helpful and when not?

Some authors have presented impressive and expanded frameworks for deeply integrating evidence in professional decision-making activities (e.g., Pearson, Wiechula, Court, & Lockwood, 2007). Parse (2008) has defined the notion of unfolding evidence. She proposed that truth in the moment emerges as persons describe their own lives and situations. Reeder looked to a future of "cosmic patterns of change in the life world" (2007, p. 208) to predict what evidence might look like decades from now. Cody (2006) suggested that evidence can play an important but limited role in professional nursing practice. He distinguished between evidence-based clinical care and values-based nursing practice. In agreement with Cody, I believe that evidence plays a relevant role in clinical care, in the procedures and protocols that nurses perform in health care settings—especially acute care. But this role, although important in the delivery of clinical care, constitutes a small part of nursing practice with clients who are, as we are, persons with freedom to make decisions and to participate in life, and who have their own value priorities, concerns, and hopes. Perhaps the differences between evidence and values can help nurses to locate and clarify when evidence might be useful in practice and when not.

It is intriguing that evidence is spoken of as elusive and difficult to integrate in practice. On the other hand, evidence is everywhere; we all integrate evidence in daily life according to our needs and interests. It is human nature to experiment with choice and consequence, and many things from childhood to old age are learned within the frame of "this causes that." Persons are bombarded with evidence every day, day after day. For instance, billboards show evidence, television commercials and broadcasters proclaim evidence, and government agencies strategically select and promote evidence according to established priorities. Most people are familiar with the powerful verbal and visual images that are presented in the interests of population health and cultural change. Messages such as smoking causes lung damage, seat belts save lives, drinking and driving do not mix, and family violence is harmful—these are powerful and important messages informed by evidence and societal values. The intentions behind the messages can be traced to desires to decrease unnecessary morbidity, mortality, and costs. Indeed, these powerful messages are effective in promoting change—at least to some degree. For instance, according to 2005 Health Canada Statistics, fewer than 5 million Canadians, only 19% of the adult population, smoke. Smoking rates dropped from 35% over two decades thanks in some part to evidence-based public health messages and societal pressures to stop the harm from smoking and second-hand smoke (retrieved from http://www.marketwire.com/press-release/Health-Canada-749424.html).

Drug testing for new pharmaceuticals is another area in which random, controlled trials—the gold standard for generating evidence—result in products, marketing, and decisions that have a profound influence on human lives, for better and for worse. Obviously, evidence is important in areas such as population health and clinical drug trials. It is also clear that evidence is constructed and influenced by societal values, government officials, ideologies, and profits. Sometimes these influences and intentions are made clear to consumers, and sometimes the real story or purpose is concealed. It is troubling and impossible to ignore the fact that some evidence, though powerful and extensive, does not influence decisions even when there is a high probability of favorable changes in population health and well-being. For instance, there is convincing evidence that poverty correlates with illness and chronic disease, yet poverty and hunger increase while billions of dollars get pumped into fuel and tertiary health care (Shawler & Logsdon, 2008; Woolf, Johnson, & Geiger, 2006). Evidence surrounds us in day-to-day life and in nursing practice. Before moving to a deeper consideration of evidence in nursing practice, I would like to suggest at this time that evidence is not the same as knowledge, and it is notably different from wisdom. First, a closer look at knowledge.

The Nature of Knowledge. There are several interesting conceptualizations of knowledge that can inform nurses and their work to develop relevant nursing knowledge. A traditional view of knowledge is that it is a substance or content that can be found or discovered and then communicated to others (Davis, Samara, & Luce-Kapler, 2000). From this view, knowledge can be transmitted, stored, retrieved, dispensed, and withheld. Some educational initiatives, in both academic and service settings, have been built on the belief that those who know can give knowledge to those who do not know and the consequence will be learning and change in a way predefined by the knower. Although there may be many instances where knowledge is delivered or dispensed, there must be an open, willing learner who is participating in the process of defining the learning, and who is not simply an empty vessel waiting to be filled (Freire, 1998). This traditional notion of knowledge as transferable content is quite limited and has shown itself to be less than satisfactory for many involved in the teaching-learning process. Fortunately, computers and other technologies can assume responsibility for dispensing information, and those interested in more participative processes can focus on developing meaningful ways of teaching-learning. Recent developments and theory about knowledge have expanded opportunities for professionals in practice disciplines such as nursing.

Clancey (1997), for example, described knowledge as more choreography than content. He suggested that knowledge is about being in the moment and knowing how to create space and opportunity for the novel, the unexpected, and the unfamiliar. Choreography involves dancers who move with fluid movement, showing a togetherness and wholeness for those engaged. Persons watching choreographed motion may see patterns and themes, yet there is openness to the novel even amid the connectedness of theme and story. Clancey speaks of activity as not merely a movement or action, but a "complex choreography of identity, sense of place and participation" (p. 7) that informs actions. So too, professional nursing practice is not merely movement or action that can be prescribed. It is also a choreography of one's theoretical identity and one's sense of purpose or intent while engaging with persons and families and their issues, concerns, hopes, and dreams. Picard (2008) related choreography to an embodied knowing that expresses wholeness. Learning how to move with knowledge and to be in the moment, in ways that help others, is informed by nursing philosophy and theory.

Feyerabend (1991) presented a view of knowledge that is experience-based and embedded in culture and history. Some things make perfect sense to one group and no sense to another; this divergence is because people experience and learn knowledge that is meaningful within their own frames of reference. Knowledge and sense, like art and philosophy, are not out there waiting to be discovered, according to Feyerabend; they are human creations. He presented a very critical view of traditional medicine and the hierarchy that places evidence or one view of rationality above other ways of knowing—the humanities and even human emotions are capable of creating a knowing that can transform a person's life. He proposed that you cannot know another's health or illness until you learn and come to know the person(s). This idea of learning about persons first, before evidence, will be addressed again in regard to nursing knowledge and practice.

Goodman (1992) offered some additional insights into knowledge and *worldmaking* that require some attention before moving to the idea of wisdom. He contended that frames of reference, or worldviews, encompass a particular description of the world such that persons can articulate how the world can be known from various standpoints or perches, so to speak. Goodman stated, "Our universe … consists of these ways, rather than of a [one] world" (p. 3). Each view of the world may be right from a certain stance. An important point from Goodman is that persons should not try to reduce these multiple and sometimes diverging worldviews. Unity comes not with reduction, but with new description that brings unity to diversity (Goodman, (1992). Human beings are capable of embracing and describing different ways of thinking or viewing reality. Langer (1997) referred to this capability as the sideways learning of mindfulness. The idea of resisting the tendency to reduce multiple views will become an important point when we later consider how evidence extends to human life. Thinking about human life and possibility inspires a brief look at wisdom.

Wisdom. The concept of wisdom has been developed in numerous disciplines of study—the humanities, philosophy, religion, and psychology, to name several. For purposes here, a few ideas about wisdom will suffice. I know wisdom as a quality of thought and action and as an ability to discern subtle distinctions. I believe that wisdom evinces an attitude of reverence and stillness. In my experience, wisdom shows itself in relations with others and the universe. Wisdom is thoughtful, open, and loving. Opportunities to learn more about wisdom provided insights about language and the arts and how they propel thinking and insight.

Zwicky (2003), for instance, wrote about wisdom and metaphor in a tantalizing and deep way. For Zwicky, wisdom and metaphor are similar in that each grab hold of connections among different meanings and contexts in ways such that insight and new meaning emerges. Insight creates meaning and carries the potential of a shift of view, a gestalt of understanding. "To get it, to understand, is to experience meaning...being able to go on" (p. 82L). For Zwicky, metaphor shows repeating patterns and meanings in our complex universe, and metaphor expands the potential for dialogue and transactions among divergent contexts. Thinking about nursing practice, one can also see the way wisdom expands the possibility for dialogue with persons, families, and others who hold diverging views. Wisdom, like knowledge, creates space that beckons understanding, meaning, and change. It will become clearer that the wisdom that emerges with experience, metaphor, art, and story is relevant to the complexities of nursing practice.

Evidence, Knowledge, And Wisdom— Nursing Practice In A Complex And Mysterious Universe

There have been increasing references that suggest a shift in global thinking about how to be with our very complex lives in an even more complex universe. Numerous voices are echoing a call to be less certain, more open, more relational, more loving, and more concerned about each other and the earth we inhabit (Senge, Scharmer, Jaworski, & Flowers, 2004; Westley, Zimmerman, & Patton, 2006; Wheatley, 2005, 2006).

Many authors inspire and some help create a leap of understanding that can shift one's view of familiar questions and
issues. I experienced this leap of understanding when reading a book called *Getting to Maybe*, by Westley, Zimmerman,
and Patton (2006). These authors presented a simple and
effective way to distinguish among notions of the simple, the
complicated, and the complex. The thoughts affiliated with
the distinctions among these notions or activities aligned
in my thinking with ideas about evidence-based practice,
multidisciplinary health care, and the nurse-person/family
process. Nurse authors such as Cameron (2006) and Parse
(1998, 2007) helped clarify my addition of two more kinds of
activities that extend those offered by Westley et al. Namely,
nurses participate in activities that hold the unspeakable and
the unknowable.

It is necessary to address activities surrounding the
unspeakable and unknowable because they represent the
realities of nurses when they are with persons who are typically living through situations that transform life. Nurses bear
witness to unspeakable suffering and change. How does one
describe with mere words the panic and awareness being
shown by a person newly diagnosed with Alzheimer's disease? Or how could one describe in words the pain and loss
witnessed by family members who watch the gradual changes overtaking loved ones living with dementia or Parkinson's
disease?

Also, nurses regularly bear witness to the fathomless
ambiguity of the unknown. Will my child's cancer return?
Will my father live through the night? How will I make it
through? How do I say goodbye to my child? Nurses know
that the unspeakable and the unknowable coexist and trans-
act within activities described here as the simple, the complicated, and the complex. If these various activities all coexist,
then nurses have opportunities to learn and develop insights
into ways that evidence, knowledge, and wisdom can help
them to better understand their place in our complex universe as well as their place in the stillness and depth of the
nurse-person relationship.

Nurses bring the *who* that they are when they engage
with others in the simple, the complicated, the complex, the
unspeakable, and the unknowable. The who that they are
is shaped by personal values, lived experiences, intentions,

family, culture, and understandings gleaned from education. Nurses are also influenced, but not determined by, their
workload, colleagues, and workplace values. Persons experience who the nurse is in all of the messages and actions
shown and not shown in the nurse-person process. There is
no question that nurses bring their learning, as well as their
values and experiences, when engaging with all clients. This
is precisely why it is critical for nurses to reflect on as many
nursing theories as possible, so that they can choose what
kind of nurse they want to be. Theories shape the way relationships develop while people engage in simple, complicated, complex, unspeakable, and unknowable activities. What
then are the roles of evidence, knowledge, and wisdom in the
unfolding experience of being a nurse?

Although presented as if they exist in separate ways,
in reality the five activities coexist and interrelate in ways
beyond a full understanding. The five kinds of activities or
affairs—simple, complicated, complex, unspeakable, and
unknowable—are fluid yet distinct enough to consider in
light of nursing evidence, knowledge, and wisdom. Seeing all
of these views simultaneously may invite the deeper learning
and heightened awareness that Senge et al. (2004) suggested
will accompany an evolving and emerging understanding of
wholeness. A closer look at all five views—beginning with
the simple—provides interesting ideas in the context of
nursing practice.

***Simpler Things in the Complex Universe of Nursing
Practice.*** For Westley et al. (2006), there are things human
beings participate in that are quite simple and replicable—
like baking a cake. One can follow a recipe with very specific
instructions and produce what is promised if steps are completed with the exact ingredients defined. Further, a person
can bake that same cake time and time again if the same
recipe is followed. Simple things that involve measurements
and objects/ingredients have a high degree of predictability.
Simple things may also be improved upon in the mixing or
baking of the cake. If there were discoveries, for instance,
that generated evidence that novel ways of heating the ingredients could produce the same quality of cake in 5 minutes
instead of 45, that new efficiency could change the recipe
and the product. People would need to get the new heat-

ing device and bake the cake with the new instructions—a breakthrough in evidence-based cooking.

The parallel with the simple, menu-driven approach that exists in health care, and that nurses participate in millions of times a day, includes all the procedures and protocols that professionals and researchers have developed and tested over the years. Procedures require specific instructions, with particular instruments, solutions, tools, and materials directed toward achieving a specific outcome. Far too many to list, common procedures and protocols include physical assessment, catheterization, intravenous insertion, chest tube removal, dressing change, and so on. Nurses and other professionals who perform these tasks typically receive instruction and learn to follow very specific techniques in order to complete the procedures with the highest quality possible. Procedures/protocols are also updated on a regular basis in order to ensure the latest and best evidence for the highest quality and lowest cost. In my experience, the procedures and protocols are updated annually by teams of nurses and other professionals as needed to achieve best practice. In the realm of the simple, according to Westley et al. (2006), evidence, protocol, and meticulous procedure and technique ensure success and replicability. Missing in this parallel portrayal of the simple activities is the reality that many procedures performed by nurses involve persons and their unique views, pains, concerns, and patterns of relating. The layers of complexity, even with the simple activities, will be addressed as we move along with this exploration.

Complicated Things in the Complex Universe of Nursing. Wesley et al. (2006) defined more intense activity by multiple players, and more complex protocols, as complicated. Complicated activities are those requiring different levels of specialization, multiple disciplines, and numerous protocols, formulae, and techniques. Westley et al. (2006) used the example of sending a rocket to the moon, or the shuttle to the space station. It takes many experts to develop and coordinate all the necessary requirements; and because there are many involved working on many steps and details, there is a much greater risk of human error. History documented the incredible cost of human error when leaking fuel rings caused the disintegration of the shuttle Challenger in 1986. We also know that it is possible to successfully replicate the complicated work to repeatedly send the shuttle into space. Planning, expertise, resources, and careful attention make prediction possible but always amid the awareness of risk, error, and the ever-present unpredictability of human activity and intentions.

One parallel for the complicated in the health care arena is the multidisciplinary team and the complicated work of medical and surgical care. The operating room bears some resemblance to the shuttle work described above. Multiple experts bring techniques and protocols together in order to replace a hip or remove a brain tumor. There is a blueprint to follow for hip replacement, and those involved must rigidly adhere to the rules governing the major surgical procedure. Medical management of chronic disease can be even more complex because it might take multiple specialists to diagnose and treat one person. Those of us in health care know that systems do not always facilitate the coordination and communication required to minimize risk and injury. The development of specialists according to body part and disease brings its own kind of risk when caring for whole human beings. Instances of reported error in health care settings have been a matter of increasing attention over the past decade, adding significant and understandable layers of fear to the complex layers of activity.

Complicated activities in both space travel and orthopedic surgery require constant evaluation and improvement. Research that develops new products and techniques generates evidence to inform complicated activities. Improvements and enhancements change quality and/or efficiency, yet history also teaches that despite convincing evidence, some persons do not change the protocol or formula or theory being followed. Hence, perhaps, the clarion call for evidence-based health care. If teams of specialists are going to be performing surgery or prescribing medications, certainly their actions should be based on the best information at hand. If nurses are participating in team activities in clinical health care, they have an obligation to ensure their contributions are sound and based on rules of evidence, where it exists. However, some authors have indicated that even when evidence is published and accessible, there are some practitioners who do not change their actions. Explanations for the lack of change include expressions of social resistance (Pope, 2003) and resistance against oppression (Davies, 2003). Resistance to change may be a topic for another paper. It is time now to move to the third activity of interest, the complex.

Complex Things in the Complex Universe of Nursing. Westley et al. (2006) offer the example of rearing a child to describe complex activity. Children, they say, do not typically respond to rigid rules and protocols. Success with rearing one child does not carry over to the next. Each child is unique and requires understanding of his or her personal reality and perspective. Parents need to be responsive to individual children rather than following a blueprint of how to parent. Uncertainty is a constant when raising a child. The parts of the child have little relation to his/her essence, which can be known only in relationship. Rearing a child also means experiencing joy, sorrow, fear, concern, care, and love.

It is interesting, and perhaps necessary, to note here that people who rear children also bake cakes, and many are involved in complicated work situations. Doing the simple and the complicated well does not ensure they are good parents. Baking a wonderful chocolate cake does not mean you are a good mother. So too, a nurse who follows procedures well and who participates in team meetings with great skill and knowledge may not know how to relate to patients/persons in ways that are meaningful and helpful—in ways that enhance health, well-being, and quality of life from the perspective of other persons. A different kind of knowledge is required for complex activities.

An example of complex activity in nursing might be pain control. Although other team members are involved, nurses bear primary responsibility for finding out specifics about persons' drug sensitivities, desired level of control, experience of relief and side effects, and desired frequency of medication. Nurses know that pain management means working with unique persons who have different expectations, tolerances, consequences, and issues. The more persons and families are involved in care decisions, the more complex they become and the more opportunity there is for both error and excellence.

The knowledge and skill required for each of the activities so far—the simple, complicated, or complex—are different and not transferable. This is true even though there are connections among the kinds of activities. The knowledge required for relating with persons and families is not of the evidence kind—meaning it is not of the kind *this* causes *that*. Rather, it is knowledge of human nature, of assumptions about reality, of values and beliefs, of intentions and purposes that shows itself in the nurse-person/family/community process.

Nursing knowledge of how to relate with persons in particular ways for particular purposes has not typically been the foundation of nursing programs, even though being with persons is the place where nursing happens. Nurses have been educated with a focus on clinical/health problems within a holistic frame of bio-psycho-social-spiritual-cultural care. Even though many schools of nursing may have required students to take courses in psychology, sociology, education, or communication, these topics have usually been structured within a problem-based, assessment-centered approach, in which experts identify problems, make normative comparisons, and prescribe interventions. It seems that complex activities with persons were collapsed or reduced to activities that are simple or complicated. Complexity science has clarified that the different activities require different processes and knowledge.

More recent developments in nursing knowledge, most notably theories concerned with unitary human beings in mutual process with the universe, offer practice methodologies (see Newman, 2008; Parse, 1998, 2007) that preserve the distinctness of layered activities. The theories of Newman and Parse inform nurses about how to be with people in participative relationships that honor the irreducibility, dignity, and freedom of persons to choose their own way in light of the values and patterns they want to live given their particular situations. Other nurse scholars are articulating relational nursing (Doane & Varcoe, 2005) and trans-theoretical nursing (Cowling, 2007; Watson, 2005; Watson & Smith, 2002) to provide knowledge for nurses looking for participative practices with unitary, whole persons.

Participative relationships require theoretical knowledge as well as communion; respect; creativity; openness; and an authentic, nonjudgmental regard for the others' wisdom and life situations. Polifroni and Packard (1993) noted that the essential nature of nursing and the knowledge required to practice nursing are not informed by "this causes that" data or evidence. We know, because of our own experiences as human beings who continuously relate, and because of research that has affirmed, that persons want to be treated with respect; to be listened to; and to be involved in honest, helpful processes with health care professionals (Crocker & Johnson, 2006). Nurses with particular theoretical knowledge understand that persons have different expectations with respect to how much they want to be involved in health care. Rather than approaching people with generalized, evidence-based interventions, a nurse with nursing knowledge provides relational care that is responsive to the needs, concerns, and wishes of persons and families. This individualized responsiveness not only improves quality and satisfaction, but it also diminishes risk and error (Beyea, 2006; Eisenberg et al., 2005).

Getting to know others and learning about their unique situations can only happen when nurses know how to commune with respect, openness, and genuine presence. Persons do not disclose in the absence of respect, openness, and listening. This may be why attempts to sever tasks from nursing and assign the tasks to persons without nursing knowledge have generated serious errors or depletions in quality of care. To return to an earlier point, just because a person can follow a recipe and make a cake does not mean they know how to be a good parent. Nursing knowledge is an essential complement to the knowledge required to complete the simple, complicated, and complex activities of modern nursing. Nursing knowledge is required for all nursing activities, and wisdom is also required for activities and situations that are unspeakable and unknowable.

The Unspeakable in a Complex Universe. The unspeakable, also called the ineffable, has been explored in philosophy and psychology in interesting ways (Heidegger, 1971; Kukla, 2005; Scharfstein, 1993). Kukla presented questions about the very idea of the ineffable. Is it possible that humans have the potential to understand truths about reality that are not utterable or represented in language? Or, asked Kukla, is the inability to articulate simply a matter of cognitive limitation that has nothing to do with knowing? I am in agreement with those who believe that persons, and in particular, nurses, do know about activities with persons that are not initially utterable or describable. Language is at times inadequate to express the reality of intimate and unusual relating (Scharfstein, 1993). Nurses have intimate and unusual relationships with persons. Even when nurses become accustomed to particular specialties of practice, human uniqueness calls nurses to attend to the unusual and indescribable.

The unspeakable has been written about by nurses trying to clarify the depth and breadth of the nurse-person relationship (see Cameron, 2006; Cohen, 1993; Eifried, 2003; Mitchell & Bunkers, 2005; Rallison & Moules, 2004; Ramey & Bunkers, 2006). These authors have addressed the reality that some things experienced in nursing are not easily spoken of or represented because they are ineffable. An insight attributed to Dienske (1985) by Cameron (2006) is that "the ineffable is that which cannot be objectified; rather it must be shown" (p. 24) Cameron stated, "We need to grope for words that take us back to the space where we can bear witness to the fullness of the human condition" (p. 26). Similarly, Mitchell and Bunkers took several years to speak and write about the intense human engagements that nurses are called to witness and experience. These authors used the metaphor of the abyss to represent the risk and uncertainty involved in being with others and engaging human truths during intense and transformative times. Mitchell and Bunkers proposed that if the unspeakable could be articulated, there would be opportunities for additional learning and insight. Indeed, Ramey and Bunkers (2006) published on how to teach nursing students about the abyss through Parse's (1998, 2007) practice of true presence. Such efforts will continue to provide ways for nurses to learn about and articulate the ineffable in nursing.

Creating space for learning about the unspeakable means thinking about ways to recognize, be with, and express nursing realities through concept and theory invention, metaphor, storytelling, or other artistic expressions that assist others to see and engage with the unfamiliar. Nurses bear witness to the incredible, the unexpected, the horrifying, and the transformative. Telling stories of unusual situations sheds light on the depth of nursing, and stories provide opportunities for connecting and for meaningful and memorable learning. Nurses often share their wisdom about experiences of caring for human beings through stories, and those who hear the stories create transactions with their own experiences and stories. These stories, like metaphor, are multiply resonant—they echo truths and bring unity in diversity. Several authors have noted the power of story in teaching-learning processes (Benner, Tanner, & Chesla, 1997; Bunkers, 2006; Yoder-Wise & Kowalski, 2003). Heidegger (1971) reminded us that once there is a word for something, we can begin to understand what it is; words give being, and being is to persist in presence. Nursing's unspeakables, like Heidegger's poetry, leave a thought-provoking residue that beckons to be spoken. Speaking is listening and saying is showing; these things promote learning and understanding.

Additional opportunities for learning about the unspeakable are possible. Trying to understand and articulate the reality, the essential nature of something is an ontological interest. Zwicky (2003) again shed light on the desire to attend to and understand the ontology of something. She stated, "Ontological attention is a form of love. When we love a thing, we can experience our responsibility toward it as limitless ... That is how much it is possible to attend; that is how large complete attention would be" (p. 57L). Linking love with ontological attention is connected to insights from Mitchell and Bunkers (2003), who stated, "In being present, in risking engaging with the explicit-tacit truth of a situation, one discovers truth and only love can abide with truth (p. 123). It is important to try to speak the unspeakable because there is truth there that nurses can come to know and benefit from. Though there are many truths to articulate, there are also things that are unknowable.

Considering the Unknowable. The unknowable relates to mystery. Parse has written about the mysterious in human becoming and in human relationships. For Parse (2007), mystery represents the unexplainable and impenetrable of human-universe relating. There is a realm of mystery in being human, and nurses open to engaging in human-to-human relationships with clients attend to mystery with a humility and deep respect for what is known and what is not known. As Parse proposed, there is always more to know about persons, situations, and even oneself. For Heidegger (1971), mystery abides in concealment as the unshowable. Similarly, Scharfstein (1993) proposed, "We are partially ignorant of what we think because, thinking with our whole person and experience, we generate ideas from a substratum that is opaque to consciousness" (p. 11). Human potential and the will to power and change are mysteries nurses engage with in every nurse-person process. Knowing how to be with human potential requires wisdom.

Wisdom in Nursing. Wisdom in nursing has been articulated in visions of expertise, artful practice, and participatory experiences that transform those involved. Nurse scholars have articulated clinical wisdom and practice wisdom (Begley, 2006; Connor, 2004; Jenkins & Thomas, 2005; Litchfield, 1999; Phelan, 2001; Zerwekh, 1997). Clinical wisdom has been linked with expert practitioners and their ability to assess and discern subtle changes in clients' health and to then act in ways that avert complications or apply effective interventions to achieve a goal. Practical wisdom has been presented as a mature ability to integrate moral reasoning, experience, theoretical understanding, and intelligence in order to provide and enable care for self and others (Begley, 2006; Phelan, 2001). Phelan went beyond the notion of wisdom as application by nurses when she included the ideas of openness and abiding with sorrow and a play between understanding and perception. Armstrong (2006) offered a compelling case for considering moral virtues and a virtue-based practice consisting of exercising moral virtues such as compassion, judgment, and moral wisdom to reestablish the contextual and relational nature of nursing. Wisdom in nursing unfolds in expert decision making, dialogue, and relationships that enhance health and quality of life.

In the presence of the unspeakable and unknowable, wisdom is expressed in moments of being with turmoil, pain, or suffering. Wisdom is seen in the courage it takes to be with ambiguity and uncertainty. Wisdom waits and shows an open reverence for what might come forth. Wisdom as an openness to the unfamiliar and the unknown is consistent with authors who linked wisdom with creativity (Phelan, 2001; Sternberg, 2001). Wisdom is a commitment to possibility in human lives and in nurse-person relationships. Wisdom emerges in moments of silence that convey or search for understanding (Senge et al., 2004): "In that special silence you can hear, or see, or get a sense of something that wants to happen that you wouldn't have been aware of otherwise" (p. 79).

Wisdom in nursing is lived out with others, even when there are no answers, no questions—just raw human experiences. Wisdom is lived in spaces that invite dialogue and that embrace the truth of the moment (Parse, 2008) with compassion and unconditional love. Truths can surface in the back-and-forth of dialogue about a matter of common interest in the context of shared history. This surfacing of truth in dialogue is emerging in the shared foundation of human science nursing theories (Newman, 2008; Parse, 1998, 2007). Relational nursing theories provide nurses with understanding about dialogue and how dialogue enables persons to articulate, reflect, and clarify truths in their own lives. Being with others as they express their own truths—their own issues, concerns, loves, and hopes—requires nursing wisdom.

It is proposed here that if nurses embrace the idea that they need knowledge and skill for all the activities they participate in, for all the worldviews they engage and help to create, then attention can begin to focus on how to extend nursing's theoretical knowledge base—especially for relational activities that are complex, unspeakable, and unknowable. Senge et al. (2005) suggested that all learning involves thinking and doing. Table 6.1 has been set up to suggest the thinking and doing for the five types of activities of interest—the simple, complicated, complex, unspeakable, and unknowable—with a focus on evidence and its place in the breadth of nursing activities. Please note that in all activities nurses bring their experiences, values, beliefs, and theories. Evidence has a place and thinking and doing with evidence happens in different ways in simple, complicated, and complex activities. Further, in the realms of the complex, the unspeakable, and the unknowable, evidence diminishes and even disappears. Indeed, applying evidence with individuals in complex, unspeakable, and unknowable situations may create harm.

Professional nursing involves context, discovery, understanding, improvisation, rhythm, meaning, and dialogue with others. Nursing knowledge and wisdom are lived uniquely with every person and family; both unfold in moments of being together with others. Knowledge and wisdom are different from information and evidence. Nursing knowledge and wisdom involve and embrace ambiguity, uncertainty, and the creativity that unfolds in all authentic relationships. Viewing knowledge as an open process that unfolds stands

6.1 Evidence & Relevance in Nursing Activities/Situations

Distinguishing Nursing Activities/ Situations	Thinking and Doing With Evidence
Simple	Evidence is relevant to thinking in simple activities. Doing with involves systematic evaluation, multidisciplinary/disciplinary reviews, and writing protocols for best practice.
Complicated	Evidence is relevant to thinking in complicated activities. Doing with involves team relating and individual/ disciplinary reviews, discussion, and updates.
Complex	Evidence may be interesting and informative in complex activities/situations. Doing with involves introduction of evidence for discussion, reflection, and consideration by persons.
Unspeakable	Evidence is less relevant to thinking in unspeakable activities/situations. Doing without evidence involves being in relationships and living theoretical and philosophical beliefs. Doing involves creating theoretical conceptualizations, philosophical explanations, and artistic expressions (including metaphor and story) that inform and enhance understanding of unspeakable situations.
Unknowable	Evidence is not relevant to thinking about the unknowable. Doing without evidence involves being open and present, showing reverence for mystery, and listening and enabling the novel and interre-lationships. Doing involves learning and living wisdom in participative relationships guided by nursing theories that invite truth, creativity, and the unfamiliar.

To all activities, nurses bring their experiences, assumptions, values, and theories that show up in attitudes, approaches, and relationships with others.

in contrast to viewing knowledge as a substance that can be delivered or contained in predefined prescriptions called "evidence." Viewing wisdom as courageous risking with truth stands in contrast to the view that wisdom is expertise exquisitely applied. These different views need to retain their differences in order to coexist; and the more nurses can embrace and articulate these different ways of seeing, thinking, and acting, the more open they can be to the novel and unfamiliar of our shared humanity.

References

Armstrong, A. E. (2006). Towards a strong virtue ethics for nursing practice. *Nursing Philosophy, 7*(3), 110–124.

Begley, A. M. (2006). Facilitating the development of moral insight in practice: Teaching ethics and teaching virtue. *Nursing Philosophy, 7*, 257–265.

Benner, P., Tanner, C. A., & Chesla, C. (1997). The social fabric of nursing knowledge. *American Journal of Nursing, 97*(7), 16BBB–16DDD.

Beyea, S. C. (2006). The value of knowing the patient. *AORN Journal, 83*(4), 825–826.

Boswell, C. & Cannon, S. (2007). *Nursing research: Incorporating evidence-based practice.* Sudbury, MA: Jones & Bartlett.

Bunkers, S. S. (2006). What stories and fables can teach us. *Nursing Science Quarterly, 19*, 104–107.

Cameron, B. L. (2006). Towards understanding the unpresentable in nursing: Some nursing philosophical considerations. *Nursing Philosophy, 7*, 23–35.

Clancey, W. J. (1997). The conceptual nature of knowledge, situations, and activity. In J. Feltovich, K. M. Ford, & R. R. Hoffman, *Expertise in context: Human and machine,* (pp. 247–291). Cambridge, MA: MIT Press.

Cody, W. K. (2006). Values-based practice and evidence-based care: Pursuing fundamental questions in nursing philosophy and theory. In W. K. Cody, *Philosophical and theoretical perspectives for advanced nursing practice* (4th Ed.), (pp. 5–12). Sudbury, MA: Jones & Bartlett.

Cohen, M. H. (1993). The unknown and the unknowable: Managing sustained uncertainty. *Western Journal of Nursing Research, 15*(1), 77–96.

Connor, M. (2004). The practical discourse in philosophy and nursing: An exploration of linkages and shifts in the evolution of praxis. *Nursing Philosophy, 5*, 54–66.

Cowling, W. R. (2007). A unitary participatory vision of nursing knowledge. *Advances in Nursing Science, 30*(1), 61–70.

Crocker, L., & Johnson, B. (2006). *Privileged presence.* Boulder, CO: Bull Publishing.

Davies, B. (2003). Death to critique and dissent? The policies and practices of new managerialism and of "evidence-based practice." *Gender and Education, 15*(1), 91–103.

Davis, B., Samara, D., & Luce-Kapler, R. (2000). *Engaging minds.* Mahwah, NJ: Lawrence Erlbaum.

Dienske, I. (1985). Beyond words: On the experience of the ineffable. *Phenomenology & Pedagogy, 3*(1), 3–19.

Doane, G. H., & Varcoe, C. (2005). *Family nursing as relational inquiry.* Philadelphia: Lippincott Williams & Wilkins.

Eifried, S. (2003). Bearing witness to suffering: The lived experience of nursing students. *Journal of Nursing Education, 42*(2), 59–67.

Eisenberg, E. M., Murphy, A. G., Sutcliffe, K., Wears, R., Schenkel, S., Perry, S., & Vanderhoef, M. (2005). Communication in emergency medicine: Implications for patient safety. *Communication Monographs, 72*, 390–314.

Feyerabend, P. (1991). *Three dialogues on knowledge.* Cambridge, MA: Basil Blackwell.

Freire, P. (1998). *Pedagogy of freedom: Ethics, democracy, and civic courage.* (P. Clarke, Trans.). Lanham, MD: Rowman & Littlefield.

Goodman, N. (1992). *Ways of worldmaking.* Indianapolis: Hackett.

Health Canada Statistics (2005). http://www.marketwire.com/press-release/Health-Canada-749424.html.

Heidegger, M. (1971). *On the way to language* (First ed.). (P. D. Hertz, Trans.). New York: Harper & Row.

Holmes, D., Perron, A., & O'Byrne, P. (2006). Evidence, virulence, and the disappearance of nursing knowledge: A critique of the evidence-based dogma. *Worldviews on Evidence-Based Nursing, 3*(3), 95–102.

Jenkins, S. K., & Thomas, M. B. (2005). Thought for application and application with thought: Issues in theoretical thinking and practical wisdom. *Advances in Health Sciences Education, 10*(2), 115–123.

Kirkham, S. R., Baumbusch, J. L., Schultz, A. S., & Anderson, J. (2007). Knowledge development and evidence-based practice: Insights and opportunities from a postcolonial feminist perspective for transformative nursing practice. *Advances in Nursing Science, 30*(1), 26–40.

Kukla, A. (2005). *Ineffability and philosophy.* New York: Routledge Taylor & Francis.

Langer, E. J. (1997). *The power of mindful learning.* Reading, MA: Perseus.

Litchfield, M. (1999). Practice wisdom. *Advances in Nursing Science, 22*(2), 62–73.

Milton, C. L. (2007). Evidence-based practice: Ethical questions for nursing. *Nursing Science Quarterly, 20*, 123–126.

Mitchell, G. J. (1991). Nursing diagnosis: An ethical analysis. *IMAGE International Journal of Nursing Scholarship, 23*(2), 99–103.

Mitchell, G. J. (1995). Nursing diagnosis: An obstacle to caring ways. In A. Boykin (Ed.), *Power, politics, and public policy: A matter of caring* (pp. 11–23). New York: National League of Nursing.

Mitchell, G. J. (1999). Evidence-based practice: Critique and alternate view. *Nursing Science Quarterly, 12*, 30–35.

Mitchell, G. J., & Bunkers, S. S. (2005). Engaging the abyss: A mistake of opportunity. *Nursing Science Quarterly, 16*, 121–125.

Newman, M. A. (2008). *Transforming presence: The difference that nursing makes.* Philadelphia: F. A. Davis.

Parse, R. R. (1998). *The human becoming school of thought: A perspective for nurses and other health professionals.* Thousand Oaks, CA: Sage.

Parse, R. R. (2007). The humanbecoming school of thought in 2050. *Nursing Science Quarterly, 20*, 308–311.

Parse, R. R. (2008). Truth for the moment: Personal testimony as evidence. *Nursing Science Quarterly, 21*, 45–48.

Pearson, A., Wiechula, R., Court, A., & Lockwood, C. (2007). A reconsideration of what constitutes "evidence" in the healthcare professions. *Nursing Science Quarterly, 1*, 85–88.

Phelan, A. M. (2001). The death of a child and the birth of practical wisdom. *Studies in Philosophy & Education, 20*(1), 41–55.

Picard, C. (2008). Creative movement and transformation to choreography: A mode of research presentation. *Nursing Science Quarterly, 21*, 112–114.

Polifroni, E. C., & Packard, S. (1993). Psychological determinism and the evolving nursing paradigm. *Nursing Science Quarterly, 6*, 63–68.

Pope, C. (2003). Resisting evidence: The study of evidence-based medicine as a contemporary social movement. *Health: An Interdisciplinary Journal for the Social Study of Health, Illness, and Medicine, 7*(3), 267–282.

Rallison, L., & Moules, N. J. (2004). The unspeakable nature of pediatric palliative care: Unveiling many cloaks. *Journal of Family Nursing, 10*, 287–301.

Ramey, S. L., & Bunkers, S. S. (2006). Teaching the abyss: Living the art-science of nursing. *Nursing Science Quarterly, 19*, 311–315.

Reeder, F. M. (2007). What will count as evidence in the year 2050? *Nursing Science Quarterly, 20*, 208–211.

Rogers, W. A. (2004). Evidence based medicine and justice: A framework for looking at the impact of EBM upon vulnerable or disadvantaged groups. *Journal of Medical Ethics, 30*, 141–145.

Saarni, S. I., & Gylling, H. A. (2004). Evidence based medicine guidelines: A solution to rationing or politics disguised as science? *Journal of Medical Ethics, 30*, 171–175.

Scharfstein, B-A. (1993). *Ineffability.* New York: State University of New York Press.

Senge, P., Scharmer, C. O., Jaworski, J., & Flowers, B. S. (2005). Presence. *Exploring profound change in people, organizations, and society.* New York: Currency Doubleday.

Shawler, C., & Logsdon, D. (2008). Living vigilant lives with chronic illness: Stories from older low-income minority women. *Health Care for Women International, 29*(1), 76–84.

Sternberg, R. (2001). What is the common thread of creativity? Its dialectical relation to intelligence and wisdom. *American Psychologist, 56*(4), 360–362.

Van Zelm, R. (2006). The bankruptcy of evidence-based practice? *International Journal of Evidence-Based Healthcare, 4*(3), 161.

Watson, J. (2005). *Caring science as sacred science.* Philadelphia: F.A. Davis.

Watson, J., & Smith, M. (2002). Caring science and the science of unitary human beings: A trans-theoretical discourse for nursing knowledge development. *Journal of Advanced Nursing, 37*, 452–461.

Westley, F., Zimmerman, B., & Patton, M. Q. (2006). *Getting to maybe.* Toronto: Random House.

Wheatley, M. J. (2005). *Finding our way: Leadership for an uncertain time.* San Francisco: Berrett-Koehler.

Wheatley, M. J. (2006). *Leadership and the new science: Discovering order in a chaotic world.* San Francisco: Berrett-Koehler.

Woolf, S., Johnson, R., & Geiger, H. (2006). The rising prevalence of severe poverty in America: A growing threat to public health. *American Journal of Preventive Medicine, 31,* 332–341.

Yoder-Wise, P. S., & Kowalski, K. (2003). The power of storytelling. *Nursing Outlook, 51,* 37–42.

Zerwekh, J. V. (1997). Wisdom and falsehoods: Naming the practice wisdom of nursing in the home and the falsehoods opposing that practice. *Holistic Nursing Practice, 11*(4), 46–55.

Zwicky, J. (2003). *Wisdom and metaphor.* Kentville, Nova Scotia: Gaspereau.

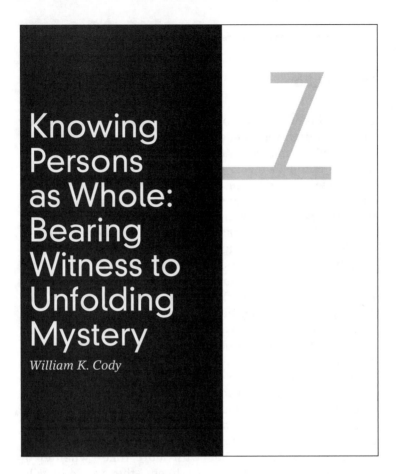

Knowing Persons as Whole: Bearing Witness to Unfolding Mystery

William K. Cody

Chapter Overview

Knowing the person as a whole is a project that emanates
from nursing's philosophical and theory base, which, historically, has referred uniformly to the wholeness of persons as a
fundamental precept of the discipline. Both older and newer
paradigms of nursing center on the wholeness of persons,
and thereby challenge practitioners to find ways of actually coming to know persons as whole. It is suggested in this
chapter that knowing the person as whole is not the same
as knowing the whole person. Rather, knowing the person
as whole is construed as venerating the other as whole and
unbounded in relation while honoring the ultimate unknowability of the other.

Introduction

For millions of nurses in practice, everyday demands on their time, attention, and intellect include the axiomatic mandate, expressed or implied, to know their patients. This mandate may be taken to mean many different things. For some, the knowledge and skills associated with pathophysiology, assessment, medicine, and technology are essential to what they do, and greater knowledge and skills in these realms equate to knowing the patient and providing better care.

For others, knowledge of interpersonal relations, cultural beliefs and values, skills in listening, and transcultural communication are essential to what they do, and greater knowledge and skills in these realms equate to knowing the patient and providing better care. These nurses and others with diverse views value this phenomenon of knowing the patient. It is engrained in the culture and tradition of Western nursing. Even nurses fully immersed in a medical model of practice pride themselves on the thoroughness and reliability of the head-to-toe assessment. In the pervasive context of today's fast-paced, impersonal, high-volume health care environments, it hardly seems possible to know the recipient of care well. Nonetheless, many nurses in such environments profess that, with more time—whether or not the prospect of more time is likely—they would be willing and able to come to know the person well, and that this knowledge would enhance care.

The very notion of the nurse's, or anyone's, knowing the person offers possibilities for explication from any number of perspectives, including even the assertion of the *impossibility* of such a project (Levinas, 1961/1969). One starting point, for example, not to be explored in depth here, could be the contrast between the views specified throughout history in various perspectives on *realism* (coming to know through the evidence of the senses) and *idealism* (coming to know through the imagination, logic, and reason of the mind). A thousand explorations of the ontologies and epistemologies rooted in these competing philosophies would not exhaust the topic. In this chapter, I will attempt to adduce for discussion several considerations in knowing the person that are salient in relation to contemporary nursing practice.

Coming to Know the Wholeness of the Person in the Nursing Discipline

Knowing the person receiving care, in some sense, is portrayed as a key process across many realms of discipline-specific and interdisciplinary health care practice—in medical models, in psychotherapeutic models, and in nursing models. Among these models, however, only nursing models, as a class, uniformly refer to the person as *whole* and seek to address the person as whole, as a fundamental precept of the discipline.

What does it mean to say that one knows a person as whole, or should know a person as whole, or can know a person as whole? Knowing in theory and research is differentiated from knowing in practice by its very purpose. The purpose of knowing in theory and research is precisely to enhance knowledge and understanding. The purpose of knowing in practice is to use knowledge in service to humankind. Unfortunately, as is apparent to any keen observer, the most commonly taught method of nursing practice, the traditional nursing process, does not derive from a body of theory or research and thus offers little hope of apprehending that which our theory base says is most central.

Theoretical frameworks of nursing have put forward numerous ideas, explicitly or implicitly, about what it means to know a person as whole. An older paradigm of nursing science, emanating from the dominant realist/objectivist ontology of mainstream general science, has posited the human as a dynamic bio-psycho-social-spiritual organism continually interacting with a complex environment (King, 1981; Neuman & Fawcett, 2002; Roy & Andrews, 1999). Within this paradigm, the goals of science in general and nursing in particular are objective knowledge of cause and effect and, ultimately, control of events for the purpose of improving objectively defined health and well-being. The preeminent metaphor for the person in this paradigm is the *system*, which is defined as a whole made up of parts. To know the person as a whole, from this perspective, one must understand the (biological, psychological, sociological, and spiritual) parts.

Knowing the person in this paradigm is construed consistently with the dominant realist/objectivist ontology of contemporary general science and is oriented toward observable conditions and events and objectively defined (preferably measured) empirical referents. The nurse's process of coming to know is construed as a knowledge- and skill-based, scientifically grounded process of collecting observations and making inferences based on expert knowledge. The empirical referents of interest are predominantly measures of status and function to be understood in relation to predefined and calculable norms. What has traditionally been known as sick care is construed as reparative or palliative, and health promotion practice is construed as educative, supporting, or empowering. The traditional nursing process has been used with these frameworks; however, nurse scholars agree that methods somewhat more subtle and complex than the basic nursing process are required for knowledge of the person that is more than a basic or technical understanding of the person's "problems."

A newer paradigm of nursing science emerged with Rogers' (1970) introduction of the science of unitary human beings, which posited the human (person) as irreducibly whole, inextricably interrelating continually with an unbounded environment with illimitable possibilities. Such views evolved within a contemporary intellectual climate influenced by existentialism and phenomenology (which had recently brought about the advent of humanistic psychology), new developments in theoretical physics, critical social theory, the infiltration of Eastern philosophies in the West, and the emergence of post-structuralism and postmodernism. Within the new paradigm, the goals of nursing are oriented toward co-participation in the ever-changing processes of living, the desired quality of life from the person's perspective, and the quality of the nurse-person (caring) process.

Knowing the person in the new paradigm, an ontology of illimitable possibilities, is oriented toward apprehending the patterns and meanings of lived experiences from the person's perspective. The nurse's process of coming to know is rooted in the beliefs and values of the new paradigm, based on the fundamental unity of person and environment, and absent any concentration on norms. It is a process of focused openness, exploration, and reflection, guided by a value for honoring, caring for, even loving the person, rather than a value for observations, facts, and expert inferences. The counterparts to empirical referents are narrative descriptions of humanly lived experiences, perceptions, and expressions. Such theory-guided practice is not approached differently whether in what has been known traditionally as sick care or in health promotion. The common conceptualizations and terminology of repair, palliation, and patient education are fundamentally inconsistent with the beliefs of the new paradigm. Rather, the new paradigm nurse is called to co-participate with persons anywhere, in any situation, with the general goals of fundamentally honoring the human dignity of those cared for, enhancing quality of life, and encouraging knowing participation in change (Barrett, 1998; Parse, 1998).

The use of the rubric of body, mind, and spirit or soul, to name the constituents of the human being, strongly associated with the self-identified movement of holism in nursing, clearly evolved from and reflects the summative ontology of the older paradigm. For this reason, the discourse associated with body, mind, and spirit often straddles the older paradigm and newer paradigms. Recently, Watson (2005), perhaps the most widely known popularizer of the body-mind-spirit rubric in past decades, has associated her work with the work of Rogers (Watson & Smith, 2002) and has adopted more consistent use of unitary language.

The paradigmatic differences in nursing today echo the historical differences, in the social/behavioral or human sciences, between objectivist and realist ontologies on the one hand and humanistic, relativist ontologies on the other. Whereas some scholars have pursued human betterment through methods of observation, measurement, and replication, others have pursued human betterment through co-participation, narrative, and non-generalizable understanding. The byword of the humanistic, relativist approach, exemplified and inspired by the phenomenological approach to human science, has been that the human being is fundamentally not an object, but rather an experiencing, self-defining, willful subject. Subject-to-subject knowing is posited as different, on a primordial level, from subject-to-object knowing.

And yet the successes of objectivist science surround us and infiltrate the health care enterprise in contemporary society. The nurse who embraces subject-to-subject knowing inspired by a more human-science, relativist, or new paradigm perspective must nonetheless also find ways to address the highly valued presence of objectivist science in the health care enterprise. If we are committed to the notion of nursing as a unique discipline, science, and profession, and if we believe that one of its unique elements is the very focus on the wholeness of the human being, then we are (nursing as a discipline is) especially challenged to explicate the value of knowing the person as a whole.

Each nurse must decide what synthesis of values among the myriad human beliefs about coming to know the person will guide her/his practice. One's practice is one's own incontrovertibly, and it cannot be subjugated to the dictates of others without one's willing cooperation. There may be costs associated with truly owning one's own practice, and each nurse has choices in this realm to make. How does the nurse, as nurse, wish to be known?

Each nurse chooses how to come to know the other, then, based on personal values. A commitment to human betterment can be incarnated in persons with any range of ideas about the nature of reality, the conditions of knowing, and the goals of health care practice. What then, to make of the axiomatic mandate for any nurse to know her/his patient (hereafter, the person), and, thus, implicitly, within this discipline, to know the person as whole?

Knowing the Person as Whole, or Revering the Person as Whole?

Being whole, unique, sentient, willful, and inextricably embedded in an ever-changing, unbounded universe, I find it self-evident that I am, as a whole, certainly unknowable. I would hasten to add that this does not mean that attempts to provide guidance for coming to know the person as a whole are without merit or purpose. For example, my cultural background, itself composed of innumerable constituent particulars over hundreds of years, obviously pervades my way of being; however, there are ways in which I have challenged, rejected, or drifted away from my cultural background. To know *well* a person's cultural background, and the ways in which she/he deviates from it, is a tremendous challenge. The attempts to inform such a project, including the works of Leininger (1995) and others, have contributed to nursing science and guided nursing practice in ways that surely lead to human betterment. In the past two decades, scores of studies of the health care needs of Latin American immigrants to the United States have appeared in the literature and have, no doubt, contributed to improvements in health care for this population. Yet even such a massive body of work could not be said, seriously, to allow for knowing any one person among that population as whole.

The several systems frameworks of nursing (King, 1981; Neuman & Fawcett, 2002; Roy & Andrews, 1999) basically guide the nurse to inventory and assess the parts of the human system and, through knowing the collection of the parts, to come to know the whole. Despite obvious and intellectually stringent attempts to be thorough, these frameworks inevitably come up short in actually guiding the nurse to fully come to know the person as a whole. Although they share in similar (systems) ontologies, they do not even inventory the same parts. Carper (1978) took a different and broader approach when she posited fundamental patterns of knowing in nursing, asserting that the knowledge needed to underpin nursing practice is so vast that it entails empirical knowing, aesthetic knowing, ethical knowing, and personal knowing. Surely it is, at least in part, nursing's focus on the whole human being that precipitated the call for such a broad-ranging knowledge base.

The birth of a new paradigm of nursing science in Rogers' (1970) work was clearly anchored in the assumption and prospect of new knowledge about unitary human beings. Much of the literature of new-paradigm nursing has addressed the need for reinterpreting the realities of human life, human health, and caregiving practices. Two famous and revered quotations have been reproduced countless times to underscore that the advent of the new paradigm was brought about by the necessity of rising to new levels of awareness and adopting new ways of thinking:

> *The dogmas of the quiet past are inadequate to the stormy present. The occasion is piled high with difficulty, and we must rise with the occasion. As our case is new, so we must think anew and act anew. (Abraham Lincoln)*

> *Problems cannot be solved at the same level of awareness that created them. (Albert Einstein)*

But it would require more than a new paradigm or new way of knowing ever to come to know, well and in full, the whole human being.

Critical social theorists, philosophers, feminists, and others have observed that different persons are known and wish to be known in different ways. They also commonly do *not* wish to be known (and indeed do not even believe) in the ways in which they are commonly known by others, such as in sexist or bigoted narratives or discourses that characterize one in an undesired way (Butler, 2005). Levinas (1961/1969) has suggested that the determination within oneself to regard the other in a chosen way is a form of violence. The ethical relation—in his thought more fundamental than ontology—is one of passivity toward the other. This conceptualization has been described as a shift from "ethics as knowledge to knowledge as ethics" (Todd, 2001, p. 69). In a similar vein, qualitative methodologists exploring narrative approaches to knowing persons through research have taken to radically passive methods of eliciting descriptions of lived experiences from persons (Parse, 1998; Jones, 2003), seeking to elicit, as purely as possible, only the story the person intends to relate. In the United States, laws (such as the Health Insurance Portability and Accountability Act [HIPAA] and the Family Educational Rights and Privacy Act [FERPA]) now limit the information that professionals are entitled to access regarding their clients and the circumstances under which a professional may divulge information to another. Increasingly, public discourse seems to indicate that persons regard the ethical warrant for others to have access to intimate knowledge of them—to say nothing of comprehensive knowledge of them—to be extremely rare and limited, with greater restrictions and controls much desired. What, then, are the implications of such a stance for a discipline that strongly identifies itself as a practice discipline and doggedly regards the human being or person as a whole and even unitary being?

Bearing Witness to Unfolding Mystery

The formal knowledge base of nursing clearly calls the nurse scholar or practitioner to know the person as whole. This tenet of our discipline need not be construed, however, to mean that the nurse must or should know the whole person. More fundamental than an ontology of wholeness, perhaps, in human affairs, is an ontology positing veneration of the other in relation as originary. For example, Watson (2005), drawing on Levinas (1961/1969), connected the concept of otherness and the ultimate unknowability of the other with the infinity of "Cosmic Love":

> *The subject as Other is an incomprehensible, infinite Other-ness. The human face is not a concept; the human heart is not a concept, it is not a figure whose message can be captured by conventional knowledge from the head. It is the Other, the face, the heart-felt call in its exposedness, its nudity, as an opening toward the infinite, the infinity of Cosmic Love that reminds us that we belong together in this life as given to us, which is beyond our control, making one responsible for the Other. (Watson, 2005, p. 81)*

Despite her recent turn toward unitary discourse, here the particulate/summative language of "head" and "heart" resurfaces. The specific rendering of the nature of human wholeness here, however, is less important than the forceful assertion of the centrality of love in human-to-human relatedness.

Placing respect for the human dignity solidly at the core of nursing practice, Parse (1998) has described the encounter of person with person as follows:

> *In the rhythm of human-human presence, individuals give messages consistent with personal valued images. The message the other receives is all-at-once, yet not complete. Full understanding of the message is not possible in light of the realms of knowing, that is, the explicit-tacit knowing, what is known and utterable and what is known and not utterable ...* No individual can fully understand another; each experiences the other from a personal perspective. *(pp. 40–41)*

From Parse's (1998, 2007) perspective, articulated in the "humanbecoming" school of thought, each human being is always an unfolding mystery, ultimately unknowable to others. Practice guided by the human-becoming theory is incarnating true presence, being with and attending to the person or persons in a unique, theory-guided, yet free-flowing and authentic way: "True presence is an intentional reflective love, an interpersonal art" (Parse, 1998, p. 71).

True presence is also bearing witness to the lived realities revealed by the person(s):

> *The nurse enters the person's or group's world as a not-knowing stranger ... Persons share with the nurse only the reality that they wish to disclose. The nurse in true presence joins the reality of others at all realms of the universe and is available to bear witness without judging or labeling. (Parse, 1998, p. 72)*

Parse's approach to practice offers a distinct, coherent, and fully articulated alternative to methods that depend on the nurse's knowing of the person, whether such knowing is characterized as objectivist or humanistic, knowing a bio-psycho-social-spiritual being, knowing a person as body, mind, and spirit, or as a field pattern. From this perspective, it is not knowing the other that is most important and central in the relationship between nurse and person, but rather it is offering true presence—which is honoring, revering, being with, and attending to the person. Attending to the person leads to some understanding on the part of the nurse, which may or may not correspond closely to the person's own original story and/or the messages given by the person in the nurse-person relation. The nurse always has a professional responsibility to articulate what she/he knows and to be able to describe in some coherent manner what transpires in the nurse-person interchange. But the nurse is not obliged in any case to know the person's whole life story or to seek to obtain a comprehensive version of whatever narrative is unfolding in the moment.

For all its apparent passivity, bearing witness is a powerful co-constituting process in human relations. Actually, bearing witness is only one half of a rhythmical, paradoxical process of bearing witness– not bearing witness. Bearing witness is attesting to the authenticity of something with one's personal presence. Not bearing witness is a choice and is equally as co-constitutive of situations as bearing witness. What one chooses to bear witness to is a realm of reality. In a caregiving situation, or any human relationship, to refuse to bear witness to the meaning of the messages put forward by the other is to disrespect or negate the other's reality, and thereby, the person (Cody, 2001, 2007).

"Attention must be paid," as Arthur Miller (1949/1981, p. 56) eloquently asserted in *Death of a Salesman*. The attention that must be paid is attention to human dignity, with reverence for humanly lived experience, regardless of one's personal ability to understand or value the particulars of that humanly lived experience. It is valued *as* humanly lived experience. At the core of the disciplinary tenet of knowing persons as whole, then, are the veneration of human dignity and the practice of bearing witness to the unfolding mystery of each person.

"Love is a practice. Love is truly a practice" – Thich Nhat Hanh, (in McLeod, 2001).

References

Barrett, E. A. M. (1998). A Rogerian practice methodology for health patterning. *Nursing Science Quarterly, 11*, 136–138.

Butler, J. (2005). *Giving an account of oneself.* New York: Fordham University Press.

Carper, B. (1978). Fundamental patterns of knowing in nursing. *Advances in Nursing Science, 1*(1), 13–24.

Cody, W. K. (2001). The ethics of bearing witness in healthcare: A beginning exploration. *Nursing Science Quarterly, 14*, 288–296.

Cody, W. K. (2007). Bearing witness to suffering: Participating in cotranscendence. *International Journal for Human Caring, 11*(2), 17–21.

King, I. M. (1981). *A theory for nursing: Systems, concepts, process.* New York: Wiley.

Jones, K. (2003). The turn to a narrative knowing of persons: One method explored. *Nursing Times Research, 8*(1), 60–71.

Leininger, M. M. (1995). *Transcultural nursing: Concepts, theories, research and practices.* New York: McGraw-Hill.

Levinas, E. (1969). *Totality and infinity: An essay on exteriority.* (A. Lingis, Trans.). Pittsburgh: Duquesne University Press. (Original work published 1961).

McLeod, M. (2001). This is the Buddha's love: Melvin McLeod interviews Thich Nhat Hanh. *Shambhala Sun.* Retrieved July 26, 2008, from http://www.shambhalasun.com/index/php?option=com_content&task=view&id=2882&ItemID=0

Miller, A. (1981) *Death of a salesman: Text and criticism.* New York: Penguin. (Original work published in 1949).

Neuman, B., & Fawcett, J. (Eds.). (2002). *The Neuman systems model* (4th ed.). Upper Saddle River, NJ: Prentice-Hall.

Parse, R. R. (1981). *Man—living—health: A theory of nursing.* New York: Wiley.

Parse, R. R. (1998). *The human becoming school of thought: A perspective for nurses and other health professionals.* Thousand Oaks, CA: Sage.

Parse, R. R. (2007). The humanbecoming school of thought in 2050. *Nursing Science Quarterly, 20,* 308–311.

Rogers, M. E. (1970). *An introduction to the theoretical basis of nursing.* Philadelphia: F. A. Davis.

Roy, C., & Andrews, H. A. (1999). *The Roy adaptation model* (2nd ed.). Stamford, CT: Appleton & Lange.

Todd, S. (2001). On not knowing the other, or learning *from* Levinas. *Philosophy of Education 2001 Yearbook (pp. 67–74).* Champaign,IL: University of Illinois. Retrieved July 26, 2008, from http://www.ed.uiuc.edu/EPS/PESYearbook/2001/todd%2001.pdf

Watson, J. (2005). *Caring science as sacred science.* Philadelphia: F.A. Davis.

Watson, J., & Smith, M. (2002). Caring science and the science of unitary human beings: A trans-theoretical discourse for nursing knowledge development. *Journal of Advanced Nursing, 37*(5), 452–461.

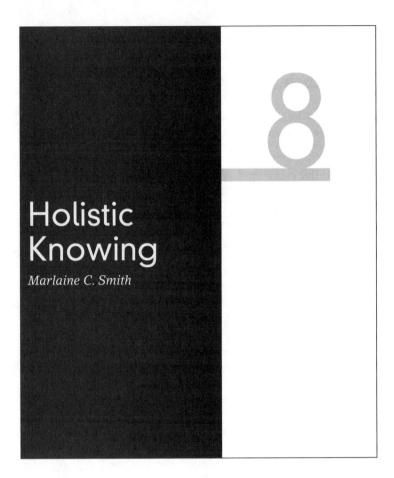

8

Holistic Knowing

Marlaine C. Smith

Chapter Overview

This chapter describes the foundations of an epistemology through which we come to know persons holistically from a unitary perspective, as elaborated through the following concepts: pattern seeing, resonant relating, caring consciousness, and integral synopsis. Key elements from these concepts will be synthesized to provide a foundation for holistic knowing with support from examples of such knowing in practice.

Introduction

All the King's horses and all the King's men
    Cannot put Humpty-Dumpty together again. (Mother Goose)

This familiar nursery rhyme rings true for those seeking and receiving health care in the current environment. Fragmentation and specialization thwart the goal of seeing the whole person and the whole picture of health or even disease. I have a cardiologist, gynecologist, endocrinologist, and gastroenterologist. They talk to my primary care provider through written reports that reflect an analysis of the systems in which they specialize. I appreciate this focus when I need diagnosis of a particular problem with my heart or thyroid gland. But it is difficult for them to look at how these different systems might be communicating with or affecting each other. Like in the story of the blind men trying to describe the whole of an elephant by feeling its different parts, we can never know the whole person and the whole picture of human health through analytical, reductionist processes of knowing.

Nursing scholars recognizing the limits of this medical model have struggled with the concept of holism and with epistemologies that facilitate coming to know humans as whole (Erickson, 2007). Some have adopted a pragmatic, summative view of holism. This is the perspective embodied by the totality (Parse, Coyne, & Smith, 1988) or interactive-integrative (Newman, Sime, & Corcoran-Perry, 1991) nursing paradigms. In this paradigm there is acknowledgement of the importance of coming to know the person as whole, and knowing as whole is accomplished through assessing all dimensions and synthesizing the analysis into a summative portrait. For example, the nurse using this approach would assess the biological, psychological, social, and spiritual dimensions and come to an understanding of the whole through understanding the relevant information gleaned from these interacting dimensions.

Some nursing scholars have disagreed with this approach, asserting that we can never come to know the whole through analysis of the dimensions or parts. Most notably, Martha Rogers (1970) argued that the whole of human life is more than and different from the sum of its parts. This perspective is espoused in the simultaneity (Parse et al., 1988) or unitary-transformative (Newman et al., 1991) nursing paradigms. The unitary perspective on holism belies an epistemology focused on the analysis of discrete parts or dimensions of personhood and embraces one that appreciates the mystery of its dynamic unity. The purpose of this chapter is to describe the foundations of an epistemology in which we come to know persons holistically from this unitary perspective. The foundations will be elaborated through exploring the following concepts: pattern seeing, resonant relating, caring consciousness, and integral synopsis. The key elements from these concepts will be synthesized to provide a foundation for holistic knowing. Examples of using this process of knowing in practice will be offered throughout.

Foundations of a Holistic Epistemology

I am not the first to grapple with the concept of holistic knowing from this unitary perspective. It is a worldview reflected in ancient civilizations. Indigenous cultures in North and South America, Australia, Africa and Asia have accessed knowledge through wisdom, intuition, and symbols acquired through interconnectedness with a larger whole: community, nature, ancestors, and the divine. Ancient Greek scholars acknowledged a holistic perspective; however, the advancement of scientific knowing with empirical-analytic supremacy colored Western thought by separating science from religion and philosophy, human interiority from nature, and mind from matter (Erickson, 2007).

This was the primary landscape of most science, and certainly nursing science, when Martha Rogers (1970) described the human being as an energy field. She later emphasized that "human beings don't have energy fields, they are energy fields" (Rogers, 1992, p. 30). A field is open, unbounded, and in a continuous, dynamic, mutual process of interaction with the environment, also described as a field. These fields are infinite, meaning that the entire universe and everything in it are interconnected. Energy fields, by their nature, cannot be divided; they are irreducible wholes. Yet each field is unique, manifesting the uniqueness of each human being. So, how can we know this unique, dynamic, ever-evolving, changing, whole person? There are four concepts that might be helpful as we attempt to answer this question: pattern seeing, resonant relating, caring consciousness, and integral synopsis. Each will be elaborated.

Pattern seeing. Pattern seeing is an essential skill needed for holistic knowing. In 1980, Marilyn Ferguson in *The Aquarian Conspiracy* predicted that pattern seeing would be a survival skill for the 21st century. Indeed if nursing is caring for the health (wholeness) of human beings, these skills are essential for holistic knowing, and arguably, all nursing practice. The term "seeing" is metaphoric in that the "sight" is perception that can involve senses and perception beyond the senses.

We have been trained from an early age to trust information that comes to us through our senses and to distrust the information that is extrasensory. We consider sensory data as primary, legitimate knowledge; whereas dreams, intuitive insights, and hunches are dismissed as interesting, but unreliable. Children often manifest signs of extrasensory awareness that are squelched as they are programmed into the traditional empirical and analytical processes of knowing.

With the assumption that human beings are energy fields comes the insight that we cannot know holistically through relying on our sensory perceptions alone. Sensory perception limits us to knowing in three-dimensional space and linear time when the universe from a unitary perspective is pandimensional (Rogers, 1992), existing beyond sensory awareness and linear time. William Blake (1960) asserted, "If the doors of perception were cleansed, everything would appear as it is ... infinite". David Bohm, (1980), an eminent physicist, described the universe as a whole consisting of implicate and explicate orders. The implicate order, the unseen pattern of the whole universe, gives rise to the explicate order, or the three-dimensional world that we access though our senses. The explicate order can provide a portal through which we can glimpse the underlying primary pattern of the whole.

Pattern is the distinguishing identifier of the whole. The whole (person, family, group, community, etc.) has a pattern that is the unseen fingerprint of the whole. Pattern manifests, or shows, itself explicitly through form, structure, time, space, and movement. These pattern manifestations can be seen, heard, felt, and perceived. Pattern was defined by Rogers (1992) as "the distinguishing characteristic of an energy field perceived as a single wave" (p. 30). Pattern provides identity to the whole while constantly changing. It is not directly observable, but the manifestations of pattern are observable or subjectively perceived. Patterning is innovative and capable of expressions that are rhythmic and limitless in diversity.

When I was a graduate student and first heard about Martha Rogers's ideas of wholeness and patterning, Dr. Mary Jane Smith, my professor, shared a story that facilitated my understanding. It went something like this:

Once there was a seasoned fisherman who was passing his knowledge and wisdom on to his daughter. He told her that the most important teaching he could impart was for her to come to know the fish. He told her to go and return to him when she came to know the fish. The young girl scampered off and caught a fish. She examined the fish carefully and then returned to her father. She told her father the details of the fish's scales, fins, eyes, and tail. Her father said, "You do not yet know the fish ... return to me when you do."

The daughter was puzzled but determined to prove to her father that she could arrive at the knowledge he was seeking. She caught another fish, dissected it, removed its parts, categorized them and described them with the utmost precision. She returned to her father and presented her findings on the fish, showing him a poster detailing her careful analysis. The father smiled and gently told her, "You do not yet know the fish. Come back to me when you do."

Now she was getting a little frustrated. This time she drew upon all the available technology. She used an electron microscope to examine the cellular structures of the fish organs. She conducted chemical analyses of the tissues. Now she returned confident of her in-depth knowledge of the fish, armed with tables, charts, and graphs. He listened calmly and said, "No my child, you do not yet know the fish. Return to me when you do." This time she was angry and hurt. She had worked so hard....of course she knew every part of that fish. What was he talking about?!

Exhausted, she collapsed by the bed of a slow-moving stream. She began to relax with the sounds of the stream, the odor of the earth and moss, and the light glistening off the water. Her eyes caught a glimpse of a beautiful trout swimming downstream. She watched for a long time as it meandered through the rocks, paused to nibble on a stone and brought its mouth to the surface of the water for a breath. She was fascinated, enthralled by the fish's beauty and uniqueness, how it thrived in its environment. For what seemed like hours, she watched and marveled.

She returned to her father, humbled by her experience. She told him that she could not know everything about the fish... only what she experienced in the time she was present on the bank. She described the water bubbling, the fish darting and stopping as it swam through the water, the vibrant colors changing in light and shadow. She told him how this fish was different from and similar to others in the stream. Her father smiled, "Now, my daughter, you know the fish." (Smith, 2008, pp. 58–59)

In this story, we see the daughter approaching her task of knowing through an empirical (through the senses)–analytic (separating a whole into elemental parts) process. Her wise father tells her that through this process she did not know the whole; one can never know the whole through more precise processes of objectification, reduction, and analysis. Instead, coming to know the whole occurs through being fully present, experiencing self as integral with the other, and seeing the other as integral with the environment. This involves using all modes of awareness in coming to know the unique and universal qualities that constitute the pattern of the whole: "Being fully present is the crux of unity consciousness and is requisite to nursing practice/research" (Newman, 2003, p. 242). The diversity of patterning isn't judged, but instead is described by, for, and/or with the other in reverence and awe.

Pattern seeing is developed through repeated, intentional efforts at shifting focus from the parts to the whole. We see pattern through apprehending expressions of (1) uniqueness and diversity, (2) connectedness with the environment (others, nature, Universe/God), and (3) meaning. These may be discerned by listening to the other's story, observing the body through space and time, and sensing and extra-sensing subtle messages. Newman (2002) reminds us that "the data of pattern are the stories of people and their connectedness with their environment, reflecting the complexity of continuing change" (p. 6).

Pattern seeing is learned through practice. I have lived in south Florida for two years. During these years I've walked the beach hundreds of times gathering shells for my collection. Without thinking about it, I've developed my skills to the point of being able to casually walk and pick out a small, rare shell among hundreds resting on a patch of sand. I've trained my attention to see something I would never have seen before.

Newman (1994) described this process of pattern seeing as pattern recognition, and Cowling (2001) called it unitary pattern appreciation. Both of these scholars have developed practice-research or praxis methods, in which the nurse-practitioner researcher engages the client participant in exploring his/her own pattern though reflecting on significant life events (Newman, 1994) or experiences, perceptions and expressions (Cowling, 2001). The practitioner researcher shares his/her own perceptions of patterning through a life-pattern diagram (Newman, 1994) or an artistic creation that captures the universal and unique aspects of the pattern (Cowling, 2001). The nurse approaches the other as a partner or participant in a journey of discovering pattern. For Newman, it is a hermeneutic-dialectic process. The nurse and client in partnership interpret the pattern together and apart; each interpretation contributes to a greater understanding of the pattern of the whole: "Meaning in a person's life is not only critical, but also a way of identifying pattern. A pattern possesses meaning" (Newman, 2002, p. 4). Pattern appreciation is synoptic with the emphasis on "sensing an emerging pattern that reflects the wholeness, uniqueness and essence of human life" (Cowling, 2001, p. 36).

The following two examples might illustrate pattern-seeing as a dimension of holistic knowing. Marta has been hospitalized for metabolic acidosis secondary to Type II diabetes. In caring for her prior to her discharge, Benjamin, her nurse, notices that her BMI is 31, up from 28, where it was 6 months ago. Her glycolated hemoglobin is 12.2.

Marta looks sad, worried, and agitated. Because she speaks very little English, Benjamin calls an interpreter so that he can communicate with her. Through the interpreter he says to Marta, "Tell me about what it will be like when you go home." Marta responds that she is very nervous about going home. She has two jobs that she needs to return to, cleaning houses and cooking in a local Mexican restaurant. She cries as she tells Benjamin that "life is hard." She is 36 years old and has lived in Florida for 8 years, having emigrated from Mexico. Marta is undocumented and has two children, 13 and 7 years old. Besides caring for them, she is the sole support of her 66-year-old mother. Her husband left her several years ago for another woman. She eats very little during the day when she is cleaning, but when she goes to the restaurant at 5 p.m., she eats "a lot" of Mexican food. When she gets home at 1 a.m., she eats even more. She says she cries a lot and is "just tired all the time."

When Benjamin asks about what is most important to her she smiles and says her beautiful children: "I need to be strong for my children."

Benjamin sees Marta's pattern as struggling with a difficult life in which she is experiencing heavy burdens and very little joy. She doesn't feel in control of her health, but she wants to feel better and be better for her children. Benjamin has engaged in pattern seeing through being in a caring relationship with Marta. He obtained a translator and pulled together all sources of information for a snapshot of Marta's pattern.

Another example is Barbara, who is seeking "help with my pain and nausea" from Dana, her holistic nurse. After talking about how she is doing with her chemotherapy for treatment of breast cancer, Dana asks Barbara to lie down on the massage table. She moves her hands over her body, holding them about 4 inches above Barbara's skin. Dana senses a prickly sensation over Barbara's left breast, left arm, and side and feels a "heaviness" as she moves down her legs. Dana shares her perceptions with Barbara. Barbara tells her that she has had some pain in the surgical site and some lymphedema lately. She says that she just can't seem to "get over this and get moving again ... Maybe this is why you felt such heaviness in my legs. I just can't make myself get out and start living again like I was." She weeps as she says, "I feel almost frozen. I guess I'm not as brave as I pretend to be." In this example, Dana has used her hands to sense the pattern of the whole. Because she has shared her perceptions, both she and Barbara have acquired deeper insight into the meaning of Barbara's health experience.

Resonant relating. Resonant relating is the second concept that may help illuminate the process of holistic knowing. Resonance is a field phenomenon defined in physics as "the tendency of a system to oscillate at its maximum amplitude at certain frequencies, known as the system's resonance frequencies (or resonant frequencies)" (Wikipedia). Rogers (1970, 1992) included the concept of resonancy as one of her principles of homeodynamics. She defined resonancy as "continuous change from lower to higher frequency wave patterns in human and environmental fields" (Rogers, 1992, p. 31). Newman identified (2008)"resonating with the whole" as the way that information is received in the nurse-patient relationship.

Resonance is tuning in to a vibrational frequency that provides critical information about the pattern of the whole. Like tuning in to a radio channel, the nurse tunes in to a vibrational frequency of the patient's energy field that contains this critical information. Attuning occurs through intention to be fully present in the moment and awareness of intuitive insights or feelings about where to place attention and focus. The nurse may pay attention to a certain feeling that she should ask a particular question or make a comment. Resonance is acquiring information through feelings, hunches, intuitions, and senses that occur simultaneously outside the boundaries of logical analysis. Resonance leads to information about the pattern of the whole. "The basic way of knowing through attunement and resonant receptivity manifests itself in intuition and revelation" (Newman, 2008, p. 37).

Resonance is contrary to rational, objective, analytical thinking. In fact, rational analytical thinking "breaks the field of resonance" (Newman, 2008), so approaching the patient with a structured assessment hampers the possibilities for gaining information through resonance. It is "simultaneous perception of the whole" rather than logical analysis and judgment (Newman, 2008, p. 39). A nurse expert in holistic knowing can focus on the whole, receiving information first through resonance, and then through inviting reflection upon more structured questions, always feeling and sensing the whole through the parts. Although the whole is not a sum of parts, the whole can be reflected or encountered in the parts (Newman, 2008). The nurse pays close attention to any messages conveyed by the patient in the moment because "everything that presents itself is purposeful" (Newman, 2008, p. 38).

Objectivity or "spectator awareness" (Newman, 2008) interrupts resonance as well. Holistic knowing requires participation in the discovery of pattern. One cannot resonate with the whole by standing back and observing it. Instead the nurse enters the world of the other as a caring companion cocreating meaning. There is no pattern of the whole apart from its interpretation within the relationship. The nurse intends to see the whole, and through engagement with the other, senses or intuits that whole: "For the intuitive mind, there is a reversal of perception: there is perception of the universal in the particular, which is a concrete manifestation of the universal" (Newman, 2008, p. 48).

Newman (2008) described resonance as the essence of information that is accessible through feelings. Consciousness is the information capacity of any system. As consciousness expands, so does the ability to access information. Information transfer is not limited to sensory information, and it is nonlocal, present everywhere. As human consciousness expands, resonant abilities will evolve. "The holistic mode of consciousness is nonlinear, simultaneous, intuitive, and concerned with relationships, rather than elements that are related" (Newman, 2008, p. 39).

Sheldrake (1983) described how resonance allows instantaneous access to information enfolded within interconnected fields. Newman (2008) asserts, "One cannot perceive the whole by standing back to get an overview, but by going further into the parts—by going further into the center of self and seeing the phenomenon anew" (Newman, 2008, p. 39).

The story of the hundredth monkey illustrates the phenomenon of resonance. Monkeys on the Japanese island of Koshima had been studied by scientists for over 30 years. The scientists were dropping sweet potatoes on the sand for the monkeys to eat, and although they liked the potatoes, they avoided eating them because the sand was distasteful. One young monkey learned to take a potato, wash it in a stream and eat it. He taught his mother to do this, and then others in the tribe learned to wash the sweet potatoes before eating them. Soon this practice grew throughout the monkey tribe. But a fascinating phenomenon occurred. Once the practice became widespread on the island, once it was embedded in the consciousness of a critical mass, it spread across the sea to other islands, where monkeys who had never been in physical contact with the monkeys on Koshima began washing the potatoes in streams before eating them (http://www.100thmonkey.com/zwebstory100th.html. Retrieved 8/19/08). Once a critical awareness is reached, it becomes encoded in the field that connects everything. The information is available to all through resonance with the field.

Holistic knowing through resonance occurs through "attunement, resonant receptivity, intuition, revelation—a direct unfiltered index of communication between the senses and the environment. This involves the capacity to become selfless through reflective silence, quiet contemplation and meditation" (Arguelles, 1984). Apprehending the whole is possible with shifting consciousness. "In the beginning of learning to grasp the whole, we may flip back and forth between the intellectual and the intuitive, between the sensorial and meaning, but we can be assured that they are all dimensions of the whole" (Newman, 2008, p. 50).

The following story reveals an example of resonance: Lucia, a hospice nurse, was caring for Mr. Williams, a 74-year-old, African American man with advanced lung cancer. Lucia was listening to Mr. Williams's lungs but focusing on the pattern of the whole.

Inexplicably she stopped, pulled the stethoscope from her ears, and asked, "Do you have children?"

Mr. Williams teared up, turned away, and said, "I have a daughter, but we don't talk anymore."

"Why not?" Lucia inquired.

"Oh, it was a silly argument over the man she married," he said.

"Well, should a silly argument keep you two from being together now?" she asked.

Lucia stayed by Mr. Williams as he dialed his daughter's phone number and told her the story of his illness. The next day Mr. Williams's daughter came to the hospice with her two little boys and continued her visits almost daily until Mr. Williams died. This was a healing experience for Mr. Williams and his daughter, and it all began with the nurse having the hunch to ask a simple question that surfaced from resonant relating.

Caring Consciousness

Caring consciousness (Watson & Smith, 2002) is described as a quality of consciousness expressed through higher frequency wave patterning and exhibiting a connection with the other that "transcends time, space and physicality and is open and continuous with the evolving unitary consciousness of the universe" (p. 459). Newman (1994) described this as absolute consciousness experienced as love. Others have referred to this as agape, or divine, love.

Knowing holistically is a spiritual act. The foundations of process spirituality and the metaphysics of love connect the ideas of apprehending wholeness through the spiritual quest. In the literature of process spirituality, human beings are created in the image of God, whole and beautiful, and Universal Intelligence or God knows human beings as whole. This knowing flows from divine love and caring. In other words, the Universe (God) loved human beings into existence.

Nursing literature affirms the centrality of caring and wholeness. Caring is a way of being in the world and a quality of consciousness that mirrors divine love. Through caring consciousness, we attune to the unitary nature of human life: "Caring is the process through which wholeness is addressed and which potentiates the emergence of innovative patterning and possibilities" (Cowling, Smith, & Watson, 2008, p. E44). Knowing the other holistically, through this quality of consciousness, is visible through listening to what matters most, listening to the person's story.

Human beings are by their nature whole, but knowing this whole is obscured by our human perceptual capabilities and our engrained reductionistic patterns of knowing. Caring is seeing with God eyes: "Caring cleanses the doors of perception so that we can see ourselves and others as we/they are…whole" (Cowling et al., p. E46). As we become aware of this unitary nature, it becomes more difficult to judge, label, objectify, fix, advise, intervene, and order (Ibid): "Knowing holistically calls for acceptance, non-judgment, appreciation, recognition, sojourning, accompanying, partnering, exploring, dialoguing, and listening" (Ibid). All of this evolves with a caring consciousness.

Unconditional love, or agape, affords us the grace to accept others as they are without the need to change them. When we experience this love, we come to know the other as holy, as the face of the Divine. When we approach others with a heart filled with love, we are grateful and appreciative for their presence and connectedness to us. This awakens us to the beauty of their nature and enables apprehension of the whole or the holy. The creativity and beauty of the Universe is present in all human life; seeing all life as a manifestation of this creativity and beauty is seeing the holy or the whole: "Our essential connectedness with God and the ambient world is … the ground of wholeness, transformation, beauty and healing" (Epperly, 2001, p. 4). Epperly (2001) argued that the spiritual evolution deepens awareness of the whole, writing, "Our deepest care for others creates a gentle matrix of wholeness and beauty from which their moment by moment experience arises" (p. 5).

Our experience of this wholeness comes to us first in sighs too deep for words. It is grasping the awesome nature of the complexity, diversity, beauty, and mystery of the human being. Each client we encounter is evolving, and coming to know wholeness is knowing for the moment because human beings are always creating and re-creating life. As Epperly wrote, "We are the artists of our own experiences, constantly bringing forth, something of unique beauty from the pigments that life gives us" (2001, p. 6). Epperly went on to say, "Each moment and encounter is an 'icon,' a window through which we glimpse the Soul of the Universe in its countless incarnations. Pain, suffering ... and brokenness are real: but they are not final. The ever-present and constantly creating Center brings forth novel alternatives that redeem and transform what appears to be mere wreckage and refuse" (2001, p. 7).

Engaging imagination and affirmation are ways to perceive wholeness in times when we are challenged to do so. Imagination can help when encountering a person that we are challenged to like. Imagine that person as a beautiful infant in the arms of his/her mother or affirm, "All are created in the image and likeness of God." Retreating in prayer or quiet meditation can help discern wholeness. Touch is an avenue to apprehending wholeness through caring consciousness. Massage, Reiki, healing touch, and hand holding can be channels of expressing caring consciousness. An ecological perspective flows from this consciousness. Seeing persons as whole and integral with the environment brings greater appreciation of the earth and the gifts of her precious resources.

The importance of caring consciousness to knowing wholeness is illustrated in the following example. Imelda, a public health nurse, receives a referral to visit an immigrant family because of suspicions of abuse and neglect of children and an elderly woman in the home. When Imelda arrives at the Makowski household, she is shocked at the condition of the home. Trash is piled in the front lawn and porch, and the grass is knee-high. The interior of the house is filthy, with dirty dishes strewn throughout; dog urine and feces soak the stained carpet. The walls have fecal material and dirt caked on them. There is so much trash on the floor it is difficult to walk through. Two preschool-aged children with matted hair and dirty clothes are staring at the television, feeding themselves from a Captain Crunch cereal box. Imelda explains to Wendy Makowski, the children's mother, that she is there to check on Wendy's children and elderly mother. Dragging on her cigarette and sipping on a beer, Wendy challenges Imelda, arguing that her kids are fine, and pointing to them on the floor. When Imelda asks to see her mother, Wendy points to a closed door. Imelda finds Mrs. Makowski, Wendy's mother, in a dark bedroom, lying in her own urine and feces. There are clothes and trash all over the floor. Mrs. Makowski is dehydrated and extremely weak.

Imelda feels indignant anger rise in her as she begins making a series of judgments about Wendy who, in her mind, is seriously neglecting her children and mother. How could she do this? How could she live like this? A flurry of stereotypes and labels dance through her consciousness. Suddenly, she recognizes these judgments and stops. Taking some deep breaths, Imelda sets an intention to care, and to see Wendy as more than and different from a drunk, a bad caretaker, a slob. She focuses on coming to know Wendy and her story.

She tells Wendy her concerns about the safety of the children and her mother. Wendy is clearly intoxicated, and her response to Imelda is abusive. Imelda tells Wendy that in her judgment Wendy is not able to care for her children and mother at this time, and that for their safety they would need to live somewhere else. Imelda calls Social Services and the police and makes arrangements for the children and Mrs. Makowski to be resettled in another home.

When they are gone, Wendy collapsed in tears, shaken to the core by the actions taken. She tells Imelda that she doesn't know where to turn or what to do next. She knows she is sick and needs help. Imelda suggests that she enter a rehab center, and when Wendy agrees she makes arrangements with the center and drives her to the detox unit. She gives Wendy her card, and tells her that she cares about her, and that she has faith and hope in Wendy's ability to turn her life around and get her family back.

Integral Synopsis

Integral synopsis is the final concept in this explication of the foundations of knowing holistically. This concept originated in the ideas of Ken Wilber and Philip Phenix (1964). Wilber (1997) described an integral vision of knowing that acknowledges the source and objects of knowing. The sources of knowing are interior (i.e., subjective, originating within consciousness) and exterior (objective, originating from sensory data from the external world). The objects of knowing are either individual or collective, knowing one or more than one. From these dimensions of sources and objects, Wilber created four quadrants representing the four faces of truth or knowledge. For Wilber (1997), knowing proceeds from whole to parts and parts to whole in a circle of understanding:

> *We move from part to whole and back again, and in that dance of comprehension, in that amazing circle of understanding, we come alive to meaning, to value, and to vision: the very circle of understanding guides our way, weaving together the pieces, healing their fractures, mending the torn and tortured fragments, lighting the way ahead—this extraordinary movement from part to whole and back again, with healing the hallmark of each and every step, and grace the tender reward. (p. 1)*

Wilber (1997) used the term *holon* to describe the part-whole unity. Holon refers to "wholes that are simultaneously parts of other wholes." From Wilber's (1997) perspective, the universe is composed of neither parts nor wholes but of whole/parts or holons: "We exist as fields within fields, patterns within patterns, contexts within contexts, endlessly" (p. 100). Therefore, we come to know through integrating multiple perspectives, examining and integrating knowledge of holons. These multiple perspectives are from the following four faces of truth: exterior (objective world), interior (subjective world), collective interior (intersubjective) and the collective exterior (inter-objective). All are equally significant and important for the understanding of human phenomena.

Knowing the whole is apprehending all the faces of truth all at once. Wilber (1997) called this the "eye of the spirit," and it can integrate these faces of truth into a holistic portrait through synopsis. Each face is tapped for the knowledge that it can provide and then interpreted through synopsis, capturing what is meaningful: "The integral vision attempts … to include the moment of truth in each of these approaches—from empiricism to constructivism to relativism to aestheticism … but, in stripping them of their claims to be the only type of truth in existence, releases them from their contradictions and places them into a genuine rainbow coalition" (Ibid, p.29).

Wilber (1997) asserted that understanding involves shifting attention to the whole and its parts. This integral epistemology takes the approach of backing "up to a level of abstraction at which the various conflicting approaches actually agree with one another" (p. ix). It is moving beyond reductionism through developing what he calls "orienting generalizations" or "sturdy conclusions," those ideas at a level of abstraction that is agreed upon. Then, the integrative method involves a phenomenology of all human knowledge conducted at this level of orienting generalizations. What does this body of knowledge tell us about the whole? The knower synthesizes a systematic vision of the phenomenon and looks for a way to represent its wholeness or coherence.

According to Wilber (1998), spiritual practice or meditation is assistive in developing skill in integrative knowing or perceiving through what he calls the eye of the Spirit. Through meditation, perceptions shift so that non-dual awareness occurs. A sense of a unity of knowing and being, self and world is experienced during meditation; one experiences the whole: "This life of yours which you are living is not merely a piece of the entire existence, but is, in a certain sense, the whole" (Wilber, 1998, p. 17). This is a direct and immediate perception of wholeness that informs and transforms the process of coming to know.

With evolving non-dual awareness, it is possible to sense the whole through the smaller whole. For example, while feeling a pulse, it may be possible to acquire synoptic understanding of the whole person. Also, through knowing the larger whole, it may be possible to gain synoptic understanding of a smaller whole. Wilber (1997) asserted that this circle of understanding might be grasped more proficiently and instantaneously through some form of spiritual practice or meditation.

Synoptic knowing (Phenix, 1964) is a transformative form of knowing that creates a synthesis from knowledge that was compartmentalized. It is creating meaning and coherence from isolated fragments in flashes of insight or recognition that apprehend how the parts come together to form the whole. It is not a summary, but an expression of essence. Through synoptic knowing, we can grasp the whole

quickly through an apprehension of what is most meaningful. It can facilitate understanding beyond the particular to
the universal, beyond the individual to the community.

According to Phenix (1964), synoptic knowing has an
integrative function, "uniting meanings from all the realms
into a unified perspective, that is, providing a 'single vision'
or 'synopsis' of meanings" (p. 235). He described a process of
"going to the limits" as one in which the limits of understanding through finite means are experienced. Through transcendent and immanent spiritual practices, a new perspective
may be illuminated from the whole (p. 247). Integration
through synopsis occurs through a process of interpretation
or gathering the expressions of meaning from many sources
and then coming to the meanings of meanings, or "meta-
meanings" (p. 253).

This practice exemplar may illustrate this process of
knowing. Malcolm is a nurse practitioner at an inner-city
clinic. He is seeing Mrs. Darcy after her hysterectomy for
advanced cervical cancer. He listens to Mrs. Darcy's story
and examines her. He wonders why Mrs. Darcy never came
in to the clinic to get a free Pap smear and asks her. She
describes what it is like to live in her apartment. There are
thugs everywhere who harass the residents, and she is afraid
to leave her apartment, so she stays there most of the time.
She only goes to the doctor if she has symptoms. For her it is
more important to stay safe than to seek preventive health
care. This insight awakens Malcolm to an understanding of
a larger whole, the community in which Mrs. Darcy lives.
He realizes that to promote health for Mrs. Darcy and others like her, the issues that kept her away from care must
be addressed.

This chapter elaborates a framework for holistic knowing. Holistic knowing is a foundation for nursing practice,
and when engaged, it can transform the traditional nursing
process phase of "assessment" into a process of coming to a
deeper and fuller understanding of the whole person (family,
community) (Potter & Frisch, 2007). Four concepts informing holistic knowing have been explicated: pattern seeing,
resonant relating, caring consciousness, and integral synopsis. This epistemological framework for holistic knowing can
provide guidance to novice holistic nurses and an explicit
rationale for those experienced nurses who have relied on
these processes in their practice.

References

Arguelles, J. (1984). *Earth ascending: An illustrated treatise on the law governing whole systems.* Santa Fe, NM: Bear & Co.

Blake, W. (1960). *The marriage of heaven and hell.* London: Trianon Press.

Bohm, D. (1980). *Wholeness and the implicate order.* London: Routledge & Kegan Paul.

Cowling, W. R. (2001). Unitary appreciative inquiry. *Advances in Nursing Science, 23*(4), 32–48.

Denslow, W. W. (1902). Humpty Dumpty. In *Mother Goose.* www.wikipedia. org. Accessed January 2, 2009. pperly, B. G. (2001). Process spirituality and original wholeness. Retrieved August 18, 2008, from www. ctr4process.org/publications/Seminar Papers/242Epperly.doc

Erickson, H. L. (2007). Philosophy and theory of holism. *Nursing Clinics of North America, 42,* 139–163.

Ferguson, M. (1980). *The aquarian conspiracy: Personal and social transformation in the 1980s.* Los Angeles: J. P. Tarcher.

Newman, M. A. (1994). *Health as expanding consciousness* (2nd ed.). New York: National League for Nursing.

Newman, M. A. (2002). The pattern that connects. *Advances in Nursing Science, 24*(3), 1–7.

Newman, M. A. (2008). *Transforming presence: The difference that nursing makes.* Philadelphia: F.A. Davis.

Newman, M. A. (2003) A world of no boundaries. *Advances in Nursing Science, 26*(4), 240–245.

Newman, M. A., Sime, A.M. & Corcoran-Perry, S. A. (1991). The focus of the discipline of nursing. *Advances in Nursing Science.* 14(1), 1–6.

Parse, R. R., Coyne, A. B., & Smith, M. J. (1988). *Nursing science: Major paradigms, theories and critiques.* New York: Wiley.

Phenix, P. (1964). *Realms of meaning.* New York: McGraw-Hill.

Potter, P. J., & Frisch, N. (2007). Holistic assessment and care: Presence in the process. *Nursing Clinics of North America, 42,* 213–228.

Rogers, M. E. (1970). *An introduction to the theoretical basis of nursing.* Philadelphia: F. A. Davis.

Rogers, M. E. (1992). Nursing science and the space age. *Nursing Science Quarterly, 5*(1), 27–34.

Rogers, M. E. (1994). The science of unitary human beings: Current perspectives. *Nursing Science Quarterly, 7*(1), 33–35.

Sheldrake, R. (1983). *A new science of life.* Los Angeles: Tarcher.

Smith, M. C. (2008). President's message. *Visions, 15*(1), 58–60.

Watson, J., & Smith, M. C. (2002). Caring science and the science of unitary human beings. *Journal of Advanced Nursing, 37*(5), 452–461.

Wilber, K. (1997). *The eye of the spirit.* Boston: Shambhala.

Wilber, K. (1998). *The essential Ken Wilber: An introductory reader.* Boston: Shambhala.

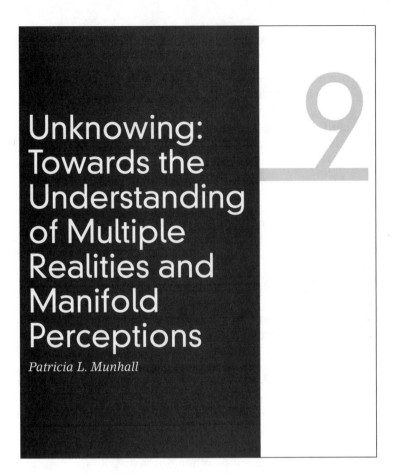

Unknowing: Towards the Understanding of Multiple Realities and Manifold Perceptions

Patricia L. Munhall

Chapter Overview

This chapter challenges the reader to understand and practice the process of unknowing as an essential component of humanistic, compassionate, and empathic nursing care. The focus is on achieving a state of mind, that of unknowing, as a condition of openness to the patient. This focus suggests that knowing or thinking we know the patient, in contrast, can lead to a form of confidence that inherently leads to a condition of closure. This closure is often premature and essential understanding of the patient and the patient's experience is precluded. Transference, countertransference, "wide-awakeness", consciousness, and the very pragmatic consideration of time are discussed. This author believes that the practice of unknowing leads to authentic human understanding where dignity, autonomy, and empathy are the outcomes for our patients. From this practice, complications in care will be significantly decreased, and the patient is authentically understood by the nurse.

Introduction

"You don't know how it feels to be me," Tom Petty sang plaintively and with frustration on his 1994 CD *Wildflowers*. This is perhaps a simple thought, though it conveys an enormous challenge. Yet we are confronted with this every day and have felt this way ourselves. The sentiment reminds me of a child trying to explain her feelings to her parents when she might not be getting what she wants, when she wants it, or of an angry adolescent frustrated with his parents' apparent inability to understand him. Adults as well can be heard saying this when they feel misunderstood, and couples are experts at this refrain. A patient lies in bed realizing, for the most part, that those caring for him do not know him very well at all. The claim becomes a lament of frustration.

I have written extensively on unknowing and will list all the references to these articles or chapters at the end of the chapter, along with other notes. If you are familiar with those referenced articles, some of this material will be very familiar to you. I am writing this chapter from notes that I have collected over the years that went into some of those works. I was inspired to write on unknowing (my first article on unknowing, "Unknowing: Toward Another Pattern of Knowing in Nursing," was published in 1993) during my education as a psychiatric mental health nurse-practitioner, from training as a psychoanalyst, and as a researcher and author on phenomenology. Unknowing is actually essential to researching from a phenomenological perspective. This perspective is aimed at understanding the meaning of experience for another person. Also a book I should mention here is *The Art of Unknowing*, by S. Kurtz (1989) for its very insightful approach to unknowing. Carper's (1978) work on fundamental patterns of knowing in nursing stirred the idea that there may be something to unknowing (the way it is described in this chapter) that will lead to knowing, thus another pattern of knowing. Unknowing what we know, or suspending belief in what we believe, is different from not knowing and will be discussed in another section of this chapter.

Attempting to understand how it feels for another may be an extended kindness and a generous act, but it is absolutely essential to caring for a patient. Verbal catharsis is known to be curative of symptoms of frustration, among them anxiety, loneliness, feelings of isolation, feelings of non-being, fear, insecurity, and defense mechanisms. Unfolding one's narrative to a caring other can lower blood pressure and stress as well as being curative of the above conditions. Additionally, being listened to has wondrous outcomes such as feeling appreciated, valued, cared about and held in high esteem.

Why Unknowing?

Doing your best to understand another person's perspective and subjectivity is an act of openness to another. You open your mind to a different way of thinking or seeing a phenomenon.

You allow yourself to become unknowing as an act of openness. You turn off the switch to premature closure. If you believe you know something, it most often prevents you from contemplating a new or contradictory thought. We often think of the things we know as equated with the truth.

Kurtz (1989) offered a profound insight: "Knowledge screens the sound the third ear hears, so we hear only what we know (p. 6)." This is why unknowing can be considered a critical path to new and undiscovered knowing for nursing and for all interpersonal relationships. This chapter then focuses on this state of mind, that of unknowing as a condition of openness.

Knowing, in contrast, can lead to a form of confidence that inherently leads to a condition of closure. Actually, I use Petty's song "You Don't Know How It Feels" as a meditative way to open my phenomenology workshops. I mention this because unknowing is part of being phenomenologically present to another human being, an authentic presence to another person. Unknowing is an acknowledgement of the infinite variations that compose the human condition.

Some Philosophy and Psychodynamics of Unknowing

Phenomenology in this context is philosophically oriented to encourage us to understand meaning in experience for another person, from that person's perspective. Simultaneously we should also reflect on the meaning of our own experience—in this instance, of being interconnected with this patient, sharing an intersubjective space. Two subjective beings are interconnected in communication and experience. From this reflection we come to know and name the reactions this patient produces in us.

Pause here and consider what patients have done that has produced anger in you, which is a completely normal response. What is critical to note here is that this transfer of anger gives us new knowledge about the patient. This alerts us to try to understand the patient's anger. This is not a luxury, as some might think. We are not psychoanalyzing a patient. Instead we are using several principles inherent in the field of human understanding to enable us to assist the patient to optimal being. Anger has devastating effects on a person's health and well-being. This richness of information is what comes from assuming this perspective of unknowing.

Of Transference and Countertransference

Called "countertransference," (Atwood & Stolorow, 1984), some of these reactions, such as anger, may be a reflection of the way the patient is feeling. The patient wants us to feel what he or she is feeling. The patient "transfers" anger towards the nurse, who responds with a countertransference of anger toward the patient. In other words, the patient may do something that makes the nurse angry precisely to let her know how he is feeling. This process is usually an unconscious one.

We experience countertransference, and the patient experiences transference toward us. Transference is where a patient has feelings or reactions toward us or about us that originate from his or her past, as with anger. Those feelings or reactions toward us have little to do with who we are but are manifestations of the patient's reactions in similar situations in the past. The patient may not trust us when we are completely trustworthy. However, with an unknowing stance, we wonder where that comes from, where did the patient lose feelings of trust?[i]

Oftentimes patients have bad memories from past experiences in what we call the health care system (is it really a health *care* system?). When we assume an unknowing position, we understand that there are lifetimes of experiences that have created these patients, these human beings. What we do not know are the context and contingencies of our patients' lives. Seeking that understanding will make all the difference in our practice of nursing. We have little knowledge of them. It then behooves us to recognize the need to hear the patients' narratives, if our nursing care reflects a humanistic perspective and reflects an individual understanding of the patients.

As nurses, we who care for others in some of the most intimate of all human experiences need to understand what the meaning of the experience is for the individual. This understanding comes when the person's subjective perception of whatever may be occurring is shared with us. When we allow and open the space for that story and the patient's own interpretation to be told, we listen with the third ear (Kurtz, 1989, p. 7).

We should not assume to know how it feels to be someone other than ourselves, yet in reality we often do just that. We make assumptions, have preconceptions and biases, and even turn to theory that tells us how individuals feel or ought to feel. Think about all our stage theories concerning development or dying (Kubler-Ross, 1973). Without asking, we assign a normative stage to individuals and assess if they are progressing as theoretically prescribed—no questions asked. Worse, if patients are not at the right stage we have often been taught as normative, we then assign the word *deficit* or judge them to be insufficient in the construct of a nursing diagnosis. In our ordinary, day-to-day world, how often do we say, "I know just how you feel" when we should simply ask the person?

Being a nurse and doing nursing at its highest ethical level is to care. Here is an excerpt from an e-mail I sent a few days back, which at the time I did not think would be placed in this chapter. This nurse friend and I often discuss complexities of situations between nurses and patients. I wrote:

Anything to do with more than one variable can be quite confounding, those damn confounding variables that make up life…We could take nursing to a higher level if we were to focus on the complexities of human nature and human understanding. Actually it is the least we can try to do when "caring" for people, is to try to understand them, but that would be a complex task, so we skip over that and make a plan of care sometimes before even meeting them. The missing link I think is the word caring; do nurses really care about the interior lives of patients?[ii] Or is their agenda driven by completing tasks in an often too demanding environment?

My good friend answered:

Take a look around you. The answer is they are not encouraged to the caring part, and yes to the completing tasks part, and you are fortunate if that is what can be accomplished with the staffing shortages. We both know that, unfortunately, nurses are not supported to care in that Jean Watson way except as students; and that, unfortunately, in most places it is all about cost-effectiveness.

I think we all celebrate the many excellent nurses who certainly do care and attempt to understand the patient's experience from the patient's perspective. However, we are also aware of the many obstacles put in nurses' ways to practice caring in the health care system that today is more like a stopwatch relay race to "get things done" and then record these tasks ad infinitum. Nurses are frustrated and complain. I have heard many say, "This is not why I went into nursing," to run relay races, so to speak and to spend hours documenting in writing that could be spent at the bedside.

We are aware that there may not be the time available for nurses to care from the perspective of seeking the unknowing, and that is a pity. We suspect that there is an unspoken and sometimes spoken norm that if the nurse is not doing something, the nurse is wasting time. Listening with the third ear or just listening is not often considered doing something. I have not attached monitors to any individuals, but in my knowing way, I believe if patients felt understood, their stress, anxiety, and fear—all portals to complications—would decrease, and in a statistically significant way (and that is always necessary!).

Feeling Understood

Feeling understood calls for the nurse to become unknowing and to hear the perceptions and feelings of the patient. What then happens is that the patient unburdens himself or herself of carrying all the psychological weight of the experience. He or she no longer feels frustrated with loneliness and is no longer so isolated or being treated as an object. The patient's personhood has been honored by the nurse, and the patient is comforted in the confidence "that someone knows how it feels to be" him or her, or someone is at least making an effort. This to me is what quality nursing practice is about. I think we also want to have a nurse who knows how to do a sterile catheterization and dispense proper medication. However, it should not be an either-or proposition: for quality nursing care and optimal patient well-being, both are essential.

The Intersubjective Space

Why we become unknowing. We become unknowing to bring to light what lies in the intersubjective space of two people, or a group of people, allowing new and different perceptions and representations of reality to be acknowledged. We also become unknowing so that the patient can experience authentic caring. The intersubjective space is created when a nurse enters a room where there is a patient. An intersubjective space is also created when you and a friend meet for lunch. Intersubjective spaces are everywhere there is more than one person. A room with one person has one subjective space, their subjectivity, and their individual perceptions.

When two individuals come together in what only appears to be a shared experience, there are actually two experiences occurring, two perceptions of the experience created, two sets of subjective feelings, and the intersubjective space created where knowing and understanding are possible, if explored!

Figure 9.1 attempts to illustrate this intersubjective space, where in this instance, two individuals are in interaction and the intersubjective space is apparent. The process of the patient's subjective space eclipsing the nurse's space is also illustrated. The intersubjective space in the world of interaction is the center for agreements, conflicts, misunderstandings, isolation, or feeling understood. This is the space for human interaction and human understanding to unfold.

9.1

Unknowing and intersubjectivity

ONE INDIVIDUAL'S SUBJECTIVE SPACE
One subjective space—perceptual field representing one individual
One knower, one knowledge holder

TWO INDIVIDUALS PRESENT; NOT IN INTERACTION
Two subjective spaces representing two individuals
Two knowers, two knowledge holders unknowing the other

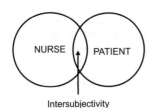

Intersubjectivity

TWO INDIVIDUALS IN INTERACTION
Two subjective spaces interact representing intersubjectivity between two individuals
Perceptual field is created with two knowledge holders
Potential to move from unknowing to knowing the other

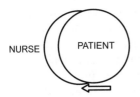

COMING TO KNOW THE PATIENT
One intersubjective space eclipses the other representing the patient's subjective space eclipsing the nurse's subjectivity
Nurse coming to know the subjective world of the patient

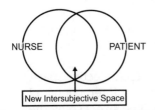

New Intersubjective Space

KNOWING THE PATIENT: CUMULATIVE PROCESS
A new intersubjective space forms representing the knowing of the patient as part of the nurse's subjective space
Nurse incorporates patient's subjectivity into care

Knowledge and subjectivity: Includes formal knowledge, assumptions, contingencies and contexts, biases, history, psychological perspective, and emotional components (including hope, fears, dreams, and desires). Intersubjective space represents all the components that make a whole of an individual's perspective in the present moment.

How we become unknowing. Caring to understand the other's subjective world requires that we suspend our presuppositions, biases, assumptions, theories, experiences, perceptions, and what is in our subjective consciousness to allow for clarity when we attempt to understand the other's subjective world of perception. The nurse, in suspending all of his or her own subjectiveness to the extent possible, is welcoming understanding of what it means to be this other person. She or he is practicing the highest level of care possible. This is not a nurse who is doing tasks; this is a nurse who is seeking to understand the patient, an act of no small consequence.

Once I heard in an analytic institute I attended that there is no greater gift that one person can give to another than understanding. There is nothing greater that a person wants than to be understood. I hear Tom Petty's sorrowful lament, "You don't know how it feels to be me." *A nurse who cares wants to know*. When the nurse understands the patient's representation of the world and subjective perceptions, there is now the possibility for empathy and care when the nurse places aside his or her own knowingness and allows the patient to be the knower. The patient has ownership of the patient's reality and through revealing and in essence, the *patient teaches the nurse what the nurse needs to know*. This new knowledge provides the nurse with the information to alter the one-size-fits-all models of many nursing interventions or protocols so that the nurse can prevent complications and facilitate healing. I would venture that almost all one-size-fits-all protocols need individual altering, which ideally comes from the knowledge the patient holds.

Pursuing the unknown of the patient is the true essence of caring, from my perspective. Reaching out with the quest of understanding the world from the other's perspective is taking nursing to the next level, to the level of individual human understanding with all its messiness and time-consuming requirements. Perhaps the hardest part is to allow yourself to be the unknowing one with your diligent study of theory, interventions, protocols, evidenced-based nursing, and the use of the nursing process all held in abeyance.

Once upon a time. Here is a little story that is true. Once upon a time, when I was a young nursing instructor (those of you from this era will remember this, and I shudder to think that this practice might still be going on), I went to the local hospital late in the afternoon and assigned patients to students for the following day. I did this from the patient Cardex, looking for specific diseases and conditions that the students were studying so they could apply the class theory to practice. This was an important learning method guiding clinical assignments. I was, in essence, objectifying patients. Without the time to check all 10 patients, I went back to the college to post the assignment. The students then picked up their assignments, noted the disease or condition of the patient, and went back to their desks and wrote a plan of care for this patient using their textbooks—those huge, 1,252-page texts that are ubiquitous in schools of nursing. They had yet to meet the patient. One could say they were truly unknowing, but in this true story they became knowing through a textbook and through applying a nursing theory. They had non-contextual knowledge, knowledge that might be considered objective because it had nothing to do with the subjective world of the patient.

What This Has to Do With Unknowing

This common practice had, at the time, everything to do with knowing and nothing to do with unknowing. The student began to fill the subjective space of his or her consciousness with seemingly objective knowledge—what to do, what the patient needs, the interventions—in other words, nursing care, the plan for nursing care, the plan for nursing tasks. The student (or practicing nurse) then could plan the day knowingly and confidently armed with the relevant theory of the patient's disease and condition.

Further complicating the pursuit of openness to an individual, subjective reality, when the nurse finally does interact with the patient, the nurse usually does so through the lens of a *nursing* theory. We can safely assume the patient does not know this nursing theory. However, the nurse will see and hear the patient through the concepts and prescriptions of this nursing theory and in the process of listening to the patient will begin to select data for the theoretical fit. The patient is asked questions as designated from the nursing theory, and the patient in fact has been defined by the nursing theory and processed through the steps of the theory.

This is not to say that we do not need nursing theory. Rather it is to suggest a different way to use nursing theory: to hold it in abeyance and become unknowing when listening to the patient. If the prevalent nursing theory does not fit the patient well, then the nurse is able to modify the theory or use a theory that is more compatible. For example, if the self-care theory does not fit the patient, perhaps because of cultural values that involve the family, we should alter our perspective, not the patient's.

In strict application of nursing theory, we have a complete overlay of the nurses' subjective perspective over the patient's perspective. When the nurse is the knowing one, the nurse understands the patient according to her objective representation of this experience. Nurses are taught to be objective, so this is an acceptable practice. However, objectivity, from my perspective, is largely a myth. Objectivity is a subjective concept and is judged subjectively (another day's discussion).

Unknowing and Phenomenology[iii] (3)

Phenomenology questions our consciousness, as we are in the world—how we experience the world and how we give meaning to experiences. Meanings and interpretations emerge from our situated context and provide for heterogeneous perspectives of life's events.

Aggregates and generalizations of cultures, race, sex, and conditions—all are questioned, as is evidence-based practice. The one-size-fits-all, the one-intervention-fits-all, and the one-protocol-fits-all conditions need critical questioning. Perhaps most of our complications in health care come from the variables within the various conditions that were not considered with the application of the one-protocol-fits-all model. Phenomenology, because it individualizes us as beings and gives us the freedom to interpret the world through our own and others' own contexts and contingencies, is where authentic understanding of another can become known. Many of these individual contingencies alter the prevailing protocols or theories.

Practicing nursing from a phenomenological perspective or doing research from this perspective calls for unknowing. In some references in the literature, the word *bracketing* is used to mean the same process. Over the years, I have found more meaning to this idea of unknowing; that is, of letting another person's subjective space eclipse our own. This interpretation is opposed to the standard meaning of bracketing, where one puts aside one's own beliefs, theories, and biases as with unknowing. However, bracketing does not speak to subjectivities and the interaction of subjective representations, so to me this is different and leans more toward phenomenological philosophy.

Unknowing, therefore, becomes a process with the potential to free us from the distorting aspects of prejudices, biases, our histories, and traditions. It indeed leads to freedom. Unknowing can liberate us from our unsubstantiated presuppositions when they are no longer of value (if they ever were of value). Freedom and liberation for oppressed groups and within the theme of this book, for our patients, becomes possible. Patients are free and liberated from our prescriptive practice because we have removed them from aggregates and generalizations and have begun to understand them as separate individuals with their own theories — and it would be good practice to understand our *patients'* theories.

Unknowing or Not Knowing?

Unknowing is different from not knowing within the meaning of this chapter. Not knowing implies that we do not know something, and that there is nothing to unknow. We do not know theories, we do not know assumptions, propositions, interventions; and we are essentially in some areas without necessary knowledge. Unknowing implies that we do know something; in fact, we may know things very well. We know theories, propositions, and assumptions underpinning knowledge. The practice of unknowing, unlike not knowing, asks of us to hold all this knowing in abeyance and allow another's subjective perspective to eclipse our own for evaluation and intervention to be individualized. With not knowing, there is nothing to hold in abeyance.

Unknowing potentially can raise and expand our consciousness and enable our understanding at the central core, from which all things can be known about another human being and that is from his subjective world. The interpretation of the meaning of this allows for congruency in communication and in nurse-patient interaction. There is a wide-awakeness to experience, in its reverence for differences and the subsequent possibilities, and in its ability to liberate us to care in specific ways for our specific and very individual patients. We awaken to the magical variety of individual interpretations. To this day I am amazed and delighted at my own experiences of surprise, disbelief, never-dreamt-about perceptions, and creative inter- pretations that occur when I suspend my knowing, letting the patient eclipse my knowing and sharing with me their interpre- tations of their experiences. I become wide-awake like a child.

Waking up Through Unknowing

Sit down before fact like a little child, and be prepared to give up every preconceived notion, following humbly wher- ever and to whatever abyss nature leads, or you shall learn nothing. (Huxley, 1982, p. 225)

Writing about wide-awakenesss, I recall delivering a paper entitled, "Drifting Without Consciousness," which depicted how many health care professionals are basically on autopilot—carrying out protocols, meting out various nursing process formulas, and formulating nursing care plans *before* meeting the patient or family, based solely on a medical diagnosis. I have called this modus operandi "fog- based nursing". The fog can be lifted through embracing the "unknowing" component of an individual, family, or any group. To lift the fog, we must uncover the "unknowing" of the patient and circumstances; we must come to know the intersubjective world of the patient. We achieve clarity, the fog lifts, and we understand the inner world of the patient. We then are different knowers; we are attempting to under- stand the other. We *see* the person, we *hear* the person, and we are honoring the person's autonomy and dignity. We open the way to empathy. We make empathy possible because only through understanding the unknown of the patient can the meaning of the word *empathy* be used accurately.

In example after example, I described how this lack of attentiveness to the consciousness of the unknowing part of what we need to know, not pursuing what we do not know, has led to critical complications. We may be knowledge hold- ers, but we must also recognize that our patients and oth- ers are also knowledge holders, and their perceptions are not in a textbook or a footnote somewhere. In the end, *the patients' perceptions will exert more power.* If we want our nursing care and caring to accomplish the patient's goals, we must step aside and let the patient be the knower. In this way we come to know what this individual patient needs; we know how it feels to be that patient, to the extent possible. We know how to deliver the care that is individualized for this person.

> *Where is the wisdom we have lost in knowledge? Where is the knowledge we have lost in information? (Eliot, 1934/1964)*

This Is You Practicing the Art of Unknowing

I know your diagnosis, but I do not know you. I am unknowing about you as an individual and about your subjective reality. I am not on autopilot with a list from a protocol, but because I am unknowing about you, that list may not be appropriate for you. I am a fallible health care professional in need of your knowledge, in need of knowing your perceptions, the meaning you attribute to this experience, the intrinsic and existential you, or the phenomenological you. I am a health care professional with presuppositions, assumptions, knowledge, biases, and my own subjective perspective of reality. Our two subjective worlds are now connected, and thus we are in the realm of intersubjectivity, the threshold for mutual understanding. I come here to care for you, a mystery before me, seeking to understand the dynamics of our intersubjective world. Then I will know through you—but only if I attempt to unknow the assumptions, the protocols, the biases and all the other clutter in my mind so I can see you in all your wholeness and not as a medical condition with nursing problems.

This attitude applies to personal relationships as well. For example, sometimes we think we know best, or we do not hesitate in answering a question without asking the other person what his or her thoughts are on the matter. Only when we know the thoughts, perceptions, and beliefs of the other can we modify, make adjustments, and give that person the respect that we would want to be known for and that we would like to receive as well.

Returning, then, to the belief that phenomenology questions the consciousness of us all, it also is calling on us to be wide-awake. We cannot drift without consciousness when we are caring for others. Our consciousness must be heightened. One way of heightening it is through the process of "unknowing".

Recall that knowing something can lead to a form of confidence and premature closure. When we already know, there is nothing more to know; thus we have a closed mind, one drifting with a low level of consciousness, hardly wide-awake.

An Excellent Illustrative Film for Unknowing

Along with songs, I also use films in my workshops. I do this because of the way a good film can illustrate an idea or process in a poignant, memorable way. Films expand our consciousness. A wonderful film that illustrates unknowing from the perspectives of five different individual subjectivities and perspectives is *Whose Life Is It Anyway?* What makes the film so compelling is that the plot and subplots all follow what goes wrong when people do not understand one another. This, for our purposes, is further enlightening because it involves a patient, a nursing student, a dogmatic and determined doctor, a nurse drifting without consciousness, and the patient's girlfriend. Each of the five main characters is experiencing the same experience in a different way, based on individual contingencies, context, belief systems, and knowledge. The patient, until the very end, is torturously in a state of despair, not understood by anyone. He is treated as though he has absolutely no autonomy or dignity. Interventions are *done* to him. His *pleas for understanding are ignored — and worse, they become a negative diagnosis* of his mental status. The nursing student in the film seems perplexed: she is wondering about the moral dilemma that she sees being enacted. (Some of you may recall the same reaction of the nurse in the book and play *Wit* (Edison, 1999), another excellent example of what happens when we do not know the subjective world of the patient.)

In the intersubjective space in which the characters engage in dialogue, there are excellent examples of how if the health care providers had practiced unknowing, they would have contributed to an understanding of this patient. Instead, the health care providers are complete and confident knowers, illustrating the idea of premature closure. The patient is completely misunderstood and "taken hostage" by the knowledge holders. This film's presentation of the devastating effects of not being understood will leave an indelible impression on you. I will not tell you the end; but watch and listen to a person being heard in a phenomenological manner as the film comes to its conclusion.

From Literature, Two Completely Different Subjectivities

You may already be a parent; if not, imagine yourself as a parent for a moment. How do you think you will perceive your children as they evolve into adults? You have your own subjective ideas of this experience. When we practice unknowing, we know these ideas belong only to us and may not belong to another parent. Here from two wonderful books are two contrasting perceptions, perspectives, and subjective representations of the same experience, watching one's adult children.

Jane Smiley wrote in *Ordinary Love and Good Will* (1989),

> *As I sit on this hard bench I suddenly yearn for one last long look and not only of the phenomenon of little Joe and little Michael, but of the others too; Ellen, four, and Annie, seven months, sharing a peach…As I watch them now as adults the fact that I will never see their toddler selves again is tormenting. (p. 120)*

Ann Beattie feels differently in *Picturing Will* (1989):

> *When you are thirty, the child is two. At forty, you realize that the child in the house, the child you live with, is still, when you close your eyes, or the moment he has walked from the room, two years old. When you are sixty and the child is gone, the child will also be two, but then you will be more certain. Wet sheets, wet kisses. A flood of tears. As you remember him the child is always two. (p. 53)*

Imagine if Beattie spoke to Smiley and said, "I know just how you feel," because they both feel sad. She would be very far off course. To understand Smiley, Beattie needs to explore the subjective space and world of Smiley, as we do with our patients and with those others that we care about.

Unknowing as a Means for Understanding

As a philosophy, phenomenology is our hope for understanding in this world and unknowing is a critical component of phenomenology. If we were to understand the meaning of events and experiences to people, we would approach them in a way that would reflect understanding of them specifically, not of theory reflecting aggregates of individuals. Our theories would acknowledge the many ways of being and acknowledge that there is not a *best* way to be in the world.

In our postmodern world, we have come to understand diversity as we never did before. That gives us great reason to hope for increased human understanding. Today we find more and more in our writings the recognition of individuals representing a wide variety of what it is like being in this world through our recognition of multiple realities and polyvocality. Our multicultural world and with it many opposing paradigms (none of which represent truth, but rather, different interpretations of reality and the world) have appeared more clearly to be representative of experience.

The health care provider would not be the author or the authority for patient care. Until the subjective meaning of an experience for a patient is known, the intervention is not contextual; and because it is not contextual, it could be the wrong intervention. Noncompliance, I believe, results from not understanding the patient and the meaning of a behavior to the patient. Because nurses are often concerned in a caring way about behavior that may be detrimental to a patient, family, or community, they need to understand meaning. At the meaning level, we can offer to patients our understanding, and perhaps this generalization is well grounded; we all wish to be understood. Unknowing implies questioning generalizations, understanding that a generalization is merely a mathematical mean.

There is a phrase that comes to mind; "the tyranny of the mean", the mathematical average. The tyranny implying the mean becomes a representative norm, where people then are judged, evaluated, and diagnosed. The sad part of this is that there may actually be no one at the mean at all; it is indeed vacuous. Phenomenology resists this homogenizing response to experiences, categorizing individuals and placing them in stages. Unfortunately, individuals are viewed as atypical or, worse, abnormal if they deviate from the "mean" of a statistical equation or the goals of a theory. They are labeled noncompliant if they do not follow our knowledge instructions.

In contrast, nurses following the path of unknowing inherent in phenomenology are interested in the particular of experience. While recognizing that there are similarities, they search for the particular, the difference, the anomaly. They see the horizon of the experience, the context in which the experience occurs, and the contingencies affecting the individual as being integrated and critical to successful outcomes. Nurses are privileged people. They are allowed into the mysteries of others being in the world.

Returning to the e-mail exchange discussed earlier, I wonder how many places there are where nurses *can* practice unknowing, and *can* have the encouragement of others to understand the experience of those they care for. How many places reward this practice, which experientially prevents complications and misunderstandings or even despair? Does it appear that nurses do not care, or is the problem that nurses are not encouraged to care? In our society and media today everyone says they care, to the point that it has become a meaningless term. If nurses, however, were encouraged to demonstrate caring through the practice of the art of unknowing, then we would achieve individual human understanding, to me the epitome of caring.

What Is Needed For Unknowing

This sounds so simple, and it actually is. The nurse needs at least an hour of uninterrupted time with each new patient, listening without the static of knowledge and theories. Each day the nurse also needs uninterrupted time to continue building upon the patient's narrative. The nurse needs to demonstrate a sincere desire to understand the patient in ways other than completing tasks. This means he or she needs a very caring and generous spirit. The nurse needs devotion to the cause of caring for human dignity and autonomy, for patient freedom and liberation. What might be the most challenging is that the nurse needs to know how to practice unknowing and what it means. This means beginning with self.

In pragmatic terms, when a patient is encountered in a health care setting—for example, a hospital—the nurse usually performs a health history: *his story*. Unfortunately the patient's story cannot be revealed as a narrative of meaning of the experience because it is largely an objective checklist of questions to which the answer is either "yes" or "no," and if the answer is yes, a date is asked.

Here is what Edmund Burke (1860) would say of this practice: "We do, unfortunately, live in an age of 'economists and calculators' who are eager to reduce all things to the *dust of numeracy.*" These people are neglecting what Burke called "the decent drapery of life".

Self-consciously modern people have an urge to reduce assessments of their lives to things that can be presented in tables, charts, and graphs. This *sharpens their minds by narrowing them.* This leaves us to conclude that unknowing as a process towards understanding, is diametrically opposed, since it sharpens our minds by opening them. We open our minds to the "wisdom lost in knowledge" and "the knowledge we have lost in information."

Concluding Thoughts

Let us not drift without consciousness of what is before us and also hidden from us. Let us be wide-awake to the possibilities of what can come from going from unknowing to understanding a human being's subjective experience. Let us realize how the subjective perceptions of experience create a reality for the patient; it is incumbent upon us to know that reality. It is from this reality known through understanding the patient's subjective world of where and how that we can effectively individualize care. The subjective space and then the ensuing intersubjective interaction is where humanistic nursing care can be actualized. To accomplish this, we must become unknowing, we must use our unknowing to the patient's advantage, and we must engage the patient so that we come to know the patient's reality. The subjective space and then the ensuing intersubjective interaction is where humanistic nursing care can be actualized. All else is not contextual. All else is robotic. All else is devoid of our humanity.

We need to bring the art of unknowing to our nursing practice. In doing so, we can answer Tom Petty and those whom we are privileged to care for: "In our acknowledgement of unknowing your subjective world and then seeking to understand it, we come close to understanding how it feels to be you." Then we will know how in the most authentic way to care for the patient: care based on the patient's subjective world, a method that provides the opening for compassion, dignity, autonomy, and empathy. Would we want less?

References

Atwood, D., & Stolorow, R. (1984). *Structures of subjectivity*. Hillsdale, NJ: Erlbaum.

Beattie, A. (1989). *Picturing Will*. New York: Random House.

Burke, E. (1860). *The works of Edmund Burke with a memoir*. New York: Harper Brothers.

Carper, B. (1978). Fundamental patterns of knowing in nursing. *Advances in Nursing Science, 1*(1), 13–23.

Edison, M. (1999). *Wit*. New York: Dramatists Play Service.

Eliot, T. S. (1964). The choruses. In *T.S. Eliot: Selected poems* (pp. of chapter). New York: Harcourt Brace Jovanovich. (Original work published in 1934.)

Heidegger, M. (1962). *Being and time*. San Francisco: Harper & Row. (Original work published in 1927).

Huxley J. H. In Dossey, L., (1982) *Time, space and medicine* Colorado: Shambhala.

Kubler-Ross, E. (1973). *On death and dying*. New York: Routledge

Kurtz, S. (1989). *The art of unknowing*. New Jersey: Aronson.

Manen, M. (1990). *Researching the lived experience*. Albany, New York: State University of New York Press.

Munhall, P. (1993). Unknowing: Toward another pattern of knowing. *Nursing Outlook, 41*, 125–128.

Munhall, P. (1994). *Revisioning phenomenology: Nursing and health science research*. Sudbury, MA: Jones and Bartlett.

Munhall, P. (2000). Unknowing. In W. Kelly & V. Fitzsimmons (Eds.), *Understanding cultural diversity*. Sudbury, MA: Jones and Bartlett.

Munhall, P. (2007a). *Nursing research: A qualitative perspective* (4th ed.). Sudbury, MA: Jones and Bartlett.

Munhall, P. (2007b). A phenomenological method. In P. Munhall (Ed.), *Nursing research: A qualitative perspective* (4th ed) (pp. of chapter). Sudbury, MA: Jones and Bartlett.

Petty, T. (1994). Tom Petty Wildflowers. CD. Warner Brothers.

Smiley, J. (1989). *Ordinary love and good will*. New York: Random House.

Watson, J. (1999). *Postmodern nursing and beyond: Redefining nursing for the 21st century*. Churchill Livingstone Title, Elsevier Health Science.

[i] In Atwood and Stolorow's excellent book, *Structures of Subjectivity*, transference and countertransference are discussed in greater detail. Also in this book, and in the unknowing article I mentioned previously, and a chapter entitled "Unknowing" that I wrote for Fitzsimmons and Kelley's *Understanding Cultural Diversity*, the concepts of intersubjective disjunction and intersubjective conjunction are described. I would encourage these readings if you are inspired to learn more about the intersubjective space, subjectivity, and unknowing.

[ii] Curricula and dialogue in nursing circles have centered on caring, thanks to so many nurse scholars and theorists, in particular Jean Watson and Madeline Leininger.

[iii] My most recent writing on this is influenced by many philosophers, primarily Heidegger, Morgan, and van Manen, and can be found summarized in the chapter on the phenomenological method in the fourth edition of the qualitative research book (Munhall, 2007a) and in Munhall (2007b). listed in the references. I urge those who are interested in furthering their knowledge of phenomenology to read the works of these three philosophers.

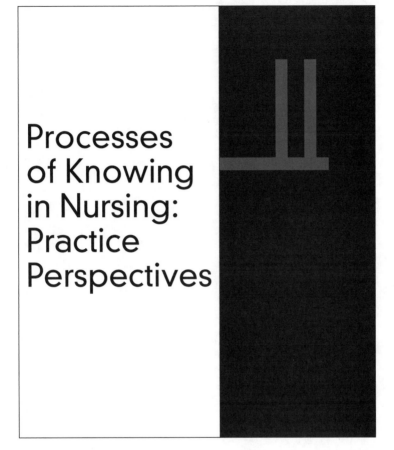

Processes of Knowing in Nursing: Practice Perspectives

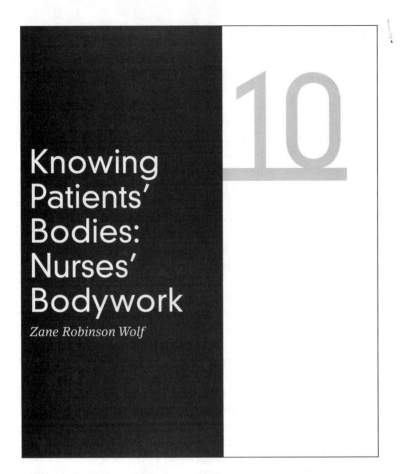

Knowing Patients' Bodies: Nurses' Bodywork

Zane Robinson Wolf

Chapter Overview

This chapter explores how nurses perform bodywork for patients. It reviews experiential, phenomenological, and empirical sources of this special, intimate, personal type of nursing care. Basic nursing care is examined in relation to direct nursing care, patient privacy, nurse and patient embarrassment, and hidden work. The interpersonal processes in which nurses and patients participate are emphasized in the context of patients' individuality and vulnerability. Also described is how nurses manage profane materials. Nurses interpret bodily cues and make clinical judgments prior to action as they attempt to learn patients' patterns and unique characteristics.

Bodywork

Nurses carry out many actions that respond to human needs as people experience developmental, situational, or health–illness transitions. They care for people who are strangers initially and establish relationships with patients. Nurses are "committed to individuals requiring care, concern, and comfort during and after the potential experiences of a transitional event" (Chinn, 1983, p. 25). The bodywork nurses provide is framed by caring theory (Watson, 1990), helping nurses who are intimately involved with patients to preserve their human dignity and humanity.

Nursing's domain of work focuses on concern for patients' welfare. In this context, bodywork can be defined as the efforts expended by nurses on behalf of patients' bodies that ideally benefit their health. Bodywork takes place during everyday nursing practice (Maeve, 1994). This embodied aspect of nursing work fits into a broader category of nursing clinical therapeutics, both interpersonal and physical, because it includes actions and activities deliberately designed to care for patients (Barnard, 1980). Bodywork implies that nurses use themselves—body, mind, and spirit—to improve patients' welfare, along with scientific (objective) and personally developed (subjective) clinical knowledge. Nurses use clinical knowledge when providing bodywork. How nurses come to know patients' bodies and know how to perform bodywork are more difficult to articulate. Clinical knowledge is "individual and personal" (Schultz & Meleis, 1988, p. 219).

Carper's (1978) model, illustrating patterns on ways of knowing in nursing—including empirics (science of nursing), aesthetics (art of nursing), personal knowing, and ethics (moral knowledge in nursing)—has provided a framework for many nurses to explain part of the scope of the discipline of nursing (Bailey, 2004). It is easy at first glance to examine bodywork and how nurses know patients' bodies. In the context of the model, nurses use personal knowledge to understand their own and their patients' bodies and to comprehend what occurs during the transactions of interpersonal encounters.

Although the four ways of knowing in Carper's model are interdependent, they may not help to understand fully how nurses develop the skills of recognizing and interpreting multiple cues and intuitions as they learn how to know patients' bodies. Other perspectives have to be acknowledged (Silva, Sorrell, & Sorrell, 1995). For example, there is a difference between *knowing that* and *knowing how* nurses know patients' bodies. *Knowing that* implies empirical knowledge, and *knowing how* includes knowledge gained through clinical experiences (Maeve, 1994), through a synthesis of nursing science and art (Silva et al., 1995). How nurses know patients' bodies is not the same as what nurses know about their bodies (Speed & Luker, 2004).

Learning Bodywork

Nursing students learn first how to provide bodywork in the laboratories of schools of nursing. They readily remember how they gave physical care to their first patients (Wolf, 1997). Students' initial self-absorption with their own performance and anxiety about patients' responses to care are replaced with increasing confidence. However, in the years that follow nursing school, many seasoned nurses may not recall how they began to understand patients' bodies.

Textbooks on fundamentals of nursing reveal indexes in which the term *body* addresses alignment, balance, build, fluids, heat, image, language, lice, mass index, odors, pressure areas, rocking, repositioning, surface area, system defenses, temperature, and weight (Berman, Snyder, Kozier, & Erb, 2008; Potter & Perry, 2009). Bodywork appears chiefly in the scientific basis and basic human needs chapters. Moreover, faculty emphasize bodywork during class and expect nursing students to study content and integrate clinical experiences into their developing knowledge base as they first bathe patients and learn to attend to signs, symptoms, and other manifestations of health and illness experiences. Basic nursing care, such as giving baths, is important bodywork because it comforts patients. Personal care is structured by patients' responses to it. Students reflect on the dignity and privacy of patients at the same time they attempt to master hygienic care. They are aghast at experienced nurses' occasional neglect and exposure of patients' bodies.

Knowing how to give body care is not limited to the hygienic care of the bath and other basic care interventions such as oral hygiene; the process is complex, involving direct recognition of patients' situations and needs through observations of cues.

Cues are integrated with textbook content and other sources as well as reports of diagnostic studies. Students also learn to detect patients' discomfort with the exposure of private body parts. They confront their own reactions to handling profane bodily products, such as feces, vomitus, urine, and sputum, because it is expected of nurses. They use medical aseptic techniques and demarcate what society and science designate as clean and dirty products and objects.

Nurses gradually learn the indicators of changes in structure and function presented by patients' bodies. As students, they begin to understand normal findings when they take assessment courses. Faculty teach them about abnormal findings (physical and physiological variables, signs, and symptoms) during classroom discussions and then help neophyte nurses contrast normal with abnormal in clinical settings. Students next study diagnostic test results and often are overwhelmed by the details, including ranges interpreted as normal. As nurses gain experience, they match test results with how patients present.

Nurses learn how to interpret signs and symptoms caused by the effects of physical illness. They combine the understanding they have gained about signs and symptoms from the literature with those that patients complain of or acknowledge when questioned and assessed. Some symptoms are expected by health care providers, since they correlate with knowledge of disease, whereas some are actually experienced by patients and differ from the typical, such as those suggesting acute myocardial infarction (Horne, James, Petrie, Weinman, & Vincent, 2000). Signs and symptoms signify the condition of patients' bodies.

A Type of Bodywork: Basic Nursing Care

Lawler (1991), a sociologist, studied the bodywork (basic nursing care or body care) of nurses and came to understand that this work was essentially about "people's experiences of embodied existence, particularly at those times when the body fails to function normally" (p. vi). Thus, nurses are witnesses of patients' bodily failures. They "invade" patients' bodies, for example, when assessing body systems, starting IVs, and irrigating wounds. They go beyond the boundaries of public space and intrude private space, touch skin, and discover personal information. They are not always able to ask permission to invade, based on circumstances. As nurses do for others unable to perform self-care, they implicitly and explicitly recognize the vulnerability of the people they care for.

Basic nursing care, such as bathing and helping patients to toilet, is interpreted as uncomplicated and commonplace. However, coordinating hygienic care with emotional and spiritual support, wound care, medication administration, intravenous therapy, and other care activities is complex, frequently overlooked, and devalued (Wolf, 1996). For many aspects of care, nurses function in the zone of patients' personal space; nursing care is often intimate and focused on keeping patients clean. By providing basic, hygienic care to those (including infected patients) viewed as unclean by society, and by managing the personal-care requirements of other patients, nurses accomplish sacred and profane work simultaneously.

Nurses' work is intimate and framed by social boundaries created by patients' dependence and level of illness. As students, nurses learn to overcome cultural barriers and control their embarrassment, touch naked male and female patients' bodies, carry out routine procedures, question patients about bodily functions, and at the same time assure patients of their privacy (Lawler, 1991). They manage embarrassment through experience and begin increasingly to understand patients' need for privacy and their vulnerability, dependence, and social discomfort in situations that involve exposing part or the whole of the body. For example, nurses are often the first health care providers to cover patients' genitalia during code situations in which nudity is largely ignored by others. They send family members and friends out of patients' rooms when exposure is required for care. Considering the need to protect patients' privacy and to understand what has happened to patients' bodies, nurses also recognize the unfamiliarity of hospitals for patients and the anxiety provoked by admission. They also protect the privacy of the bodies of dead patients from curious health care workers and others during postmortem care. Exposure or nakedness is reduced, controlled, and protected.

Nurses manage to convey to patients that they are not embarrassed when performing bodywork, for example, when checking incisions and changing dressings following breast and testicular surgery or asking about bowel function. At the same time, they recognize patients' embarrassment by interpreting cues such as when patients joke or cover themselves up quickly following exposure. Nurses redefine embarrassment for themselves and patients so that clinical situations are manageable. "Bathing male and female genitals has been a source of discomfiture for some female and male nurses for decades. Nurses bathe these parts in privacy... [they] do not shun these necessary contacts" (Wolf, 1986a, p. 31). Nurses may always be uncomfortable about bathing patients' genitalia or exposing patients' nakedness during personal care, procedures, or surgery. They themselves would be mortified if disrobed in others' presence.

Lawler (1991) represented the social ecology of the nursing situation, pointing out the following rules: "(1) the compliance and control rule, (2) the dependency rule, (3) the modesty rule, and (4) the protection rule" (p. 147). The rules fit some of nursing practice. "Good" patients give up control and are cooperative. They try to help nurses get the work done. Patients are, on occasion, completely dependent on nurses for bodily care. When physically able to perform self-care, nurses expect patients to do for themselves, every so often in dramatic conflict with patients' cultural expectations. Nurses anticipate that patients will be somewhat embarrassed as nurses control uncomfortable situations. At the same time, they protect patients' privacy and expect them to cooperate with the nursing agenda (Lawler). However, excessive modesty may hinder nursing care. A female patient who is so embarrassed that she refuses to allow a nurse to insert an indwelling urinary catheter may suffer from very uncomfortable sensations and problems associated with bladder distention.

Nurses touch male and female patients' genitalia as part of their work. Once again, nurses handle this contact in a matter-of-fact manner (Lawler, 1991). They expect patients not to define body care of sexuality-linked areas as sexual. Although tolerant of patients' sexual arousal during nursing care, as in the case of erections, they do not want physical care to be perceived as primarily sexual. Overt sexual behavior, body exposure, or harassment are not tolerated and may violate the modesty rule or could be more serious. Nurses interpret patients' unnecessary exposure of their bodies as sexual, even as a form of sexual harassment. Patients are judged harshly who exceed the boundaries of proper behavior by displaying seductive behavior, intentionally exposing themselves, joking about nurses being seductive, or making sexual overtures. Nurses manage these scenarios by making their intolerance known, trivializing the behavior, or avoiding patients. Their contact with patients' nakedness places them a position that may be misinterpreted by some patients and the public (Fagin & Diers, 1983).

Certain parts of patients' bodies are considered dirtier than others. A patient's face is cleaner than his or her hands and feet; hands and feet are cleaner than the genitals and perianal areas (Wolf, 1986b). The hierarchical organization of body parts ranging from cleanest to dirtiest is signified by the manner in which nurses are taught to bathe patients and continue that sequence over the course of their careers.

Another aspect of nurses' bodywork is the dirty or profane work that they perform (Wolf, 1986a, 1986b). The way nurses view secretions, excreta, infected products such as wound drainage, and blood can be pictured in a hierarchy of lesser to greater repugnance as "the hierarchy of yuck." Sputum is more repugnant than feces; feces are more repellent than urine. One status issue for nursing is that cleaning up body wastes is a nursing task, "and the wider cultural ambivalences around these substances undermines, or at least destabilizes, the status of the work" (Twigg, 2002, p. 427). Nonetheless, hand washing, bathing patients, wearing gloves, using other barriers, carrying out isolation techniques and infection-control bundles, and performing other standard clinical practices prevent cross contamination and control potentially dangerous products and situations. Nurses are expected to perform this work, handle profane materials, control contagion, and prove that they can handle it.

Nurses deal with bodily products fatalistically, accepting what is often viewed as repugnant aspects of nurses' work. For example, nurses help patients deal with invasive, malodorous wounds (Wilkes, Boxer, & White, 2003). They also minimize situations or bring them into control verbally or behaviorally. That is, they treat embarrassing situations as business as usual. This strategy has been used to protect patients from negative perceptions and feelings.

As nurses carry out bodywork, they learn more about each patient's bodily functions. Nursing's bodywork involves assessing private bodily functions, such as bowel and bladder function. Symptoms of disease are revealed in changes in skin; characteristics of urine, sputum, and stool; and breath odor. Nurses learn what is normal or typical and compare this with changes that signal deterioration.

Nurses maintain patients' privacy by draping body parts, drawing curtains, and closing doors. They also contain wound drainage and incontinence as they try to keep bodies and bodily products hidden from outsiders (Wolf, 1989). For privacy work to be socially permissible for the occupation of nursing, it may be contextualized by nurses' uniform (signaling identity and image) and professional manner (being clinical, matter-of-fact, and in control and giving the appearance that you know what you are doing) (Lawler, 1991). Nurses are "overtly concerned with protecting the patient's vulnerability and privacy" (Ibid, p. 153). Even though for some time traditional uniforms have been replaced by a variety of scrubs and lab coats, the clothing worn and the equipment (such as stethoscopes) used by nurses still signify the difference between nurses and patients.

Examining the body, the illness experience, and nursing, Lawler (1991) emphasized the importance of the relationship between nurses and patients during hospitalization. The social climate of the relationship allows nurses to behave professionally and accomplish bodywork. Nurses' physical accessibility, readiness to listen, and nonverbal communication are carried out in the presence of patients (McCabe, 2004). Attending behavior encompasses open/honest communication, genuineness, and empathy. Nurses see patients as persons and consider their personalities and circumstances.

Nurses practice somologically: they observe and act on signs and symptoms (focus on pathology); they attend to patients' feelings and treat symptoms and integrate pathological problems within patients' lived experiences. *Somology* is defined as nurses' knowledge and learning about the body (Lawler, 1991). Nurses who practice somologically are concerned with the body as object and its associated social symbolism, as well as the lived body in patients' illness experience (Ibid).

Nurses care for hospitalized patients who will recover or die. They take over bodywork from patients whom they expect to recover and gradually hand it back as patients get better (Lawler, 1991). This illustrates their control. Nurses gauge their expectations by whether they think that patients' recovery is typical or slow. They exhort patients to perform self-care and seek independence as they recover from stroke or learn to walk following lower-leg amputation. Dying patients, on the other hand, negotiate how much they can do for themselves, and nurses try to encourage them to do so. The care of dying patients is gradually taken over by nurses as they interpret indicators of physical decline.

Learning Bodywork: Learning About Patients

Nurses and patients are connected to each other as human beings. Their affinity allows them to create a special space in which patients' experiences in health care settings become familiar and manageable: "Within the context of caring, the nurses were ordinary people perceived as being extraordinarily effective by the very ways in which their humanness shone through their knowledge and skills to make their whole being with patients something more than just professional helping" (Taylor, 1992, p. 34). Nurses learn bodywork through the human connections and the basic physical care they provide.

Like that of other health care providers, nurses' work with patients involves bodywork on a consistent basis, interpersonal exchanges that are sometimes emotional, and outcomes that are contextualized by patients' dependency on nurses for care (Lupton, 1997). Bodywork exemplifies nurses' access to "private knowledge about care of the body" (Tanner, Benner, Chesla, & Gordon, 1993, p. 279) in clinical situations where patients need to preserve their dignity when they are very vulnerable. Direct, physical contact gives nurses access to the bodies, emotions, and social milieus of patients and families (Wolf, 1999). This access is owned by nurses and is extraordinary, intimate, and personal. It is extraordinary because few possess this proximity to patients' lives. It is intimate because it entails activities of a very private nature with patients. It is personal in that it is developed by nurses and often involves undisclosed information about patients. The fact that nurses and others may take the work for granted does not negate its complexity.

Just as nurses respond to patients' vulnerability, they should also consider their own vulnerability to the suffering patients endure (Johnson & Scholler-Jaquish, 2007). Nurses and patients are mutually vulnerable. Remaining vulnerable as a nurse can be achieved through reflective practice (Johns, 2004; Maeve, 1994). Developing self-awareness helps nurses to consciously act in a therapeutic way (Burnard, 1988; Cooper, 2001). By listening to patients and paying attention to what they are thinking, feeling, or doing, nurses pay attention to their own cognitive and emotional states as they reflect. Again, patients' vulnerability takes precedence over nurses'. Nurses "must also be prepared to experience the range of subjective experiences any patient might be having" (Maeve, p. 13), including pain and suffering.

Nurses care for patients using their own bodies in direct contact with patients' bodies (Shakespeare, 2003). Shakespeare maintained that nursing bodywork is taken for granted and inferred but seldom reported, and that nurses' bodies are the tools of the profession. Nurses' bodywork is physically challenging, as evidenced by reports of back pain and injury (Shakespeare, 2003). Nurses use their hands to accomplish instrumental or practical, expressive or affective, procedural, non-procedural, caring/social, spontaneous, and other types of touch. They see, listen, speak, and smell when communicating with patients. They lift, turn, and position patients. Moreover, Shakespeare contended that male and female nurses use their bodies differently. Perhaps embodiment or having a body involves nurses' and patients' bodies, minds, and spirits as they relate to one another. Nurses

> Tell about how they come to notice and understand the meanings of the small gestures and facial movements of people who are unable to speak. They are attuned to the patients and notice small changes in the normal pattern of sounds, for instance, when someone's breathing pattern is changing. They are familiar with the normal smells of wounds and notice almost imperceptible changes. (MacLeod, 1993, p. 187)

Nurses use their bodies by constructing the hospital unit as a domestic space, and consequently they shape the way in which nursing care is delivered (Savage, 1997). Nurses' presence in patients' personal space is considered by them to be incontestable. They "own" the territory, often speaking of "my" patients. They sit physically close to patients; the way they position their bodies brings them to the same physical level as patients. Nurses often teach this strategy to new nurses by stating, "This is how I get on their level," suggesting physical body positioning. Topics of a private nature are discussed in close and shared physical, emotional, and spiritual space.

Nurses learn that patients differ as unique individuals during the time spent with them in clinical and community settings. Although limited by the snapshot opportunities afforded by short patient stays, as in the case of most hospitalizations, nurses quickly gauge patients' individuality and needs. Nurses go out of their way (Gramling, 2004) or determine the "little things that count" (MacLeod, 1994). They are available and vigilant, know patients personally, understand patients' suffering, and pay detailed attention to basic functions in ways interpreted as artistic (Gramling, 2004). They honor patients' bodies, expressing respect during bodywork episodes (Ibid). They time and pace their intentional actions and match them to specific patients and contexts (MacLeod, 1994). Everyday nursing practice is "purposeful, complex, multifaceted and patient centered" (Ibid, p. 365).

During personal-care situations, even in critical-care settings, nurses re-create the "primacy of the intersubjective frame" (Gramling, 2004, p. 389). Each person's contribution to the care provided is paramount, but the welfare of patients supersedes nurses' needs. Patients also value knowing the nurses who are caring for them.

Nurses may not always recognize that patients try to figure nurses out and learn about their individual characteristics. For example, elders gained insights about caregivers during care episodes (Russell, 1994). They acted in ways to increase their chances of obtaining desired care. Elders used past interactions to predict future care encounters. The power relationship existed between elders and caregivers, illustrating elders' vulnerability in care situations, along with the power-laded interactions among care recipients and caregivers (Russell, 1996). Seniors wanted to be active participants in their care and used problem-solving skills when seeking care. They did not differentiate among lay and professional caregivers. Formal caregivers, such as nurses, should listen to elders' preferences and provide the amount of information they think they need.

Patients' preferences about the bodywork nurses provide must be framed by ethical principles. Regard for the autonomy of patients and the need to comfort them predominate nursing care (Doutrich, Wros, & Izumi, 2001). Nurses comfort patients by meeting physical, psycho-spiritual, environmental, and sociocultural comfort needs (Kolcaba, 1992, 1995; Kolcaba & DiMarco, 2005). They try to view patients' experiences holistically, even if physical needs and associated bodywork sometimes prevail. As nurses perform bodywork, they hope to prevent unnecessary and uncomfortable procedures and treatments if possible. Nonetheless, in the process of caregiving, they may cause patients to experience pain.

Nurses are obligated to pay careful attention so that they "see behind the words" (Doutrich et al., 2001, p. 453) when attempting to learn patient preferences. Careful listening, understanding, and eliciting more information continues the ongoing process so that nurses grasp the wants, needs, preferences, responses, and situations of patients. As a result, they learn patients' distinguishing characteristics just as they respect their autonomy to make decisions, as in the case of adolescents and adults. However, infants, children, and other patients, such as those with Alzheimer's or in coma, continue to challenge the notion of "what is best" for patients.

Nurses must avoid treating patients and patients' bodies as objects. They should regard them as subjects, free to "transcend all categorizations and expectations" (Gadow, 1989, p. 539). As advocates for silent patients, nurses should avoid viewing their own bodies as objects. They should instead revive their own human vulnerability by experiencing patients' pain and recognizing that some patients want to die. Sometimes they are unable to avoid causing and feeling patients' pain. For example, patients who are burned are in pain when receiving basic care, during dressing changes, after skin grafting, and when trying to avoid stiffness and contracture. Their suffering is shared by nurses as painful procedures increase misery. Advocacy for silent patients requires "nurses to enter patients' worlds through embodiment... [and] ... infinitely personal devotion to the most mundane intimacies of physical care" (Ibid, p. 540). Nurses will then know where boundaries lie between harm and benefit for patients (Gadow, 1989). As nurses enter patients' worlds, they connect not only to their bodies and minds, but also to their spirits.

Knowing and Clinically Engaging Patients to Understand Their Bodies

"Knowing is the weaving of threads of conceptions, perceptions, remembrances, and reflections into a fabric of meaning" (Smith, 1992, p. 2). Knowing patients involves nurses' knowing enough about patients to identify their needs and to know what can be done to improve the situation (Gaut, 1983; Jenny & Logan, 1992). They develop skill in understanding patients' subjective perceptions and objective clinical status. Spending time with patients helps nurses to understand their concerns about fears and anxieties, their personal preferences, their styles of coping, their stressors, and how to gain their trust (Jenny & Logan, 1992; Macdonald, 2008). Knowing patients and their bodies requires nurses to know themselves.

Nurses have cultivated specific ways to care for patients during clinical encounters (Ellefsen & Kim, 2005). They most likely learn these subtle ways through imitating the techniques of other health care professionals and by their own ever-expanding repertoire of experiences with patients. Patients are their best teachers (MacLeod, 1994) as nurses learn the art of nursing. Expert nurses explain their art to neophyte nurses by sharing, "This is how I do it."

Nurses' involvement involves a process of knowing patients and a dialectic synthesis with three phases, through which they integrate subjective and objective data (Ellefsen & Kim, 2005). They process information subjectively from direct observations of patients and from patients' representations of their situations. The first encounter may occur at any point on the health care continuum when nurses care for patients (Ibid). Textbook learning combines with clinical experiences in this process of synthesis. Nurses obtain data about patients' bodies directly during encounters with patients and through medical data from records, tests, and examinations. Furthermore, Macdonald (2008) argued that technology can help nurses know patients through information provided by electronic health records, personal digital assistants, blood glucose monitors and pumps, medication-dispensing systems, and various monitors.

Nurses continue to expand and revise their knowledge about patients as they give nursing care. Shift reports, hand-offs, and information provided by other colleagues add to how they know patients. Nurses appreciate the value of data gained from direct patient care as they meet and engage in patients' lives. As patients experience medical processes and treatments, nurses revise their knowledge of the clinical and patient-centered picture. For example, signs and symptoms, clinical test results, and specific patient requests add to their sources of information about patients' bodies and to the complexity of nurses' knowledge about patients. They also possess a private knowledge base about patients that is very much "in the moment." Each nurse is both a presence and a witness.

Knowing patients has been described as a complex, interpersonal process requiring a number of nursing actions. The process of perceiving/envisioning patients helps nurses actively transform observations of patients' behavior into a direct "perception of what was significant in it" (Jenny & Logan, 1992, p. 256). Their communication with patients is complex, relies on perception, and at times is not easily seen. Nurses interact with patients and pay attention to feedback as they ask questions, listen to answers, and perform nursing care. Nurses present themselves to patients as they attempt to gain patients' trust. They are honest, truthful, knowledgeable, dependable, available, and visible, and they keep their promises as they follow the plan of care. They recognize fear, anxiety, depression, hopelessness, and other problems. They listen to patients and interpret body-language cues; they notice discrepancies or inconsistencies in patients' countenances or patterns (MacLeod, 1993, p. 192). Such changes help nurses focus on patients' emerging clinical picture. The social processes nurses learn are intricate, coordinated, and interactive and can be described as patterns (Strauss, Fagerhaugh, Suczek, & Wiener, 1984).

The bodywork of nurses involves judgments about patients' tolerance for work and need for rest (Jenny & Logan, 1992). Nurses monitor patients' emotional states and determine when to push them to work harder and when it is necessary to help them manage fatigue. Nurses achieve this by attending to symptoms, evidence of illness shown in patients' bodies. If they care for patients over time, they are able to recognize patients' habitual response patterns, such as physical and emotional behaviors, and make "fine qualitative distinctions between acceptable and problematic patient attributes and responses" (Ibid, p. 258). Paying attention to emotions and physical and physiological cues assists nurses to know patients' bodies (MacLeod, 1993).

Not only do nurses work to gain patients' trust, but also patients expect nurses to give clinical care (physical, technical, and procedural) and personalized care (Henderson, 1997). Both parties need to have positive attitudes about each other, although this is not always realized. Positive relationships most likely facilitate patients' disclosure of personal information and shared perceptions of pain, stiffness, nausea, and other symptoms. Such expressions help nurses to know patients' bodies. Mutual trust and rapport facilitate patients' participation in their care when making decisions about "activities of daily living, pain management, and treatment plans" (Ibid, p. 113). Patient participation in physical care and decisions also helps nurses to know patients' bodies. Nurses probably need prolonged contact with patients to achieve this end. Consequently, shorter time periods for care most likely require nurses to achieve knowledge more rapidly and skillfully. It is essential that nurses spend quality time with patients, enough that meaningful interaction is realized. Knowing patients' bodies, therefore, calls for enough time to develop this knowledge. At the same time, nurses must avoid seeing patients as "recorded bodies" (Ibid, p. 114), where little is known about their emotional state but much is known about their physiological status.

Knowing Patients' Bodies and Clinical Judgment

Tanner (2006) proposed a perspective on clinical reasoning, the "processes by which nurses and other clinicians make their judgment, and includes both the deliberate process of generating alternatives, weighing them against the evidence, and choosing the most appropriate, and those patterns that might be characterized as engaged, practical reasoning (e.g., recognition of a pattern, an intuitive clinical grasp, a response without evident forethought)" (pp. 204–205). She positioned clinical judgment in the context of each patient's situation and each nurse's relationship with each patient. Tanner recognized that the context of the situation and nurses' relationships with patients influence what nurses pay attention to and how they interpret cues and respond to patients.

Knowing patients and their pattern of responses influences clinical judgment and directs action. Engagement with patients' concerns involves knowing typical patterns of responses, especially salient aspects, how qualitative distinctions compare to patients' typical pictures, and nurses' ability to individualize responses and interventions (Tanner, 2006). Because the interpretation of the cues displayed by patients' bodies involves the complex processes of clinical judgment, it is important to acknowledge some of this complexity. Tanner's model of clinical judgment includes noticing, interpreting, responding, and reflection.

Knowing patients helps nurses make clinical judgments about patients and select the most therapeutic nursing approaches. They are aware of patients' resources and try to respect their preferences as much as possible. This work takes place as they interact with patients and family members.

Barral (1984) cited Merleau-Ponty and allowed this interpretation: nurses find meaning at the intersection of their experiences with others. Nurses are enmeshed with others (patients) and inseparable from the subjectivity and intersubjectivity which form unity by incorporating past experiences into present experiences and those of others in our own (Barral, 1984, p. 29). The assumption is that nurses may know patients' bodies when they recognize how they use their own bodies while caring for those of their patients, as they interact and interpret each other's worlds. It is doubtful that nurses are always able to ask for consensual validation from patients as they seek to understand the cues that mean that patients are in pain, anxious, fatigued, or hopeless. Patients do not always act independently, yet they are separate from and independent of nurses. Some are unconscious or so dependent on nurses that they require total care; interpretation of cues is very difficult, as in the example of critically ill patients (Bassett, 1993). To some extent, patients' physical bodies overpower other concerns in such situations because nurses must rely on physical and physiological cues to determine problems and plans of care and when patient participation, interpersonal engagement, and responses are absent or limited. How nurses learn, respond to, and act in response to patients' bodily cues is worth examining.

Bodily Symptom Experience

Bodies suffer from the burden of symptoms. Symptom burden is defined as "the subjective, quantifiable prevalence, frequency, and severity of symptoms that place a physiologic burden on patients and may produce multiple negative, physical, psychological, and emotional patient responses" (Gapstur, 2007, p. 677). There exist many terms that describe patients' symptom experience, for example, symptom distress, symptom burden (Gusick, 2008), symptom clusters

(Kim, McGuire, Tulman, & Barsevick, 2005), sensation infor-mation (Clark & Gregor, 1988), and symptom load. Nurses are concerned about how best to assess and relieve bodily symptoms (Gapstur, 2007), and oncology and palliative care nurses have wrestled for a long time about how best to care for patients' symptom experience. For example, guidelines for dyspnea were developed in an effort to improve can-cer patients' care (DiSalvo, Joyce, Tyson, Culkin, & Mackay, 2008). Additionally, staff of long-term-care facilities rely on resident behaviors to gauge symptom severity and treat-ment efficacy (Hanson et al., 2008). However, more stud-ies are needed in the area of symptom burden and related symptom experiences to meet the needs of long-term-care residents and patients who are cognitively impaired, chroni-cally ill, or dying.

Somatic awareness, or "sensitivity to physical sensa-tions and bodily activity secondary to physiological change" (Jurgens, 2006, p. 75), is essential knowledge for some patients. Heart failure patients might benefit from recognizing heart failure symptoms through somatic awareness and certainty of the symptoms (Jurgens, 2006). Not only do patients need to monitor their heart failure symptoms, but nurses also need to teach them to identify and pay attention to normal and abnormal bodily sensations so that patients seek treatment and avoid exacerbation and hospitalization (Ibid). Often patients are unaware of any but the classic signs and symp-toms (Zuzelo, 2002) of myocardial infarction.

Nurses routinely teach preoperative patients the likely sensations and discomfort to anticipate following surgery, along with procedural information, patient expected behavior on the part of providers, and support (Bernier, Sanares, Owen, & Newhouse, 2003). Information about bodily sensa-tions prepares patients for the surgical experience. Know-ing patients' bodies during acute and chronic illnesses and symptoms of exacerbation requires knowledge of patients' individual patterns, the best literature available on signs and symptoms of diseases, and what has been learned from the care of previous patients.

Clinical experiences also help nurses to recognize changes in patients' conditions. For example, experienced nurses com-prehend patterns of deterioration early (Cioffi, 2000; Smith, 1988). Sometimes they do this before physiological, physical, psychological, and spiritual cues are evident. Recognizing changes in patients' conditions is classified as a gut feeling and a sixth sense. Nurses can recognize that something is going to happen by knowing the specific patient, comparing the current situation to past experiences with similar patients, and remembering patterns built up (Cioffi, 2000). Nurses make clinical decisions, correct or incorrect, based on this knowledge, despite the assertion that systematic approaches to clinical decisions are considered by some to be better than intuitive knowledge (Lamond & Thompson, 2000).

Nurses recognize patients' patterns of responses (Tanner et al., 1993). Specific clinical episodes with previous patients frame later clinical experiences. They carry the memory of former patients and transfer knowledge and skill to the care of current and future patients. Nurses interpret current situations based on knowing former patients' experiences, knowing about disease, and bringing current patients' experience into focus (Bishop & Scudder, 1990). They know patients' responses to therapeutic measures, their routines and habits, their coping resources, their physical capacities and endurance, and their body typology and characteristics. Knowing the patient is central to skilled clinical judgment involves the nursing skills of seeing and engagement, creates the possibility of advocacy, and sets up learning about patient populations through individual patients (Tanner et al., 1993). These themes emphasize the importance of clinical practice, the nurse-patient relationship, and the necessity for nurses to be attentive to the subtle differences among patients and in individual patients themselves.

Hidden Work

Knowing how to execute bodywork is passed from expert nurses to neophyte nurses in many instances by role modeling during direct patient care. Knowing how to do bodywork seems to be more automatic for expert nurses and under less cognitive control (Hampton, 1994). It is displayed at the bedside, in the home, chair side, or wherever nurses care for patients. Chiefly because of the intimate nature of direct or hands-on patient care, much bodywork is hidden. It is hidden work that warrants description and explanation. Interestingly, the strategies nurses use to learn how to care for patients' bodies are developed as they practice nursing. Most likely this is the way nurses develop their art.

Bodywork is frequently performed simultaneously with technical and assessment skills and may not be described in detail or measured, just documented on a checklist. For example, hygienic care often comforts patients, yet comfort is not often measured as an outcome of care. It appears in narrative nurses' notes if recorded at all.

Nurses are required to speak about patients' suffering and what nurses do as they care for them (Kahn & Steeves, 1994). Telling stories will help others understand nursing work and the effect patient suffering has on nurses personally (Ibid). Patients suffer physically, psychologically, and spiritually; and, as firsthand and expert witnesses, nurses are obliged to speak for them. The relative invisibility of much of this work makes it difficult for nurses to explain just what they do as they perform bodywork. One nurse's account illustrates the relationship established between a patient and nurse:

> *There was an immediate connection between us the moment I recognized how important it was for both of us to have him direct and guide me in my caring. He made me feel the intimacy of nursing so intensely. No one knew him the way I knew him that night. We were part of one another. (Anonymous).*

Nurses witness some of the most difficult situations that patients experience, such as pain, mental anguish, dying, and dramatic changes resulting from illness, trauma, and surgery. Nurses have not spoken often of the distress witnessed in patients or that they have experienced personally as clinicians. Their collective knowledge builds over a career and is occasionally revealed in accounts of patients' suffering, chiefly through narratives (Baker & Diekelmann, 1994), poems, and exemplars (Grant, Giddings, & Beale, 2005). A story of a new nurse follows, illustrating a lesson for her career that brought her past procedural bodywork.

I Thirst

I worked in a developing intensive care unit. It was one large room with seven beds separated by curtains. The doctors, residents, interns, and nurses worked in a small area to the side.

Chester came to this unit after being involved in a traffic accident. He had critical injuries to his abdominal and pelvic organs. We all worked very hard trying to mend Chester's broken body. Many times he asked us for a drink of water. But, because of his injuries, he could not have any thing to drink. We said no.

I can remember to this day how Chester looked at me, asking for a drink. I acted as a "good" nurse and followed the physician's orders and said no.

I changed Chester's dressings, gave him pain medication, and timed his IVs correctly. I gave him mouth care but nothing to care for his thirst. It was a very busy place and much had to be done. I was off for the weekend and returned on Monday morning. Chester was not in his bed. He had died during the night. I remember looking at his bed and knowing that Chester had died thirsty.

God revealed a truth to me at that time. Chester had been thirsty for cool water to quench his dry mouth and painful throat. I had cared for his body with the skill I believed made me a "good" nurse. But he had a greater thirst.

He needed to have been touched with gentle hands, given words of comfort, someone to have listened to his fears, and to be held by love. This was how I was shown to care for the sick.

Besides skillfully following orders, knowing the right way to change a dressing, and giving the right amount of pain medication, I needed to touch *my patients with gentle hands, I needed to* speak *words of comfort and be present to* listen *to fears.*

If Chester was given to my care today, I hope I would hold a cool,wet cloth to his mouth. My hands would gently touch h im, my words would be comforting, I would listen to his fears and hold him in love ... There are more than the skills in caring for the patient, there is the art of caring. I try to teach ... that. (Anonymous).

Knowledge of patients' health and illness experiences and the care provided by nurses are only partially revealed in progress notes, written in a shorthand way. Progress notes reveal bodywork more than patients' feelings and emotions about illness, surgery, and suffering (Parker & Gardner, 1991/1992). Furthermore, the reality of nursing care is not evident in medicolegal patient records. Only minute proportions of nursing care are documented. Examining the "shadows and

silences" (Ibid, p. 4) that are not written in notes might reveal
a great deal about the culture and politics of health care and
nursing care. Unless this changes, bodywork remains largely
silent, invisible, and minimally documented.

Keeping bodywork and other hidden work of nursing invisible has continued to devalue the everyday details
of nurses' work (McWilliam & Wong, 1994). Nurses' and
patients' bodies have been silenced since the mind or cognitive work has dominated nursing texts and discussions
(Cheek & Rudge, 1994). Bodywork can no longer be secret or
undervalued. Similar to other areas of nursing work, bodywork is silent because it is tacit, implicit, and taken for granted. Silence no longer serves patients or nurses. Accounts of
the body care given to physically changed and seriously ill
patients need a voice. Also, "The silence and weakness of
the nursing voice generally is worthy of further exploration"
(Parker & Gardner, 1991/1992, p. 8).

The everyday experiences that make up nurses' bodywork should not be taken for granted. Even though the
clinical situations of this kind of nursing work may render it
anonymous or hidden, it is not commonsense work. Expert
bodywork is an accomplishment. It involves artistic and
technical skill, useful knowledge, and procedural knowledge (Rogers, 1981), and it is framed by the nursing role.
Exquisite caregiving is "a kind of delicious delicacy and discipline which are among nursing's province and special skill"
(Diers, 1990, p. 55). Bodywork is developed through direct
experience and follows the work of present colleagues and
nurse predecessors. It takes place in the shared, social world
of nursing practice.

Special Type of Intimacy

Much of nurses' bodywork is not often witnessed by outside
observers, including other health care providers: "It is the
presence of the nurse with the patient during the intimate,
frequently vulnerable times of illness and recovery that
make it possible for nurses and patients to share many of
the meanings inherent in the illness experience" (MacLeod,
1993, p. 195). Nurses perform bodywork "...behind closed
doors" (Fagin & Diers, 1983, p. 17) when healthy persons are
unable to do it for themselves.

Nurses often perform bodywork alone with patients. In this way, access is restricted. It is not only the proximity of nurses' and patients' bodies during care episodes, but the nature of the work itself. As students, new nurses learn to "transgress their internalized social and cultural taboos" (Grant et al., 2005, p. 498).

Nurses know the secrets of patients and are with them during times of great vulnerability. They recognize the changes in patients' bodies because of proximity. This intimacy positions nurses to explain the benefits of caring, how much they enjoy doing for and with others, and the "pleasure associated with helping others from the position of a peer," or as a nurse, a member of the working class (Fagin & Diers, 1983, p. 116).

Nurses and nursing students alike need opportunities to reflect on the body care they give to patients. They will no doubt realize the privilege that this access provides. Some argue that only nursing students and nursing assistants give basic care and that experienced nurses have moved from "dirty work on bodies to clean work on machines" (Twigg, 2000, p. 390). Nurses need to examine this assertion. By sharing accounts verbally or in writing, colleagues at work and nurse educators may assist students and seasoned nurses to reflect on their everyday work and come to realize one of the many gifts of nursing practice. The poem "Dehiscence," written by Amy Haddad (1995) illustrates the complexities of the wisdom nurses develop as they gain expertise in knowing patients' bodies.

Dehiscence
By Amy Haddad

You have come unstitched.

Holes appear on your threadbare abdomen.
Tunnels develop and connect bowel, liver, pancreas.
Enzymes ooze out and digest your skin,
No matter how hard we try to stem the flow.
Mounds of dressings,
miles of tape—a jury-rigged system to
hold together our mistakes.
The stench is overwhelming, ever present,
reminding everyone, but especially you,
that you have come undone.
Since I cannot bear your suffering,

since the truth is too horrible to grasp,
since I can offer you nothing else,
I clean you up.
I wash your face,
brush your teeth,
comb your hair,
turn you gently on your side,
push soiled linens away,
roll clean sheets under you,
remove layers and layers of damp, disgusting dressings,
and replace them with new dressings and tape.

Since I am helpless in the face of your tragedy,
I give you the certainty and calmness of my motions,
the competence and comfort of my touch
as I smooth the top sheet over my work.
Done.
For a few pristine moments, we allow ourselves
to be caught in the illusion of your wholeness.
(Haddad, 1995, p. 86)

References

Bailey, S. (2004). Nursing knowledge in integrated care. *Nursing Standard, 18*(44), 38–41.

Baker, C., & Diekelmann, N. (1994). Connecting conversations of caring: Recalling the narrative to clinical practice. *Nursing Outlook, 42*(2), 65–70.

Barnard, K. (1980). Knowledge for practice: Directions for the future. *Nursing Research, 29,* 208–212.

Barral, M. R. (1984). *The body in interpersonal relations.* Merleau-Ponty. Lanham, MD: University Press of America.

Bassett, C. C. (1993). Communication with the critically ill. *Care of the Critically Ill, 9*(5), 216–219.

Berman, A., Snyder, S. J., Kozier, B., & Erb, G. (2008). *Kozier and Erb's fundamentals of nursing: Concepts, process, and practice* (8th ed.). Upper Saddle River, NJ: Pearson.

Bernier, M. J., Sanares, D. C., Owen, S. V., & Newhouse, P. L. (2003). Preoperative teaching received and valued in a day surgery setting. *AORN Journal, 77,* 563–582.

Bishop, A. H., & Scudder, J. R. (1990). *The practical, moral, and personal sense of nursing: A phenomenological philosophy of practice.* Albany, NY: State University of N ew York Press.

Burnard, P. (1988). Self awareness and intensive care nursing. *Intensive Care Nursing, 4*(20), 67–70.

Carper, B. A. (1978). Fundamental patterns of knowing in nursing. *Advances in Nursing Science, 1*(1), 13–23.

Cheek, J., & Rudge, T. (1994). Nursing as textually mediated reality. *Nursing Inquiry, 1*, 15–22.

Chin, P. L. (Ed.). (1983). *Advances in nursing theory development*. Rockville, MD: Aspens Systems Corporation.

Cioffi, J. (2000). Nurses' experiences of making decisions to call emergency assistance to their patients. *Journal of Advanced Nursing, 32*(1), 108–114.

Clark, C. R., & Gregor, F. M. (1988). Developing a sensation information message for femoral arteriography. *Journal of Advanced Nursing, 13*, 237–244.

Cooper, C. (2001). *The art of nursing: A practical introduction*. Philadelphia: W. B. Saunders.

Diers, D. (1990). Learning the art and craft of nursing. *American Journal of Nursing, 90*(1), 64–66.

DiSalvo, W. M., Joyce, M. M., Tyson, L. B., Culkin, A. E., & Mackay, K. (2008). Putting evidence into practice: Evidence-based interventions for cancer-related dyspnea. *Clinical Journal of Oncology Nursing, 12*, 341–352.

Doutrich, D., Wros, P., & Izumi, S. (2001). Relief of suffering and regard for personhood: Nurses' ethical concerns in Japan and the USA. *Nursing Ethics, 8*, 448–458.

Ellefsen, B., & Kim, H. S. (2005). Nurses' clinical engagement: A study from an acute-care setting in Norway. *Research and Theory for Nursing Practice: An International Journal, 19*, 297–313.

Fagin, C., & Diers, D. (1983). Nrusing as metaphor. New England Journal of Medicine, 309 (2), 116–117.

Gadow, S. (1989). Clinical subjectivity: Advocacy with silent patients. *Nursing Clinics of North America, 24*, 535–541.

Gapstur, R. L. (2007). Symptom burden: a concept analysis and implications for oncology nurses. *Oncology Nursing Forum, 33*, 673–680.

Gaut, D. A. (1983). Development of a theoretically adequate description of caring. *Western Journal of Nursing Research, 5*, 313–324.

Gramling, K. L. (2004). A narrative study of nursing art in critical care. *Journal of Holistic Nursing, 22*, 379–398.

Grant, B. M., Giddings, L. S., & Beale, J. E. (2005). Vulnerable bodies: Competing discourses of intimate bodily care. *Journal of Nursing Education, 44*, 498–504.

Gusick, G. M. (2008). The contribution of depression and spirituality to symptom burden in chronic heart failure. *Archives of Psychiatric Nursing 22*(1), 53–55.

Haddad, A. (1995). Dehiscence. In C. Davis & J. Schaefer (Eds.), *Between the heartbeats* (p. 86). Iowa City, IA: University of Iowa Press.

Hampton, D. C. (1994). Expertise: The true essence of nursing art. *Advances in Nursing Science, 17*(1), 15–24.

Hanson, L. C., Eckert, J. K., Dobbs, D., Williams, C. C., Caprio, A. J., Sloane, P. D., et al. (2008). Symptom experience of dying long-term care residents. *JAGS, 56*, 91–98.

Henderson, S. (1997). Knowing the patient and the impact on patient participation: A grounded theory study. *International Journal of Nursing Practice, 3*, 111–118.

Horne, R., James, D., Petrie, K., Weinman, J., & Vincent, R. (2000). Patients' interpretation of symptoms as a cause of delay in reaching hospital during acute myocardial infarction. *Heart, 83,* 388–393.

Jenny, J., & Logan, J. (1992). Knowing the patient: One aspect of clinical knowledge. *Image: Journal of Nursing Scholarship, 24*(4), 254–258.

Johns, C. (2004). *Becoming a reflective practitioner* (2nd ed.). Oxford: Blackwell.

Johnson, N. E., & Scholler-Jaquish, A. (Eds.). (2007). *Meaning in suffering: Caring practices in the health professions.* Madison, WI: University of Wisconsin Press.

Jurgens, C. Y. (2006). Somatic awareness, uncertainty, and delay in care – seeking in acute heart failure. Research in Nursing and Health, 29, 74–86.

Kahn, D. L., & Steeves, R. H. (1994). Witnesses to suffering: Nursing knowledge, voice, and vision. *Nursing Outlook, 42,* 260–264.

Kim, H. J., McGuire, D. B., Tulman, L., & Barsevick, A. M. (2005). Symptom clusters: Concept analysis and clinical implications for cancer nursing. *Cancer Nursing, 28,* 270–282.

Kolcaba, K. Y. (1992). Holistic comfort: Operationalizing the construct as a nurse-sensitive outcome. *Advance in Nursing Science, 15*(1), 1–10.

Kolcaba, K. Y. (1995). The art of comfort care. *Image: Journal of Nursing Scholarship, 27,* 287–289.

Kolcaba, K., & DiMarco, M. A. (2005). Comfort theory and it application to pediatric nursing. *Pediatric Nursing, 31,* 187–194.

Lamond, D., & Thompson, C. (2000). Intuition and analysis in decision making and choice. *Journal of Nursing Scholarship, 32*(4), 411–414.

Lawler, J. (1991). *Behind the screens: Nursing, somology, and the problem of the body.* Edinburgh: Churchill Livingstone.

Lupton, D. (1997). Consumerism, reflexivity and the medical encounter. *Social Science & Medicine, 43,* 373–381.

Macdonald, M. (2008). Technology and its effect on knowing the patient. *Clinical Nurse Specialist 22,* 149–155.

MacLeod, M. (1993). On knowing the patient: Experiences of nurses undertaking care. In A. Radley (Ed.), *Worlds of illness: Biographical and cultural perspectives on health and illness* (pp. 179–197). London: Routledge.MacLeod, M. (1994). 'It's the little things that count': The hidden complexity of everyday clinical nursing practice. *Journal of Clinical Nursing, 3,* 361–368.

Maeve, M. K. (1994). The carrier bag theory of nursing practice. *Advances in Nursing Science, 14*(4), 9–22.

McCabe, C. (2004). Nurse-patient communication: an exploration of patients' experiences. *Journal of Clinical Nursing, 13,* 41–49.

McWilliam, C. L., & Wong, C. A. (1994). Keeping it secret: The costs and benefits of nursing's hidden work in discharging patients. *Journal of Advanced Nursing, 19,* 152–163.

Parker, J., & Gardner, G. (1991/1992). The silence and the silencing of the nurse's voice: A reading of patient progress notes. *Australian Journal of Advanced Nursing, 9*(2), 3–9.

Potter, P. A., & Perry, A. (2009). *Fundamentals of nursing* (7th ed.). St. Louis: Mosby Elsevier.

Rogers, M. F. (1981). Taken-for-grantedness. *Current Perspectives in Social Theory, 2,* 133–151.

Russell, C. K. (1994). Older adult care recipients' insight into their care-givers: 'Beware the stone-face elephants!' *Geriatric Nursing, 15*(6), 308–312.

Russell, C. K. (1996). Elder care recipients' care-seeking process. *Western Journal of Nursing Research, 18*(1), 43–62.

Savage, J. (1997). Gestures of resistance: The nurse's body in contested space. *Nursing Inquiry, 4,* 237–245.

Schultz, P. R., & Meleis, A. I. (1988). Nursing epistemology: Traditions, insights, questions. *Image: Journal of Nursing Scholarship, 20*(4), 217–221.

Shakespeare, P. (2003). Nurses' bodywork: Is there a body of work? *Nursing Inquiry, 10*(1), 47–56.

Silva, M. C., Sorrell, J. M., & Sorrell, C. D. (1995). From Carper's patterns of knowing to ways of being: An ontological shift in nursing. *Advances in Nursing Science, 18,* 1–13.

Smith, M. C. (1992). Is all knowing personal knowing? *Nursing Science Quarterly, 5*(1), 2–3.

Smith, S. K. (1988). An analysis of the phenomenon of deterioration in the critically ill. *Image: Journal of Nursing Scholarship, 20*(1), 12–15.

Speed, S., & Luker, K. A. (2004). Changes in patterns of knowing the patient: The case of British district nurses. *International Journal of Nursing Studies, 41,* 921–931.

Strauss, A., Fagerhaugh, S., Suczek, B., & Wiener, C. (1984). *Social organization of Medical work.* London: University of Chicago Press.

Tanner, C. A. (2006). Thinking like a nurse: A research-based model of clinical judgment in nursing. *Journal of Nursing Education, 45*(6), 204–211.

Tanner, C. A., Benner, P., Chesla, C., & Gordon, D. R. (1993). The phenomenology of knowing the patient. *Image: Journal of Nursing Scholarship, 25*(4), 273–280.

Taylor, B. J. (1992). Relieving pain through ordinariness in nursing: A phenomenologic account of a comforting nurse-patient encounter. *Advances in Nursing Science, 15*(1), 33–43.

Twigg, J. (2000). Carework as a form of bodywork. *Aging and Society, 20,* 389–411.

Twigg, J. (2002). The body in social policy: Mapping a territory. *Journal of Social Policy, 31,* 421–439.

Watson, M. J. (1990). Transpersonal caring: A transcendent view of person, health and healing. In M. E. Parker (Ed.), *Nursing theories in practice* (pp. 277–288). New York: National League for Nursing.

Wilkes, L. M., Boxer, E., & White, K. (2003). The hidden side of nursing: Why caring for patients with malignant malodorous wound is so difficult. *Journal of Wound Care, 12*(2), 76–80.

Wolf, Z. R. (1986a). Nurses' work: The sacred and the profane. *Holistic Nursing Practice, 1*(1), 29–35.

Wolf, Z. R. (1986b). *Nursing rituals in an adult acute care hospital: An ethnography.* University of Pennsylvania. (UMI No. 8614888).

Wolf, Z. R. (1996). Bowel management and nursing's hidden work. *Nursing Times, 92*(21), 26–28.

Wolf, Z. R. (1997). Nursing students' experience bathing patients for the first time. *Nurse Educator, 22*(2), 41–46.

Wolf, Z. R. (1999). Making nursing work visible inside and outside the profession. *The Pennsylvania Nurse,* (January), 22–24.

Zuzelo, P. R. (2002). Gender and acute myocardial infarction symptoms, *MEDSURG Nursing, 11,* 126–135.

Questions that Advance the Discussion and Knowledge

1. What do you recall about the first time you performed bodywork for a patient, specifically bathed a patient?
2. How do the expert nurses you have known skillfully carry out bodywork for their patients?
3. How do you perform bodywork?

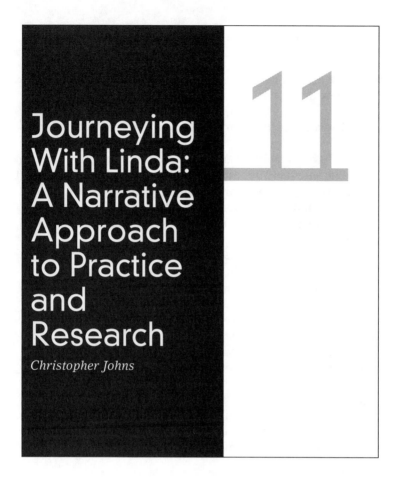

Journeying With Linda: A Narrative Approach to Practice and Research

Christopher Johns

Chapter Overview

I work as a palliative care nurse and complementary therapist in hospice and community settings. In this chapter I present a narrative of my practice with Linda, a woman with multiple sclerosis, who was admitted for respite care at the hospice. In doing so, I illuminate the value of reflective practice and narrative to both reveal and develop caring practice.

Reflection

Reflection is concerned with learning through everyday experiences toward realizing one's vision of practice as a lived reality. Reflection is being mindful of self, either within or after experience, as if looking in a mirror in which I can view and focus self within the context of a particular experience. That way I can confront, understand, and move toward resolving the contradiction or tension between my vision of practice and my understanding of my current reality. Through the conflict of contradiction, the commitment to realize one's vision, and understanding why things are as they are, I gain insight into myself and am empowered to respond more congruently in future situations within a reflexive spiral, realizing my vision of easing suffering as a lived reality.

Learning through reflection may be difficult for a number of reasons: power, tradition, and embodiment. Therefore I may require guidance to be empowered to respond more congruently with my vision in future situations (Johns, 2006).

As a nurse and therapist, my vision is to ease suffering and enable the other person to grow through the health–illness experience. Hence my reflection is a journey of self-inquiry and transformation to develop my ability to know and ease suffering so that, over time, I may perceive and respond to suffering in more effective ways. I need to become aware of my own attributes and limitations as a person and the conditions of practice that seem to influence my ability to ease suffering.

Narrative Construction

I construct narrative through six dialogical movements:

1. Dialogue with self as a descriptive, "spontaneous" account paying attention to detail—to produce a story text
2. Dialogue with the story as an objective and disciplined process to gain insights—to produce a reflective text
3. Dialogue between tentative insights and other sources of knowing to inform and position insights within the wider community of knowing
4. Dialogue with guide(s) and peers to cocreate meaning and deepen insights
5. Dialogue with the reflective text to weave a coherent and reflexive narrative text that adequately plots the unfolding journey
6. Dialogue with new experiences and with others to further develop insights; doodles in my journal

I usually write my description of an experience within 24 hours of the experience, writing spontaneously, drawing on all my senses as I pay attention to detail. Writing is awakening to self, a creative coming into conversation with self. Having written a story, I can then stand back and move into a more objective relationship to it, as if reading a text. I can ask questions of the text using the model for structured reflection (see Figure 11.1). These cues guide me to look back at the situation to make sense of it and anticipate new experiences by fantasizing about how I might respond differently if given the situation again. In looking back, I am guided to consider my empathic and sympathetic response as well as the ethical and empirical basis of my practice, and to take a hard look at myself.

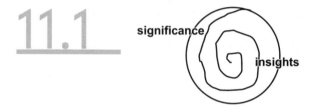

The reflective cues lead me from what I perceive as significant in the text to gaining insights. Insights are not obvious. They are often deeply enfolded within the experience. Gaining insights is a creative and imaginative journey that requires dwelling patiently within the text.

I often break the story into single lines, as if opening up the text, to read between the lines where meaning is often hidden. Holding tentative insights, I then dialogue with relevant theory and philosophy to inform and deepen my insights. I may decide to share my story with my colleagues or with my guide in formal clinical supervision. Guidance can help me see beyond myself, as if I am too wrapped up in the situation to see myself within the situation clearly. The guide is a listening board reflecting back my ideas and cuing me to explore issues more laterally, more deeply. Without guidance, it is difficult to see things that are embodied as normative, things about ourselves and the world that are generally taken for granted.

However, guidance can be problematic, as with Gladys in the following narrative. She responded to my story by surfacing her own prejudice. She could not suspend her prejudice in order to dialogue. It was too emotionally charged. Hence we could not engage, and the supervision was flawed. Guidance is underlined by *thick* trust (Cope 2001). I sensed any trust melt in the face of prejudice. It was not a space to explore intimacy. The guide is a facilitator, not an authority or judge on my practice or an imposer of favored solutions.

Reflective Model for Clinical Practice

The hospice uses the Burford NDU Model: caring in practice to structure a reflective and holistic approach to patients (Johns, 2004). The model was developed at Burford Hospital, United Kingdom, in 1990 in response to a new collaborative vision of holistic practice that valued reflective and holistic practice. The Burford practitioners decided that existing models of nursing were either reductionist or complex, so in order to appreciate the life pattern of the patient/family, a series of reflective cues were designed that tune the practitioner in to the patient, the self, and the vision (See Table 11.1). These cues are internalised and available moment to moment, enabling a narrative approach of journeying with patients that eschewed the nursing process. These cues ripple through my narrative.

11.1 The Burford NDU Model Reflective Cues to Appreciate the Patient's Life Pattern

- Who is this person?
- What meaning does this illness/health event have for the person?
- How is this person feeling?
- How has this event affected this person's usual life patterns and roles?
- How do I feel about this person?
- How can I help this person?
- What is important for this person to make his or her stay in the hospice comfortable?
- What support does this person have in life?
- How does this person view the future for himself or herself and others?

Being-Available Template

How might I recognize my learning to ease suffering? Or, put another way, how might holistic practice be known? My response to the second question was to inductively construct the being-available template (Johns, 2004). The being-available template claims that the core therapeutic of holistic practice is the practitioner being available to work to guide the person to find meaning in their illness/ health event, to help them make good decisions about their health, and to assist them with skillful action to meet their health needs.

The extent to which practitioners can be available seems to be determined by six integrated forces, listed below.

The extent to which the practitioner:

- Intends to realize a vision of practice (e.g., easing suffering and enabling growth)
- Is concerned for the person (compassion)
- Knows the person
- Responds to each situation with appropriate skillful action (practical wisdom)
- Is poised
- Can create a practice environment where being available is possible (e.g., being assertive)

Although space prohibits an in-depth exploration of these factors, the reader can discern the way these six factors are in play through the narrative.

Journeying with Linda

Day 1. A cold February day. Lying on her bed in the four-bed ward, a youngish woman catches my eye. She smiles. I interpret the smile as an invitation to engage. Kneeling beside her bed, I say, "I'm Chris, the complementary therapist."

She replies, "I'm Linda. I've been hoping to meet you."

A first step toward intimacy. "Here I am," I say. "Would you like some complementary therapy?" Always the tradesman.

She says, "I have reflexology at home with a friend; we do each other's feet. It helps to keep my hands active. It's very beneficial."

We share a common world. A second step to intimacy.

She continues, "What treatments do you offer?"

I talk through my repertoire—reflexology, body massage, Indian head massage, therapeutic touch …

"Um, I don't think I'll have reflexology, and I'm not really comfortable enough to have a massage. I used to do massage with aromatherapy, but it is too difficult now. I would like something different, maybe therapeutic touch?"

Mindful of creating a relaxing environment, I comment, "It's noisy in here."

The four-bedded ward is not a private space. Women surrounded by relatives and friends occupy the other beds. One person is close to death. It is a public space where death is on display. Yet Linda has multiple sclerosis. Death is not on her radar. Perhaps *noisy* is a metaphor for inappropriate—a word altogether more judgmental.

Linda, as if confirming my sense of the inappropriate, responds, "When I was here 2 years ago for respite care, I had a single room. I had hoped I would be offered that again."

Picking up the vibe, I ask, "Why not ask the staff?" I pause, sensing her reluctance to assert herself. "Would that be difficult?"

She again confirms my perception: "I don't like to make a fuss."

I know from experience that patients seek to fit in without making a fuss, and yet they suffer unnecessarily for loss of voice. Perhaps, as Barber (1993) suggested, it is a fear of rejection or persecution, a fear that pulls adults into child mode.

However, I don't push the issue. I inquire, "Tell me about yourself. I know you suffer from multiple sclerosis." (Why do I say "suffer from"? Perhaps she doesn't suffer at all.)

Linda takes my comment in stride. "Well, I'm 38 years old, and I do have multiple sclerosis. I have pain in my right hip and also have a urinary tract infection that's very unpleasant." She defines herself as symptoms.

"Is the infection a recurring problem?"

"Yes, but that's not why I am admitted. It's to let my family have a holiday."

I don't pursue this thought, not wanting to reinforce any idea that Linda might be a burden that her family needs a break from.

"Are *we* on top of your pain?"

"Not quite, but that's a good reason to be in here, to get that better managed."

A moment's pause. "Shall I set up an aroma stone and burn some oils?"

"That would be great."

I begin to play "What oils shall we use?" We become conspirators plotting her oils. It's fun, a lifting of the spirit. The noise evaporates. Time is transcended. Another step toward intimacy. Linda suggests clary sage and lavender. I suggest sandalwood or perhaps bergamot because both are renowned for combating urinary tract infection and easing stress. She thinks sandalwood is a good idea but is less keen on the bergamot.

I comment, "Clary sage is a good stress buster!"

"Just what I need. My shoulders get so tight. I don't like ylang-ylang."

I joke, "An aphrodisiac. It's not my favorite aroma either."

She laughs, "That would make little difference to me. I've had multiple sclerosis since my early twenties."

Her reaction makes me wonder about the impact of this degenerative illness on her body image and sexuality. Meaning hinted at. Signs on the surface that I don't pursue for deeper meaning, at least not at this time. For the moment we can ripple along the surface of things rather than explore the deeper currents.

As I go to fetch my aromatherapy kit, I inquire of Kirsty (a staff nurse) about the possibility of a single room for Linda. Kirsty says she will see what she can do. Two vacant single rooms are booked for men. On my return I inform Linda of my action. No reaction.

Linda shuffles from her right side onto her back, wincing with pain. Her pain management is clearly not well engineered. I lower the head of the bed, and she finds a comfortable position.

"That's true," she laughs.

A fan lies idle on her bed table. "Would you like it on?"

"Yes, on low."

The fan's cool air calms the room as I give her therapeutic touch for about 30 minutes. I visualize blue, cool waves taking the heat from her. *Serpent Mound,* by Rusty Crutcher, adds a haunting drone that resonates in perfect pitch with my movements.

Afterward Linda is very still. Slowly she opens her eyes. I sense she is on another level of consciousness.

She murmurs, "That was very relaxing. I still have pain but it's eased and I feel so much cooler."

I notice her dry feet. "Would you like me to moisten them for you?"

She accepts my offer. "It's been a problem. I've had some foot infections. I have some cream in the drawer."

"You might prefer my reflex cream with patchouli and frankincense added." I am a tempter, knowing her weakness.

"That sounds better."

She likes the aroma and appreciates my foot massage. She has such small, delicate feet with long, thin toes. I am a poet in motion shaping therapy with my hands.

Before I bid farewell, I urge her to ensure that her aroma stone does not run dry and remind her that she can choose her own essential oils as she wishes to suit her mood. Mindful of her reluctance to assert herself, I say, "I'll write that in your notes so the staff will expect that. I'll be here again on Friday—would you like another therapy?"

"Can I? That would be great. Can you leave the curtains around my bed, and can I have some more relaxation music?"

No problem. I take her hand and feel the connection flow between us. Touch—a further step toward intimacy.

Later, writing my journal, I wonder if I was self-conscious treating another therapist. Yes, I had been, yet it was good working *with* her. Both being therapists opened a gate to mutuality and play, an intimacy that enhanced her treatment.

I also wonder if my paternal action of inquiring about a single room was appropriate without first asking Linda if she would like me to act for her. Respecting and creating the conditions for Linda to exercise her autonomy is, according to Seedhouse (1988), the highest ethical principle. Did I insult her autonomy?

It's all too easy to render disabled people incompetent and act in their best interests, thus further undermining their autonomy and competence (Charmaz, 1983). Yet Linda didn't want to make a fuss. Perhaps she has learned that it doesn't pay to make a fuss and risk being labeled a "difficult patient" (Kelly & May, 1982), with its predictable consequence of being rejected. The staff are not positive toward Linda. It is shocking to suggest that staff label people negatively in a hospice, where expression of anger and despair should be encouraged. Perhaps there are subtle distinctions and social judgments made between people dying of cancer and those living with a chronic illness such as multiple sclerosis. Contradictions are littered everywhere.

I burn ylang-ylang essential oil and appreciate its sweet, exotic aroma. Lawless (2002) quoted Moncrieff: "The writer, working with odorous materials for more than twenty years, long ago noticed that ... *ylang-ylang* soothes and inhibits anger born of frustration" (p. 194). That sounds like a perfect remedy for someone so young who lives with multiple sclerosis and its ravaging impact on her life. Creating the essential oil mix can either be a very complex balance of factors or simply an intuitive response that stems from experience.

Day 5. Linda has not moved into a single room. She has been to the general hospital for an IVP (intravenous pyelogram) to investigate the kidney and urinary tract this morning. Over lunch, I read her notes. Her pain management has been reviewed. She is now on methadone 30 mg, diclofenac 50 mg, and mexiletine 150mg (increased yesterday from 100 mg three times daily. She was previously prescribed amitriptyline for neuropathic pain, which I perceive her pain to be. I mention this, but Gladys, one of the hospice sisters, thinks Linda's pain is due to her urinary tract infection radiating through her pelvis and down her left leg. She is prescribed trimethoprim for the infection. I don't press my opinion, yet I'm mindful that it is easy to lose sight of Linda behind a screen of symptom management.

Linda's notes reveal that she has a 17-year-old daughter named Zöe. I am surprised that the notes reveal that sexual relations with her husband ceased some time ago. It feels remarkably intrusive, as if putting her on public display. And yet, on another level, it acknowledges her as a sexual being, something I rarely see reference to within patient notes. Sexuality is integral to the person's identity and is a major factor in perceived sense of loss of self (Charmaz, 1983). Linda had thrown me the cue when discussing ylang-ylang. I hadn't pursued the cue, rationalizing that she wouldn't have wanted me to pursue it. Yet maybe I interpreted it that way because I am uncomfortable talking with women about their sexuality.

I wonder—do other staff explore this with her or is the topic avoided?

Linda lies on her bed with her back to the door. Her eyes are closed. I do not want to disturb her, so I move to visit another patient. As I move, she opens her eyes and catches my own. She reciprocates my soft smile and waves. Turning over, she says she is tired and uncomfortable but is looking forward to the reflexology. I notice the aroma stone is dry.

"The aroma stone is dry?"

"Yes. I didn't like to ask the staff to replenish it."

Linda's passivity reflects her learned patient behavior not to be demanding. To reiterate, she doesn't like a fuss, and yet I feel her frustration.

"I know you don't want to make a fuss, but I would have expected the staff to observe it was dry and replenish it."

My frown deeply furrowed at such carelessness. This neglect is a constant thorn in my side. Yet I have been unable to shift this pattern of neglect, as if aroma stones are outside the gaze of nurses despite their known benefit.

I say, "I'll replenish it in a moment and wag my finger at the staff later."

I wish I hadn't said that. My frustration leaks out.

I do not want to draw Linda into warfare.

Shifting the topic, I say, "I've read your notes and plotted the pattern of your pain management."

She laughs as she tells me her story of getting big boxes of methadone from the chemist. She requires regular break-through doses besides her regular medication.

I say, "I noticed that you're not on any neuropathic pain analgesia."

"I was on gabapentin, but it didn't suit me, but I feel I may have to go back on it. That shooting pain down my leg is sciatic on top of my normal pain." She has confirmed my perception.

"So, what oils shall we add to the reflexology cream?"

Once again we dwell in playtime like conspirators while plotting which oils to add to the reflexology cream. I ask her if she likes playing.

She laughs, "I like engaging in 'oil talk.' The aroma of neroli is intoxicating!"

I do not know how Linda feels about her multiple sclerosis. She hides her surface signs even as I intuitively probe her body signs without disturbing her calm surface. I imagine that a disease like multiple sclerosis hangs heavily over an uncertain and disabling future and that such thoughts drain her positive energy. I imagine that complementary therapy must be a powerful comforter, especially for someone such as Linda who is also a therapist.

As I apply the reflexology cream to her feet, I notice the hard skin on her big toes. Her toenails are a rich vermillion color. A red mark along the sciatic line. She has picked some hard skin. I guide her through my relaxation routine, mindful of the noise of the busy day that drifts behind the pulled curtains that separate us from the outside world.

I play *Ocean Eclipse*, by Rusty Crutcher. The album features cascades of waves breaking on the shore recorded during the longest total eclipse of the sun. Evocative music written with a deep reverence for the spirit. The water flowing and cleansing the torn spirit, moving through creative chaos until it finds lyrical form and enters a space of stillness.

Conversation outside the curtains distracts me. But that's another story.

Later, at the shift report, I again comment on my observation of Linda's pain. I ask the gathered nurses if they explore sexuality with Linda. The general response is that it's not relevant to her care. I am struck dumb. Linda's care is framed by her presenting symptoms, and sex is a taboo topic. Linda disembodied.

As I write in my journal, I wonder about intimacy and sexuality. What do I know? I sense I move toward intimacy but shrink from sexuality. Is that a contradiction? I am held by the word *intimacy*. I realize I have little idea of what this means in practice. The signs of intimacy are evident—touch, the choosing of oils, eye contact, smiles, waves. These are surface things that spring from the well of intimacy, or perhaps it is the universal well of compassion. Perhaps intimacy is itself the expression of compassion—the dwelling with another in suffering. I imagine intimacy is always something reciprocated. Did I assume intimacy through my interpretation of surface signs or through my need for intimacy? Do I doubt myself because of others' labeling of Linda as manipulative?

Are there risks to intimacy that demand professional boundaries? Menzies-Lyth (1988) wrote of necessary professional detachment as protection from emotional entanglement. I prefer to write of necessary professional involvement. Being creative rather than defensive. Being on the front foot, not the back foot.

There is no prescription for intimacy. It cannot be conceptually analyzed despite attempts to know it as a thing in itself, as if it were something out there we might all use in our practice.

The key to intimacy is being mindful, being sensitive to the rhythm between us. As Newman (1999) noted,

> *This rhythm is an indicator of the pattern of interacting consciousness. If we want to get in touch with this pattern, we need to listen to the silence, to listen with our hearts, as we attune ourselves to the rhythm of the other person. (p. 227)*

I know that Linda has an impaired body image and diminished view of herself as a (sexual) woman. As a therapist, I need to develop a strong sense of my own sexuality in relation to others.

Lemieux, Kaiser, Pereira, and Meadows (2004) noted,

> *For patients in this study, sexuality was an important aspect of their lives, even in the last weeks and days of life. Sexuality encompassed many things but was centered on emotional connectedness. Their experience of sexuality changed over time, from expressions that usually included sexual intercourse prior to the disease, to one of intimacy through close body contact, hugging, touching of hands, kissing, "meaningful" eye contact and other non-physical expressions of closeness and companionship. These expressions were a key component of their quality of life. (p. 634)*

These words resonate. I feel an emotional connection flow between Linda and me reflected in our smiles, touch, and eye contact. Lemieux et al. (2004) noted the therapeutic impact of the study in creating a space in which the participants could talk about sexuality. Considering the staff comments, we fail our patients. I will post Lemieux et al.'s paper on the staff notice board with a sign saying, "Please read."

Day 9. Linda has moved into a single room. I glance round the door. She's on the phone and does not catch my eye. A few minutes later, I glance again. This time her bed is empty. I suspect she is in the toilet. Did she get there by herself? I am conscious of not knowing about her mobility. Waiting for Linda to return, I talk to Michael's wife in the room across the corridor. I met her last week.

That is another story.

A few minutes later, Linda walks back to her room. She walks awkwardly, as if her pelvis were rotated. I give her a few moments to settle before I glance again into her room. She beckons me in and I sit in the chair beside her bed.

She is relaxed and thankful for her time in the hospice: "It was what I needed. My pain has also settled. So that's good."

"I see you have your single room!"

She laughs, "Yes, the doctor came to see me and said it was noisy in here. I agreed and said I'm not as rested as I hoped. He arranged for the single room and I was moved in half an hour. I have brought my essential oils in."

I ask about her mobility.

"I have a relapse-remitting form of the disease. I have attacks and regain about 80% of the loss. I never get back to what I was before."

"You seem so accepting of the disease."

"I get great support from my husband and daughter. I am a passive person and don't really get angry. What's the point? Better to live for each day."

So much revealed in a couple of lines. I want to ask about her family, but something stops me. Perhaps her words *better to live for each day* are a message I interpret as "don't dig too deep." What purpose would it serve? I sense it would make little difference to her care except that her story would be heard. This is a contradiction—clearly that would make a difference to her care. I know that my nature is not to intrude, but she has given me this cue.

"How are your husband and daughter?"

Another smile. "Having a good break, I hope."

Again her words constrain my inquiry. I sense the limits of my role.

I write Linda a poem.

> you say you are rested
> but it could have been more
> with kinder faces
> and with a room overlooking the gardens
> where birds danced along the fountain's edge

and preened their wings
or perched on heron's beak;
a space for healing:
instead you were closeted
in a room of death
whose noise penetrated your drawn curtains
and your smiling mask.
you didn't ask but at last were heard.

Day 11. I share my experience of working with Linda with Gladys, the unit sister, in the clinical supervision session we have every 4 weeks. Gladys met Linda 3 years earlier when she was admitted to the hospice for pain relief. Then Linda commenced taking methadone. Her mobility was severely compromised. On this admission, Gladys felt that Linda's behavior was incongruent, for example asking for break-through medication when eating a Danish pastry. She now feels Linda is abrupt and unfriendly.

I sense that Gladys is clearly hostile to Linda's plight. I wonder if Linda reads Gladys's hostility? How can she not? I find myself speculating why Gladys has such difficulty with Linda. Perhaps Linda is addicted to methadone and we haven't seen this because of our palliative care lens, where such issues are played down because of the "dying" tag. Perhaps Linda exploits our lack of understanding. It is intriguing to observe how some patients, such as Linda, evoke feelings of anxiety and hostility in caregivers as if they presented an existential threat. Gladys has judged Linda as manipulative and unfriendly. Even if Linda were manipulative, it would be for reasons that demand a therapeutic response. I know that Gladys shares her judgment with other staff and that Linda is viewed as a "bad" patient.

Kelly and May (1982) wrote of good and bad patients, where *good* is defined as a consequence of interactional pattern rather than anything inherent in the patient's behavior. Johnson and Webb (1995) termed this social judgment, that Linda has transgressed some unspoken rule and poses a threat to normal hospice life. The idea that staff can unwittingly heighten suffering is disturbing. I sense the dark side of nursing, whereby caring is diminished (Corley & Goren, 1998). I am disturbed that Gladys's use of a word *manipulative* can evoke doubt in myself but no doubt others. Like a shock, it has rattled my use of the label *intimacy*. Perhaps Gladys should be labeled as a "bad nurse"? I sense the tension between being human and being professional (Hem & Heggen, 2003) and the way practitioners retreat behind the boundary of professional distance to manage their vulnerability. No chance of intimacy.

Gladys is locked into her hostility and is not available to Linda. Radiating rejection, she isolates Linda and reinforces her loss of self. Yet her behavior is also self-alienating. Perhaps putting her into the four-bedded ward was a form of punishment? How is it that the doctor could so easily move her into a single room? Reiterating her negative view of Linda, Gladys says the doctor was easily manipulated. She suggests that perhaps I too have been manipulated. I recoil against Gladys's labeling of Linda. It is perverse, offensive. I feel a ripple of anger. I must confront her if I am to take my therapeutic responsibility seriously, but I sense it would be futile in this moment. I don't, caught up in the culture of conflict avoidance within the hospice.

Later, I share the situation with Maud, another sister whom I respect. She shares my concern. As we talk it through, I decide to ask staff at the support group meeting how they felt about Linda. Gladys will be there. I visualize moving from avoidance of conflict to collaboration (Thomas & Kilmann, 1974). I am anxious about this, but Maud encourages me to find my voice. My boldness will help others also to express suppressed feelings. Finding one's voice is a powerful metaphor for empowerment (Belenky, Clinchy, Goldberger, & Tarule, 1986).

In her single room, Linda is packed and ready, waiting for her family.

Linda remarks, "Home tomorrow. Back to the real world."

I smile. "It's been good to meet and play with you. We must do it again sometime. Was your experience at the hospice good?"

"Yes, it was. Restful. It's hard to rest at home."

She takes my offered hand. I gaze at her and wonder if her stay was really restful. What is her real world? I sense that I have little impression of that despite our conversations. Is she using her smiling face and affirming words as a mask? What does she really think and feel? I sense she has learned through her chronic illness to pay select attention, filtering out the negative gestures. Is that how she copes? I find myself making assumptions, judgments based on flimsy ground. I have only scratched at the surface of this woman.

The notion of *restful* strikes me. I didn't appreciate enough the significance of the hospice as a restful place apart from the hassle of her everyday life. Indeed, looking back, I see the hospice as a disturbing place that disrupts the restful flow.

Reflection

What started as "doodles in a journal" is transformed into the narrative text, written to unfold like a serial drama, holding the reader in suspense.

I ask myself, Could I have better responded to ease Linda's suffering? Could I have been more available to her? There is much conflict in the text. I am challenged in terms of my ability to confront what I see as attitudes and practices that seemed to increase Linda's suffering during her stay at the hospice. Scrolling down the text farther, subtle things emerge. Issues of intimacy and sexuality are challenging. For whose benefit is intimacy? Do I assume she wants it, or do I want her to want it? Does she use intimacy, as Gladys suggested, to manipulate men? Issues of privacy, noise, and public display of death all emerge as significant factors in our response to her suffering.

Each idea within the whole pattern slowly emerges and ripens until it is transformed into its potential narrative form like pieces of a complex jigsaw.

As Wheatley (1999) noted,

> To see patterns, we have to step back from the problem [text] and gain perspective. Shapes are not discerned from close range. They require distance and time to show themselves. Pattern recognition requires that we sit together reflectively and patiently. I say patiently not just because patterns take time to form, but because we are trying to see the world differently and there are many years of blindness to overcome. (p. 126)

As I constructed the narrative, I was conscious of tensions playing themselves out within me, the tensions between finding an adequate expression for my voice in relationship to those I work with and finding an adequate expression to engage readers in ways that might be meaningful. Narrative resonates with chaos theory in the sense that clinical practice is deeply complex in its wholeness, and yet within that apparent chaos there is order or pattern recognition. Narrative is movement; like a stream it manifests pace and rhythm as it deepens, widens, and is shaped by the landscape as it flows toward the sea. I can tune in to and flow with the inherent order rather than resisting the flow of energy by forcing ideas into boxes. This is a vital insight in constructing narrative. Narrative form does not demand allegiance to any specific form beyond the reflexive demand. Indeed, it is a demand for a liberation of self from oppressive forms of censorship and expression (Cixous, 1996).

I resist an urge to structure my narrative by resorting to generalizations and reducing it into an explanatory scheme, what Clandinin and Connelly (2000) described as the formulaic and reductionist boundaries of narrative inquiry. Yet, in a world largely governed by professional texts written in a formulaic and reductionist vein, it is a difficult pull to resist. Elaborate concept identification and analysis obscures rather than illuminates possible meanings when the narrative needs to be open to the reader for potential dialogue.

Narrative needs to engage the reader as if it were a drama unfolding. Feedback from public readings informs me that narratives enable listeners to sense they are more present in the drama than by simply reading it. Perhaps the narrative should be presented as an audio CD? Would it "read" better as a visual performance, a play? Such ideas currently tease me and have led me to work with drama and dance teachers, photographers, and artists. I work more with poems and images because I feel they better capture meaning in less obvious ways. I sense that insights should lie just below the surface for the imagination of the reader rather than the reader being told what is significant within the text. I try to leave signs, both obvious and subtle, about the place alongside the many signs that I am unaware of. Ben Okri (1997) strongly influences my narrative style—the idea that stories should always be transgressive, for why else write them? He talks of beauty and horror lying side by side, and indeed hospice work seems like that—the beauty of caring amidst the suffering of dying. He talks of enchantment and planting seeds to explode in the reader's mind. He says that the truth should shriek!

Narrative is never completely formed. It is always evolving through dialogue with curious readers. The written narrative is a snapshot, a moment in time, for experience continues and narrative insights are constantly being tested and developed. I must emphasize that the central issue of narrative research is not methodology but validity or coherence, a consideration of the adequate representation of experience in response to the claimed narrative plot; or put another way, a persuasion that the narrative can be trusted or is worthy (Mishler, 1990).

The worthiness of the narrative is open to the reader's interpretation. There are no fixed rules to be rigidly applied; these need to carefully considered in response to the particular project or as "actual inquiries" (Smith & Deemer, 2000, p. 889). I am drawn toward Lather's (1993) notion of rhizomatic validity as an organic approach to coherence —the idea that coherence is grown through the narrative as a complex contradictory network in ways that mirror the complexity and contradictions of everyday practice. Nothing is neat or simple within the vastness of human encounter. I know I have blind spots, have prejudices, and make unjustified assumptions. Some I have become aware of. Others lie thick on the surface or buried within the words. Such is the nature of narrative.

Laurel Richardson, quoted by Flemons and Green (2002) sums up the issue nicely: "I would argue very strongly that the self that is writing the story is changed by the process of writing it" (p. 91).

References

Barber, P. (1993). Developing the "person" of the professional carer. In S. Hinchliff, S. Norman, & J. Schober (Eds.), *Nursing practice and health care* (2nd ed.) (pp. 344–373). London: Edward Arnold.

Belenky, M. F., Clinchy, B. M., Goldberger, N. R., & Tarule, J. M. (1986). *Women's ways of knowing: The development of self, voice, and mind.* New York: Basic Books.

Charmaz, K. (1983). Loss of self: A fundamental form of suffering in the chronically ill. *Sociology of Health and Illness, 5*(2), 168–195.

Cixous, H. (1996). Sorties: Out and out: Attacks/ways out/forays. In H. Cixous & C. Clément (Eds.), *The newly born woman* (pp. 63–134) London: Tauris.

Clandinin, D. J., & Connelly, F. M. (2000). *Narrative Inquiry: Experience and story in qualitative research.* San Francisco: Jossey-Bass.

Cope, M. (2001). *Lead yourself: Be where others will follow.* London: Momentum Books.

Corley, M. C., & Goren, S. (1998). The dark side of nursing: Impact of stigmatizing responses on patients. *Scholarly Inquiry for Nursing Practice: An International Journal, 12*(2), 99–118.

Flemons, D., & Green, S. (2002). Stories that conform/stories that transform. A conversation in four parts. Part 1: Autoethnographies: Constraints, openings, ontologies, and findings. In A. Bochner & C. Ellis (Eds.), *Ethnographically speaking* (pp. 87–94). Walnut Park, CA: AltaMira.

Hem, M., and Heggen, K. (2003). Being a professional and being human: One nurse's relationship with a psychiatric patient. *Journal of Advanced Nursing, 43*(1), 101–108.

Johns, C. (2004). *Being mindful, easing suffering.* London: Jessica Kingsley Publishing.

Johns, C. (2006). *Engaging reflection in everyday practice: A narrative approach.* Oxford: Blackwell.

Johnson, M., & Webb, C. (1995). Rediscovering unpopular patients: The concept of social judgment. *Journal of Advanced Nursing, 21,* 466–475.

Kelly, M. P., & May, D. (1982). Good and bad patients: A review of the literature and a theoretical critique. *Journal of Advanced Nursing, 7,*147–156.

Lather, P. (1993). Fertile obsession: Validity after post-structuralism. *The Sociological Quarterly, 34*(4), 673–93.

Lawless, J. (2002). *The encyclopedia of essential oils.* London: Thorsons.

Lemieux, L., Kaiser, S., Pereira, J., & Meadows, L. M. (2004). Sexuality in spiritual care; patient perspectives. *Palliative Medicine, 18,* 630–637.

Menzies-Lyth,I. (1988) A case study in the functioning of social systems as a defence against anxiety. In Containing Anxiety in Institutions: Selected Essays. London: Free Association Books,

Mishler, E. G. (1990). Validation in inquiry-guided research: The role of exemplars in narrative studies. *Harvard Educational Review, 60*(4), 415–442.

Moncrieff, R. W. (1970). *Odours.* London: Heinemann Medical.

Newman, M. (1999). The rhythm of relating in a paradigm of wholeness. *Image: Journal of Nursing Scholarship, 31*(3), 227–230.

Okri, B. (1997). *A way of being free.* London: Phoenix House.

Seedhouse, D. (1988). *Ethics: The heart of healthcare.* Chichester: Wiley.

Shikpo, R. (2000). *Openness clarity sensitivity.* Oxford: Longchen Foundation.

Smith, J., & Deemer, B. (2000). The problem of criteria in the age of relativism. In N. Denzin & Y. Lincoln (Eds.), *Handbook of Qualitative Research* (2nd ed.) (pp. 887–896). London: Sage.

Thomas, K., & Kilmann, R. (1974). *Thomas Kilmann conflict mode instrument.* Toledo: Xicom.

Wheatley, M. (1999). *Leadership and the new science: discovering order in a chaotic world.* San Francisco: Berrett-Koehler.

Caring for "Not-so-Picture-Perfect Patients": Ethical Caring in the Moral Community of Nursing

12

Marian C. Turkel
and Marilyn A. Ray

Chapter Overview

The ethical way of knowing has been firmly established in the discipline and practice of nursing (American Nurses Association [ANA], 2001; Carper, 1978; Roach, 2002). The ethics of caring in nursing is a complex and dynamic issue. It illuminates the good of nursing: holism (integration of body, mind, and spirit); compassion; responsibility for the other; and loyalty to principles such as respect, beneficence (doing good), non-maleficence (doing no harm), autonomy (allowing choice), and justice (Ray, 1987, 1994, 1998, 2007; Watson, 2005). The purpose of this chapter is to shed light on the complex ethical dynamics of caring and ethical decision making when nurses are engaged with the "not-so-picture-perfect" patient: the patient whom we may think of as the difficult patient; the

one who looks and smells bad; the patient who is noncompliant; the one who won't listen; and the one who is angry or
frightful—who steals, plots revenge, acts violently, or has killed
or raped. Many of the nursing situations related to caring for
the not-so-picture-perfect patient are not discussed in standard curriculum or textbooks. Registered nurses rarely have
the opportunity to dialogue and reflect on the reality of caring
for this vulnerable patient population. The ethical expressions
of moral distress, moral conflict, and moral paradox are highlighted and discussed. Specific nursing situations from registered nurses in various practice settings illuminate each one
of the ethical expressions and give voice to their experiences,
values, emotions, and practice.

Introduction

The ethical way of knowing guides clinical nursing situations
(Carper, 1978). Nursing associations, such as the American
Nurses Association (2001) and the Canadian Nurses Association (2002) have devised Codes of Ethics for Nurses that
facilitate the guidance of nursing practice and show that the
first level of responsibility for the nurse is compassion and
respect for the inherent dignity of the patient and family. The
nursing philosopher Roach (2002) claimed that the ethics of
caring was imperative in nursing by naming conscience as
one of her six C's of caring. The others are commitment, compassion, confidence, competence, and comportment. Each one
of Roach's six C's contributes to awareness of the moral relationship of human beings with others, and to nurse caring as
holistic, the integration or synthesis of body, mind, and spirit.
    According to Ray, ethics is defined as "a code of conduct
[principles or rules] developed and reinforced in terms of what
is good and right (or moral) in character and behavior" (Ray,
1997, p. 72). Morality is difficult to define but primarily deals
with obeying codes of conduct or rules and, thus, how one ought
to live in society or culture or the moral community (Rachels,
2003). The good is defined as a societal good that expresses
the moral ideal and right choices for the protection of human
dignity within the moral community (Schultz & Schultz, 1990).
There is also an Infinite Good, the invisible other, an I-Thou
relationship that exists in individual conscience and speaks as
the ethical imperative (Buber, 1958, 1965; Levinas, 1981). The

ethical imperative of conscience is considered an inner or divine attraction to or love for what is good and abhorrence of evil. Because of this understanding of what is good, conscience centers on recognizing, witnessing, and judging (Ratzinger, 2007). In health care, the good as described by Pellegrino (1985) is threefold: the biomedical good (interventions and treatments); the patient's concept of his or her own good; and the human good—what is most proper to being human, making choices, and determining one's goals for a satisfactory life (pp. 20–22). The ethics of caring in nursing is complex and dynamic.

To address the moral dilemmas that arise from the realities of nurse caring practices, this chapter will include discussion of ethical caring, the ethical caring approach, caring emotions, technology and ethics, ethics and formation, and the ethical demand of caring. Three ethical expressions in the practice of ethical caring will be highlighted: moral distress, moral conflict, and moral paradox. Specific stories or case studies in nursing practice will follow that illuminate each one of the ethical expressions.

Ethical Caring

Many scholars of nursing have conveyed the meaning of caring. These interpretations have ranged from intentional acts or transpersonal meanings (Boykin & Schoenhofer, 2001; Davis, 1990; Gadow, 1988,1989; Roach, 2002; Watson, 2005) to contextual meanings of caring where the organizational, cultural, and technological play a significant role in the structure and expressions of meaning (Barnard & Locsin, 2007; Leininger & McFarland, 2005; Ray, 2007; Schultz & Schultz, 1990). In the ethical and moral caring sphere, nurses are called to act responsibly to seek the "good" of the other.

According to Roach (2002), ethics can be approached in three ways: first, as a discipline of knowledge; second, as relational responsibility; and third, as a process of discernment.

As a relational responsibility, ethics highlights the responsibility of the nurse not only in terms of faithfulness to duties and obligations of respect for persons, but also in terms of faithfulness to a covenant between the one caring and the one to whom one is responsible. For example, in nursing, we respond to the call from the patient to care without discrimination in terms of who the person is (race, culture/ethnic group, or religion), what the person has done, or what the person exhibits—that is, going the extra mile and helping a person in his or her need, suffering, and pain.

As a process of discernment, ethics encompasses listening to the story of the patient and family and moving back and forth among values, principles, and moral norms with a focus on responsibility to the other in a life world situation. In nursing situations the nurse is facilitating choices, while addressing human caring in terms of being ethically responsible to self and other (Levinas, 1981; Logstrup, 1997). That process means understanding the self; seeking the good of the patient in the nursing situation; and being responsive to the moral community, the family or significant others, the health care organizational community, or the cultural community (Ray, 1994, 1998; Roach, 2002; Schultz & Schultz, 1990).

The moral community in health care conveys a moral tone that reflects the degree to which dimensions of morality are integrated collectively through philosophy and standards and policies, and the degree to which they are enacted individually in ethical situations (Roach, 2002): "Thus, ethical qualities, ethical conduct [moral caring], and the moral tone of communal moral experience are the reference points for problem solving [and decision making]" (Ray, 1998, p. 72).

Within nursing, issues constantly arise in relation to the ethical demand of caring within the moral community. What do we do when we encounter a person who frightens us by how he or she looks or behaves, the not-so-picture-perfect patient—the patient who is a victim of his or her bad decisions, the patient who has just been taken off the street and smells bad and is swearing, the patient who reeks of alcohol and is abusive, the patient who just stole money from his elderly mother to get illicit drugs, the homeless patient who is full of maggots, the patient with gaping wounds crying out for help after having just murdered someone, the patient who is brought into the emergency department by police after having just raped a child? How do nurses practice holistically—body, mind, and spirit? What do nurses do when technology plays a greater role in ethical decision making, such as when technology is used as an aid to patients in the form of survival, as a computerized communication tool and an electronic record (Beidler & Chase, 2007)? Or what about when technology acts as an extension of a professional's work, in forms such as robotic applications that are mechanical, reprogrammable, and controlled by a computer (Campling, Tanioka, & Locsin, 2007)? How do we as nurses recognize that every thought and action (intentional acts) carries with it what we believe about caring; our feelings, attitudes, values, and beliefs; and our transformative energy for good or, in some situations, even bad?

Caring Emotions

In her analysis, Griffin (1983) highlighted not only clusters of meanings of caring that address concern, helping, attention, protection, guidance, and serving needs, but also other meanings that have particular relevance for this presentation of the not-so-picture-perfect patient. They refer to the attitudes and feelings underlying the activities of caring—attitudes and feelings such as attachment, inclination, and empathy; liking or not liking a person; desiring to be near someone; or not wanting at all to know about the person and his or her life. These emotions have generally been considered nonmoral (Fry, 1990). In her distinction between moral and nonmoral in human caring, Fry stated that moral aspects of caring involve human motivations or character traits, the idea of character and moral agency of the nurse caring rather than individual tastes, feelings, or preferences.

Many philosophers of caring, however, would not distinguish elements of caring in quite the same way. Caring is relational. Liking someone or the idea of a caring attitude in nursing carries strong moral tones, qualities, and actions. A nurse is always a moral agent, whether or not he or she expresses feelings for or about a patient, and whether or not he or she enacts the obligations related to his or her ethical responsibility while in a privileged, professional relationship. The privileged relationship is twofold, being there in the fullness of one's humanity and responding to one's ethical responsibility to the other. Caring presents the nurse with an awesome moral responsibility. The nurse as a moral agent should convey compassion and respect in the carrying out of moral responsibility. As a compassionate being, the nurse is involved in a compassionate "we," a process of seeking understanding the meaning of "suffering with," bearing with, or beholding the other (Ray, 1994). In the clinical nursing situation, by being there or present with the patient, the nurse is exposed to the wounds of the patient and through the relationship is present also to his or her own wounds. Thus, the nurse is a wounded healer (Nouwen, 1979). The significance of being present or being there in relationship to the other justifies all commitment to respect human dignity, to care, and to heal (ANA, 2001; Levinas, 1981).

Caring Ethics and Technology

Does the same accountability that applies to the human world apply to the technological world? The human-humanoid relationship is a certainty. We are aware of technology as an ethical nursing practice. Concepts such as technological caring (Ray, 1987, 2007) and technological competency as caring (Barnard & Locsin, 2007; Locsin, 2005) highlight this reality. Can the notion of presence as ethical responsibility extend beyond the human being to a new area arising in nursing education and nursing practice; that is, with the use of the simulated person for educational purposes, or robots for augmentation of clinicians' professional practice? Is technology more than an instrument? Can a robot be authentically wounded? In essence, can a robot be moral?

Philosophers of technology have interesting insights. Technology as instrument, property, or practice is not an individual, not a culture; but it can be a presence, and through our relationship with it, there is also co-responsibility. In other words, we fashion something from technology; it can become an art form, or we can engage with it as a programmed or programmable object (Heidegger, 1977; Smith, 1998). Smith (1998) remarked that technology lives in what is called the "middle distance"—an in-between realm of attachment and connection to the world, and a more remote disconnection, a form of separation that defines the subject-object division (p. 3). Heidegger (1977) stated that technology is both a means to an end and a human activity. For example, as both a means to an end and a human activity, when a technology is programmed by individuals or when an individual relates to the technology, the individual is present and co-responsible.

In nursing, ethical caring is implied because nursing focuses on presence and responsibility, respectively; being there for the other; and being accountable for the care of the other. But what truly differentiates the ethical activity of a person from a robot or simulated patient that has been programmed? Heidegger (1977) stated that technology must reveal a truth; technology is a mode of revealing—coming to presence in the sphere where revealing takes place, where truth happens (p. 13).

Still, what makes a technology moral or truthful? Computers, ventilators, or robots are only as truthful as the people who construct or program them. Engineers, as yet, have not created real intelligence. To reconcile the problem between technological presence and co-responsibility, subjectivity and objectivity, instrumentality and human activity, Ratzinger (2007) claimed that the key dimension is conscience. Conscience asserts the right of subjectivity (the individual person) over objectivity (detachment from the individual) because there is a voice within an individual. It asserts that something is given to each of us. It belongs to our essence; internally, each individual has a knowledge of good and evil that requires understanding of relationship, willingness, intentionality, formation, education, and judgment. Thus, conscience is the ultimate ethical quality of humanness; and, as Roach (2002) declared, as one her six C's of caring, conscience is imperative in nursing. Engaging with computers or other technologies (such as simulated patients and robots), either developing, programming, or using them for nursing practice, always will be a challenge in terms of ethical meaning. There is a fundamental commitment to the new technological reality, and thus, commitment to understanding how meaning is revealed in all human-humanoid activity.

Ethical Formation

To respond to this notion of commitment, the ethicist MacIntyre (1981) stated that humans are formed primarily by stories and metaphors: "We become through our history, tellers of stories that aspire to truth" (p. 20). Stories help us to discover the reality that gives expression to our commitments (Knowlden, 1990; Smith & Liehr, 1999). As a moral caring agent, a wounded healer, the nurse is an interpreter of meaning of the patient's story in the nursing situation. The story is often of fear, pain, or dying; and often it is of moral trauma, chaos, and confusion because of life circumstances such as sexual abuse, family breakdown, drug and alcohol addiction, and so forth. In her book *The Suffering Human Being*, Eriksson (2006) stated that we can try to eliminate suffering, alleviate it, or find its meaning. While trying to eliminate or alleviate suffering through medication and healing therapies, the nurse and the patient often find possibilities for transformation in and through interpretation of the meaning of suffering within the context of religion. Suffering is infused with a divine purpose, the idea of the ultimate Good. Thus, in a Christian sense, suffering is considered a mystery and is used for redemptive purposes or for eternal reward, recognizing that divine love alone gives meaning to life (Eriksson, 1994/2006; Ray, 1998). From a Jewish standpoint, Roach (2002), quoting Victor Frankl (who endured the Holocaust), pointed out that misery or agony can be a call to a person's liberty and that the act of freedom itself can be capable of transforming suffering, of investing it with meaning. From a Muslim perspective, giving meaning to suffering is understood within the belief of *inshallah*; that is, priority always given to God's will (Jaoudi, 1993). The creative and transforming act of interpreting the meaning of the patient's story synthesizes the nurse's ethical responsibility to the patient.

Conversely, some actions of the nurse may not be ethically responsible. Some may seem to be immoral on the surface, or the morality of the nurse in the situation may be in question. Sometimes a nurse's action may be impossible to fully discern; however, underlying everything that a nurse does, there is something significant in terms of what is happening in the world of the complex and dynamic nursing situation, and in the moral community of a health care organization. Whether or not there are extenuating circumstances in nursing practice, as a professional, the nurse (at all times) is ethically responsible for the lives of others.

The Ethical Demand of Caring

The ethical demand of caring is an intimate portrait of copresence and love (Ray, 1981, 1997; Watson, 2005). Levinas (1981), the Russian/French philosopher, used the metaphor "face to face"; and Logstrup (1997), the Danish ethicist, used the metaphor of "holding another person's life in one's hand" to reveal the intimate portrait of copresence and love as ethical responsibility for the other (Watson, 2005). Using the metaphors of face to face and holding another person's life in one's hand, the force of emotional power in the caring moment is revealed and gives direction to the life world experience.

As an ethical and spiritual meeting place, the caring moment (Watson, 2005) is a dialogical encounter within which a nurse and a patient bring their whole beings, revealing their genuine selves (Buber, 1965). This genuineness first uncovers strong emotions through the presence of each other. The nurse and the patient read the story of each other, the story where compassion, love, joy, trust, and faith, or the opposite—fear, anger, distrust, disgust or even hate—are disclosed. In a sense, the caring moment makes a demand before either nurse or patient has the absolute freedom to affirm or deny what is happening in the relationship. We have already experienced, through copresence and through our feelings and senses, a truth: the wholeness of self and other.

Although many philosophers of ethics have not claimed the emotions as a significant factor in ethical conduct (Fry, 1990), we see that emotions play a major role in the nurse ethical caring relationship. By seeing the other face to face and having a sense of holding the person's life in one's hand, there is instant recognition—a direct apperception or intuitive recognition of the truth of the relationship, the intricacy of feelings prior to the responsibility to and for the other. If the nurse is committed to holism (body, mind, and spirit), the exposure places a nurse and a patient in a human-spiritual realm, a connection where there is a living relationship between goodness and the transcendent Good, a dynamic unity. As Buber (1965) stated in his book *Between Man and Man*, this unity is a mystery that is both hidden and revealed at the same time. In other words, the nurse who believes in holistic nursing and is engaged in a compassionate "we" relationship, through caring presence, helps to bring the patient to his or her own unity of meaning, an understanding of the meaning of what is happening, body, mind, spirit. The compassionate "we," then, is an emotional and intellectual force. Its power, ethical responsibility, determines the direction of the life world for the one caring and the one cared for. The unity experienced by the emotional power of presence thus transforms the nursing situation or the caring moment. Responsibility with and for each other becomes evident and symbolizes deep meaning, both human and spiritual.

To explain this situation more fully, according to Levinas (1981), we are exposed beings; in a sense, this exposure is at first passive. When we are present with another, we expose the truth of our being; there is the exposure of the self to the other and vice versa *prior* to any decision. As exposed human beings, we communicate who we are; we are always in the language of relationship, the language of authenticity. This language reveals each person's own feelings of the joy and compassion or pain, agony, and suffering and is especially evident when a nurse sees the other (the patient) in pain, agony, and suffering. The genuineness of the dialogic encounter thus causes strong emotions in someone reading the story of the encounter; they can be sympathy, trust, joy, even love; or fear, anger, distrust, disgust, even hate. As a consequence, the nurse who is responsible in the caring moment may know about the positive elements of caring in the presence of the other but at the same time feel the emotions of, for example, fear, disgust, horror, embarrassment, or guilt (Taylor, 1985). The emotional power always conveys a moral stance. Even if nurses have not appreciated or recognized the intrinsic wholeness of the other and the force of the emotions that may motivate a nurse to struggle, err, or become negligent, nurses know that they are answerable to the other. When the compassionate response falls short of full engagement with the other, ethical problems emerge. Central to this presentation are the following:

Moral conflict is defined as blurring of nursing values of compassion, respect, and patient dignity maintenance based upon dimensions of the meaning of the wounded healer. Varied emotions, virtues, and behaviors appear when nurses encounter complex patients, families, the moral community, and even diverse technological or economic interventions. Reconciliation of moral conflict requires acknowledgement of the constant struggle of nurses, who are responsible for authentic ethical caring in nursing practice, by first recognizing nurses as wounded healers—professionals who experience pain and suffering not only in others, but also in the self and in the whole moral community during the ethical decision-making process.

Moral distress is defined as confusion about accepting or seeking understanding of the way of being of a patient or how a patient behaves. Reconciliation of moral distress requires acknowledging feelings and engaging in moral interactions to analyze problems and find creative ways to deal with the comportment of the other to support good health and facilitate the well-being of the moral community.

Moral paradox is defined as being compassionate and morally repulsed at the same time. In this situation, one knows that one should be compassionate but chooses to be "morally blind"; or one does not want to know the patient, or the painful or violent history of a person in a challenging nursing situation. Reconciliation of moral paradox is integration and acceptance of one's own feelings and suffering over not wanting to know a patient or the circumstances of why a patient is admitted. Reconciliation means seeking understanding through authentic dialogue with members of the moral community so that transformation can take place in the lives of the self, patients, and other professionals.

When the ethical caring relationship is tense and irreconcilable in the caring moment, the nurse begins to experience his or her own suffering, misery, agony, and pain. The nurse may show contempt for the suffering of the patient by fleeing interiorly and treating the patient as an object. The actual pain of the moral trauma prevents the nurse from infusing the relationship with meaning. Meaning, however, is being revealed. To help in understanding this idea of the revelation of meaning in the dialogical encounter of the caring moment, Logstrup (as cited in Watson, 2005) stated the following:

> *By our value/attitude to the other person we help to determine the scope and hue of his/her world; we make it larger or smaller, bright or drab, rich or dull, threatening or secure. We help to shape his world not by theories and views but by our very being and attitude [feeling] toward him. Herein lies the unarticulated and one might say anonymous demand that we take care of life which trust has placed in our hands. (Watson, 2005, p. 184)*

This revelation of the sheer thought of being there with the patient must motivate us to act ethically responsibly on behalf of the other.

Ethical Caring Nursing Situations in Practice

The following nursing situations reflect actual practice examples. Colleagues were very willing to share ethical struggles they encountered while caring for patients who are not so picture perfect. One participant shared, "We are never given a

chance to talk about ethical issues and nursing practice other
than learning about the Code of Ethics in school." Working
in an urban hospital setting with a vulnerable, underserved
patient population is the practice reality for these participants
and their peers. In the hospital, the professional practice
framework is Watson's Theory of Human Caring. Although
the nursing situations are defined as moral conflict, moral
distress, and moral paradox, the domains are not mutually
exclusive. At times, the moral issues and resolutions overlap.
The moral concerns and struggles arise because the registered nurses are caring, yet they are humans with their own
emotions, experiences, and frames of reference.

(The actual names of the nurses are used in the following
stories to honor each of them for their willingness to share
their experiences as professional nurses working in challenging practice settings. All quotes in the case studies are
from personal interviews conducted in 2008.)

Moral Conflict

Maryann Malloy, RN, MSN, neonatal intensive care unit
(NICU), shared her experience of caring for infants born to
mothers who have a history of drug addiction. The mothers
are addicted to either prescription medications or illegal
street drugs. At times, they have been in a treatment program
and are taking methadone. No matter the source or circumstances, registered nurses working in the NICU face ethical
conflicts when caring for the infant while establishing a
relationship with the mother. As the infant is in the process
of withdrawal, the infant's cry is constant and high pitched.
Maryann expressed the ethical caring:

> *It rips your heart out; you know the infant is hurting but you*
> *can't fix it. We become very attached to the infants, carrying*
> *and comforting them. They love to be carried and enjoy con-*
> *stant movement, so often we rock them in a chair. Usually,*
> *they stay in the unit for 2 weeks to 2 months. We become*
> *much attached; the nurses who care for these "special babies"*
> *really love them.*

Not every registered nurse is able to care for this type of
infant. The nurses who cannot are those who experience
ethical conflicts with the mother's choice making and who

cannot establish a relationship with the mother. Maryann shared the following:

> *These infants have skin breakdown because of the chemical excrement in their stool and urine. They require constant changing. When the mothers come in, they feel the nurses are causing the baby pain and think the nurses are looking at them funny or talking about them. Their behavior is a combination of drug paranoia and mommy guilt.*

In this nursing situation, the nurses are conflicted because they know the cause of the infant's pain is the mother's addiction. Knowing this makes it difficult to be compassionate toward the mother and see her as a caring person.

Registered nurses who choose to care and love the infants resolve their ethical conflict with the mother. Maryann explained,

> *We may need to set boundaries, and mothers with drug-seeking behaviors are not good with authority, so this can be challenging. As we form a relationship with the mother, a bond of trust is created and they share more. Some of the stories make your head turn. They tell you about trips to the street to buy drugs, how they cheated during their treatment, or the personal experience of going through methadone withdrawal to come clean. So as we are bonding with the mother, we are also conflicted, knowing she will be taking her baby home.*

Another ethical conflict that arises is the disconnection or lack of knowledge about what happens after the infant is born. When the infant is born, the mother thinks the infant is perfect. The registered nurses know the harsh reality of the withdrawal process: the signs and symptoms can start any time in the first 5 days of life, though we typically begin to see the symptoms around day 2. Breast-feeding presents an ethical conflict. Depending on the drug, the evidence says it is acceptable to breast-feed; however, the pumped breast milk is not able to be tested for drugs. If a mother chooses to breast-feed upon discharge, we support the mother's decision but still worry about the infant.

All of the registered nurses working in the NICU become very attached to the "special babies." The Department of Human Services almost always clears them to go home because the mother is clean or getting clean. However, Maryann expressed the following: "We worry if they can stay clean. Often their significant other is still involved. We know the surroundings they are going home to and are very concerned if they can handle the peer pressure."

The day an infant is discharged is full of emotion. Registered nurses are happy to see that the infant is physically able to be discharged, but as Maryann stated,

> *It is still hard for us. We worry about what will happen and don't want to read about our infant in the paper or see something in the news. Often, the mothers are so attached that they will call us on the third or fourth day post-discharge to say everything is OK or to ask us questions about feeding. Some even bring in pictures or baby albums for us to see. All of this is very rewarding. At times, we are conflicted, especially when the parents do not know where they will live and need to depend on the Woman, Infants and Children program for food. I remember one time, a mother called 1 to 2 months post-discharge because she had no money, so I gave her formula from our closet.*

In closing, Maryann reflected on how the caring and love made a difference for an infant girl and her family. She shared this personal experience (I remember this little girl from 4 years ago; she was in the unit for 3 months):

> *Mom was on a program. It was the worst baby I have ever seen, born at 35 weeks. We worked with the mother to leave her environment. The mother and father made a personal decision to come clean together. They rented a small apartment and left the neighborhood. The mother sends us pictures of this happy beautiful girl. This makes it all worth while and is what NICU nursing is all about.*

Moral Distress

Gene Spross, RN, BSN; and June Smith, RN, BSN, shared their personal experiences with Denise (assumed name). Denise is a well-known patient to their particular hospital. She has been a patient on and off for the past 10 years. She has a history of drug abuse, asthma, and COPD. Because of her manipulative personality and history of stealing belongings, Denise was always admitted to various nursing units. The moral distress of caring for her was exhausting and frustrating to many registered nurses. A solution was to rotate units and nurses every time the patient was admitted to the hospital. As time went by, June and Denise formed a "professional" relationship. When June was a staff nurse, she began to develop a trusting relationship with Denise. Now June is a clinical manager and Denise has found a home. She is always admitted to June's unit, and other registered nurses working on the floor have come to know and understand her as a person.

June's reflection on coming to know and understand Denise follows:

> When I first met her 10 years ago, she was addicted to street drugs, and this caused her to have a very manipulative personality. At times, she was nice and sweet and would say, Yes, ma'am. Next, she would be screaming and yelling. She knew just how to push the right buttons to send the nurses out of control.

Denise's personality caused such emotional and ethical/moral distress for the nurses that according to June, "No one wanted to care for her. However, we had no choice. As nurses we had to care for her, so she was moved from floor to floor." Denise's behavior of stealing belongings from other patients and even the gift shop contributed to the moral distress. According to June, "We knew she was doing it and assumed she was selling the items to support her drug habit."

June continued with her story:

> No one wanted to care for her. For the first few days, she would be quiet; but as soon as she was able to breathe better, she became more abusive. I remember one day she was discharged and the doctor wrote her a prescription for a controlled substance. First she told us the doctor did not give her the prescription. Then she said she lost it and refused to leave the floor until the doctor gave her a new prescription. We all knew she would fill the second prescription and sell the drugs on the street, but we did not say it. When the doctor refused to write a second

prescription, she tried to make me angry. Denise told me I was fat and ugly and should do something about my hair. I chose to listen in silence and not respond.

No nurse could deal with her for long time periods. We always put Denise in a private room so she would not steal from her roommate. One admission she even took a plant from the visitors lounge. I began to treat her with courtesy and respect, set rules and boundaries, and involved her in the plan of care. When she became short of breath, I placed oxygen on her. When she became stronger and left the floor to start to roam, I called security and she knew I knew what was happening.

I started taking care of her 2 or 3 days in a row, and she started to trust me. I would say, I know you are upset, but this is what needs to be done for you. In the past, she would bring in pills and then accuse us of taking her pills. I did a valuables form immediately on admission and counted the pills in front of her. We continued to build a relationship and she trusted me.

June was promoted to clinical manager and no longer served as Denise's primary nurse. The experienced nurses learned how to care for Denise, but she still liked to use insulting language to fluster novice nurses. June's story continued:

I remember one weekend, Denise was trying to get what she wanted with a new nurse and was really performing. By now, Denise was in a rehabilitative program and was receiving methadone in the hospital. A novice nurse was caring for her and as she went to give her the methadone pill, she spilled water on the floor. The nurse left to get equipment to clean the spill and left the methadone in the room. Denise promised to take it, but later the nurse heard Denise tell her son that she "played a trick on the nurse and still had the pill." The nurse felt her trust with Denise was violated.

Our hospital policy is to never leave medications in a patient's room. We all agreed not to be distracted by possible tricks while administering medications. A few days later, Denise tried to play the same game with an experienced nurse, whom she trusted and had formed a relationship with. The nurse refused to leave the medications in the room and Denise became verbally abusive with the nurse. However, later she came and apologized to the nurse. We have made a difference. The last time Denise was admitted to the unit, she was hot and wanted a fan. I borrowed one from my manager's office, and the day she was discharged she returned it to me. This was a major accomplishment in my eyes!

Moral Paradox

The concept of moral paradox is revealed in the following nursing situations. A group of registered nurses discussed the practice realities of caring for patients who are either in police custody or have been involved in suspect activity that is being investigated. Although it may be easier to not know the circumstances that brought the patient to the hospital, it is impossible not to see the policeman with the patient, hear information on the news, or read a story in the newspaper.

One could also say that not coming to know the patient as a person is a form of moral blindness. However, part of ethical caring for patients means hearing their experiences, questioning why they choose to be involved in illegal activity, and then struggling to resolve ethical dilemmas while providing care to this patient population.

Benita McCann, RN, BSN, has worked for 8 years in the surgical intensive care unit (SICU). She shared the following:

What my patients did on the outside doesn't matter to me. I treat all my patients the same, regardless if they are a VIP, CEO, or homeless. It is difficult when we have the victim and perpetrator in the unit at the same time. You know, it is hard when the victim doesn't do well.

As the conversation evolved, Benita explained how she provided care to her patients and experienced ethical struggles:

The patient is in need, so I take care of him. I listen; I don't ask—it is not my place. I hope they can turn their life around. It is difficult: you hear what they did on the outside and the action was bad, evil, or even heartless. Yet they are in bed being polite and showing their human side, and I show it back to them. I question why it happened, but I can't change what happened. I am not here to judge as they share their side of the story. My patient is in need and I give the care, but my emotional attachment may not be as strong.

Benita reflected on how her presence may have a small impact with the patient:

I look for the good. I try to maintain belief. My colleagues are the same. Some of the circumstances surrounding why they are in the hospital stop your heart, but we don't judge. When we have a patient in the unit who shot an officer, it is almost surreal; it is a true disregard for authority. If this is a real issue for a nurse, we can change the assignment. We provide emotional support to each other and give breaks to allow the nurse time away from the bedside.

Karen Niewood, RN, SICU, related personal experiences of what it is like to hear stories of patients wanting to get even or seek revenge or caring for patients who are her son's age. She shared the following:

When we know the circumstances surrounding the shooting, we will restrict visitors. Often, the patient is intubated and unable to communicate. However, as he gets better, I have heard a patient say, this is not going without punishment. I will follow up.

Hearing a patient say this is an ethical dilemma. Nurses wonder, Does he mean it? Is it a way of being street tough, or will he really do it?

Many of the nurses Karen works with experience frustration with the reality of nonstop violence. She explained,

A patient will come in after being shot, and we all show them compassion when they are sick, but the frustration starts. You hope and want them to go home, but you wonder. Will it happen again? Is the home environment really safer? It seems as though the violence is worse than ever, and the injuries more severe. It is sad. The patients are so young."

Karen acknowledged that working with the SICU patient population can be a very stressful experience for nurses. This is especially true when caring for a perpetrator of a violent crime on a police officer who has been shot. "Nurses helping other nurses, being there to let each other talk, and giving each other a break makes a difference. It is harder to open up to outsiders who have not had the experience," Karen said.

Vickie Jackson, RN, BSN, manager; and Gina Daniel, RN, BSN, clinical manager of Tower 4, shared their understanding of the paradox of moral blindness. Tower 4 is a forty-eight bed medical surgical unit. Patients on this unit are, at times, in police custody. This means a policeman with a loaded gun is in the room at all times. According to Vickie, "We would prefer not to know what the patient did to have police custody, but the reality is you know it is a violent crime." This is a true ethical conflict for nurses as they balance the practice reality of the crime committed, the possible personal threat or danger, and the ethical need to care for the patient. Vickie and Gina both expressed, "On Tower 4 – the rule is 'we care – no matter what.' But often, nurses close their heart and become detached because the experience is so emotionally draining and can wear you down. Our role is to help nurses keep their morale up."

Caring for this patient population presents a "shattered practice reality" that is rarely discussed. Registered nurses have a moral obligation to provide care and many strive to do so in a compassionate manner. Police officers have a moral obligation to society and need to keep the staff, visitors and other patients safe. At times, their behavior towards "a patient" resembles behavior towards "a prisoner." Registered Nurses witness this with mixed feelings. The behavior of the officers is often perceived as brutal, yet the registered nurses know the harsh reality of their world, working the streets, and dealing with violence on a daily basis. Attempting to reconcile this dichotomy is an ethical struggle and one that is not talked about in ethical case studies or experienced by many registered nurses in practice.

Conclusions in Ethical Nurse Caring for the 'Not-so-picture-perfect patient'

The dynamic interactions of co-presence and compassion as love shape the direction of the life of ethical caring and decision-making in the life of the not-so-picture-perfect patient in a complex hospital organization. In any organization, the ethical caring of patients and others is determined first by presence and being there for the patient, second, by individual beliefs, values and attitudes and emotions, and third by the moral interactions of nurses, physicians, families, administrators and other professionals in the moral community (Watson, 2005; Ray, 1987; 1994, 1998). The ethics of responsibility for the other is the focus of nurse caring ethics. Meaning emerges from experience and moral interaction—the synthesis of presence, compassion (love), emotions, spiritual insight, reason, and dialogue in the moral community. Ethical responsibility as the ground of caring in complex nursing interactions often brings forth moral distress, moral conflict, and moral paradox in terms of one's responsibility to the other. If, by our presence we see a person face to face; if we hold a person's life in our hands; if we are to direct the care of another; that is, to be ethically responsible for the other, what do we do? Do we feel compassion for, love for, and commitment to the other? Or do we feel bad and fearful, not wanting to care or wanting the patient to just go away? Nurses in many clinical environments are conflicted; they agonize over patients and their ethical responsibilities to care and to have compassion for people who cause so much pain and suffering to others or who are victims of their own bad decisions. Nurses fall victim to moral challenges that demand responsibility and reconciliation of moral distress, moral conflict, and moral paradox. The stories/case studies above illuminated the moral trauma and chaos that many nurses encounter when they are in the presence of difficult patients. The stories, however, not only illuminated the ethical dilemmas, but also provided compassionate and reasonable problem solving. Many implications for nursing, medicine, other professionals (such as the police), and health care systems have emerged and laid the foundation for additional ways to establish transformative covenants with patients and professionals in the moral community.

Implications for Nursing Practice

Following the exposition of moral dilemmas in the stories/ case studies, emotions played a significant role in moral interactions. As we understood at the outset of this presentation, morality, although difficult to define, helps us recognize and understand how we ought to live in the moral community. Ethics and morality as significant in nurse caring and within the sphere of nursing practice is an ethical mandate of moral responsibility for the other. The ultimate goal of the ethics of responsibility in nursing is the unity of the I-Thou relationship (Buber, 1965); that is, seeking understanding of the meaning of the good in one's own life and in the lives of others. Due to the many challenges in nursing practice, in reality, the I-Thou relationship often shows itself more as an I-it relationship—an objectifying of the patient or others rather than engaging in an intimate, compassionate, we relationship. The moral conflict, moral distress, and moral paradox of the nurse caring relationship expressed in the stories reveals how critical it is to create a moral community with genuine dialogue.

An authentic caring practice environment manifesting participatory decision making must be cocreated (Turkel & Ray, 2004). First nurses need to engage in self-care. Helping nurses to meditate and center, participate in exercise, engage in reflective writing or journaling, or use art as a medium of expression will release the emotions that may be pent up in relation to moral trauma in nursing practice. Second, nurses need to have the opportunity to be involved in caring dialogues with other nurse clinicians, administrators, and physicians to understand the burdens and joys associated with caring and being responsible for patients who are not so picture perfect. Third, frequent meetings and debriefing sessions that emphasize openness, flexibility, and dialogue about the meaning of caring, expressions of positive and negative feelings, and the potential for change within the moral community on different units in the organization should be encouraged. Fourth, extending hands to other participants, such as social workers or police officers, should be facilitated. Interdisciplinary teams of nurses, physicians, administrators, other professionals, and even some patients should be part of the caring dialogue.

Cocreating the Ethical Caring Dialogue

Ethical caring is cocreated by interaction of the moral community. It is necessary that continuing innovative educational opportunities be available and become a forum for participation and sharing to understand the complexity of

nursing, especially as ethical caring; that is, being responsible for the direction of the lives of others. Engaging in relationship building and listening to the stories of nurses and
other professionals will advance understanding of how the
people within the moral community think about and practice ethical caring. This type of listening and communication,
in contrast to teaching codes of ethics or just "knowledge
dumping" (Rollnick, Miller, & Butler, 2007), will not only
transform the organizational culture but also encourage
commitment to cocreate new caring practices that will allow
continual transformation to take place.

Another vital activity to cocreate a caring dialogue is
mentorship. Knowledge enhancement and nurturing of the
caregiver can be achieved through one-on-one communication and assistance. Each registered nurse should have
a peer, clinical nurse manager, or administrator as a guide
to facilitate direction. Mentors provide the face-to-face
support and the holding of one's colleague in one's hands,
similar to the ethical directive for nurses caring for patients.
As we have experienced in this presentation, nurses need
help with their own woundedness, their own suffering, pain,
anguish, and agony, and even the joy of caring for patients.
Thus, ethical caring relationships based on good mentoring
are essential to nurturing each other and cocreating healing
and caring practice environments. The recommendations of
a caring dialogue can facilitate a healthy workplace, caring
environment, and moral community within which to work
and practice nursing.

Preparing for the Future

The virtual world of robotics, patient simulation laboratories, and other technologies is continuously being advanced
to help provide care in the moral community. Although this
world is not a reality in all practice settings, it is advancing
rapidly. When reflecting on the future of nursing practice and
the development of the human-humanoid relationship, it is
necessary to give pause for thought in terms of the meaning
of moral commitment or its opposite nonmoral interaction. We
have dealt with the question of whether a robot can be moral
and came to the conclusion that it is subjective conscience
that answers the question. In the virtual world, when dealing
with computers and robots, we, as nurses, will always have to

question how a computer or a robot is programmed, be aware of who may have programmed it, and know what is programmed. We must remember that a robot cannot tell human stories that aspire to truth. Only humans can tell stories and at the same time hear the voice within that distinguishes good from evil, bear witness to suffering, facilitate choices, and make ethical judgments in nursing practice. Therefore, only humans can respond authentically and compassionately to the call, as in face-to-face encounters that have been shared in this presentation of the ethics of caring in the moral community of the hospital.

References

American Nurses Association. (2001). *Code of ethics for nurses with interpretive statements.* Washington, DC: Author.

Barnard, A. & Locsin, R, (Eds.). (2007). *Technology and nursing: Practice, concepts and issues.* United Kingdom: Palgrave McMillan.

Beidler, S., & Chase, S. (2007). Ethical implications of technology on the patient-nurse interaction. In A. Barnard & R. Locsin (Eds.), *Technology and nursing: Practice, concepts and issues* (pp. 41–59). United Kingdom: Palgrave McMillan.

Boykin, S., & Schoenhofer, S. (2001). *Nursing as caring: A model for transforming practice.* Sudbury, MA: Jones and Bartlett.

Buber, M. (1958). *I and Thou.* New York: Charles Scribner's Sons.

Buber, M. (1965). *Between man and man.* New York: Macmillan.

Campling, A., Tanioka, T., & Locsin, R. (2007). Robots and nursing: Concepts, relationship and practice. In A. Barnard & R. Locsin (Eds.), *Technology and nursing: Practice, concepts and issues* (pp. 73–90). United Kingdom: Palgrave McMillan.

Carper, B. (1978). Fundamental patterns of knowing in nursing. *Advances in Nursing Science 1*, 1–13.

Canadian Nurses Association. (2002). *Code of ethics for registered nurses.* In M. Burkhardt & A. Nathaniel (2008). *Ethical issues in contemporary nursing* (3rd ed.). New York: Thomson Delmar Learning.

Davis, A. (1990). Are there limits to caring: Conflict between autonomy and beneficence. In M. Leininger (Ed.), *Ethical and moral dimensions of care* (pp. 25–32). Detroit: Wayne State University Press.

Eriksson, K. (1994/2006). *The suffering human being* (K. Olsson & C. Peterson, Trans.). Chicago: Nordic Studies Press.

Fry, S. (1990). The philosophical foundations of caring. In M. Leininger (Ed.), *Ethical and moral dimensions of care* (pp. 13–24). Detroit: Wayne State University.

Gadow, S. (1988). Covenant without cure: Letting go and holding on in chronic illness. In J. Watson & M. Ray (Eds.), *The ethics of care and the ethics of cure: Synthesis in chronicity,* (pp. 5–14). New York: National League for Nursing.

Gadow, S. (1989). Clinical subjectivity: Advocacy with silent patients. *Nursing Clinics of North America, 24*, 535–541.

Griffin, A. (1983). A philosophical analysis of caring in nursing. *Journal of Advanced Nursing, 8,* 289–295

Heidegger, M. (1977). *The question concerning technology and other essays* (W. Lovitt, Trans.). New York: Harper & Row.

Jaoudi, M. (1993). *Christian and Islamic spirituality.* New York: Paulist Press.

Knowlden, V. (1990). The virtue of caring in nursing. In M. Leininger (Ed.), *Ethical and moral dimensions of care* (pp. 89–94). Detroit: Wayne State University Press.

Leininger, M., & McFarland, M. (Eds.). (2005). *Culture diversity and universality: A worldwide theory of nursing* (2nd ed.). Sudbury, MA: Jones and Bartlett.

Levinas, E. (1981). *Otherwise than being or beyond essence* (A. Lingis, Trans.). The Hague: Martinus Nijhoff.

Locsin, R. (Ed.). (2005). *Technological competency as caring in nursing: A Model for practice.* Indianapolis: Sigma Theta Tau International Press.

Logstrup, K. (1997). *The ethical demand.* Notre Dame: University of Notre Dame Press.

MacIntyre, A. (1981). *After virtue.* Notre Dame: University of Notre Dame Press.

Nouwen, H. (1979). *The wounded healer.* New York: Image Books.

Pelligrino, E. (1985). The caring ethic: The relation of physician to patient. In A. Bishop & J. Scudder (Eds.), *Caring, curing, coping: Nurse, physician, patient relationships* (pp. 8–30). Alabama: University of Alabama Press.

Rachels, J. (2003). *Elements of moral philosophy* (4th ed.). New York: Random House.

Ratzinger, J. (2007). *On conscience.* San Francisco: Ignatius Press.

Ray, M. (1981). A philosophical analysis of caring in nursing. In M. Leininger (Ed.), *Caring : An essential human ingredient.* Thorofare, NJ; Slack.

Ray, M. (1987). Technological caring: A new model in critical care. *Dimensions of Critical Care Nursing, 6,* 166–173.

Ray, M. (1994). Communal moral experience as the research starting point for health care ethics. *Nursing Outlook, 42*(3), 104–109.

Ray, M. (1997). Illuminating the meaning of caring: Unfolding the sacred art of divine love. In M. Roach (Ed.), *Caring from the heart: The convergence of caring and spirituality* (pp. 163–178). New York: Paulist Press.

Ray, M. (1998). A phenomenologic study of the interface of caring and technology in intermediate care: Toward a reflexive ethics for clinical practice. *Holistic Nursing Practice, 12*(4), 69–77.

Ray, M. (2007). Technological caring as a dynamic of complexity in nursing practice. In A. Barnard & R. Locsin (Eds.), *Technology and nursing: Practice, concepts, and issues* (pp. 174–190). United Kingdom: Palgrave McMillan.

Roach, M. (2002). *Caring, the human mode of being* (2nd rev. ed.). Ottawa: Canadian Hospital Association Press.

Rollnick, S., Miller, W., & Butler, C. (2007). *Motivational interviewing in health care: Helping patients change behavior (Applications of motivational interviewing).* New York: Guilford Press.

Schultz, P., & Schultz, R. (1990). Noddings' caring and public policy: A linkage and its nursing implications. In M. Leininger (Ed.), *Ethical and moral dimensions of care* (pp. 81–87). Detroit: Wayne State University Press.

Smith, B. (1998). *On the origin of objects.* Cambridge, MA: MIT Press.

Smith, M., & Liehr, P. (1999). Attentively embracing story: A middle range theory with practice and research implications. *Scholarly Inquiry for Nursing Practice, 13*(3), 3–27.

Taylor, G. (1985). *Pride, shame, and guilt: Emotions of self-assessment.* Oxford: Clarendon Press.

Turkel, M., & Ray, M. (2004). Creating a caring practice environment through self-renewal. *Nursing Administration Quarterly, 28*(4), 249–254.

Watson, J. (2005). *Caring science as sacred science.* Philadelphia: FA Davis.

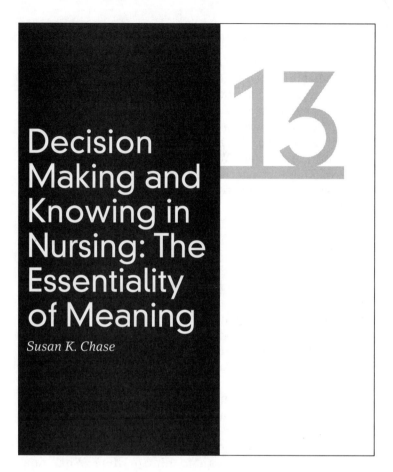

Decision Making and Knowing in Nursing: The Essentiality of Meaning

Susan K. Chase

Chapter Overview

Nurses engage in assisting persons with health concerns in a wide range of settings, from critical care units and acute care hospitals to long-term-care residential, home, and community settings. Nurses engage in a range of activities that may involve the use of sophisticated technology as well as attending to daily concerns such as diet, sleep, medication management, progressive activity, and safety; and providing health-related teaching, direct care, and comfort activities. They also work in the complex health care system with regulations and guidelines as well as standardized care systems and emerging technology.

How does an individual nurse know what to do for an individual patient in a particular moment? How does the nurse decide what information is important to know, what activities the patient needs, and how to communicate about that care? Is knowledge of anatomy and physiology or of medical-care approaches sufficient to direct nurses' activities? Nurses make decisions as part of their interactions with patients and the health care system. What thinking processes do nurses use in making those decisions? How do those thinking processes support the nurse in carrying out a contemporary nursing process?

Introduction

This chapter will present a view of the decision-making processes used by nurses as they care for patients. This chapter will also present a new look at the nursing process and will examine what happens when a nurse and a patient meet in space and time. Nurse thinking is guided by a series of questions. These include the following:

- Who is this person (the patient), and what does this health pattern mean to him or her? What is at stake for the patient?
- Who is this person (the nurse), and what does this health pattern mean to him or her? What does responding in caring as a nurse require of the nurse?
- Do the nurse and patient want the patient's health patterns to change, and if so, how?
- What will it take to achieve a chosen health pattern?
- Now that a new health pattern is established, what comes next?
- What aspects of this process can and should be documented?

The chapter will argue that the important question is, What meaning is made during and after an encounter between a nurse and a patient? Further, the chapter will examine the conditions necessary for nursing decision making to occur and for nurses to grow in their abilities to nurse.

For the purposes of this chapter, the concept *patient* can mean an individual, a family, a group, or an entire community. This reflects the scope of nursing practice as delineated in Nursing's Social Policy Statement, published by the American Nurses Association (2003). Nurses from other countries may refer to their grounding documents but will likely find references to the recipients of nursing care as including all these elements.

The word *patient* is chosen purposely to reflect the waiting presence of the person entering an encounter with an expressed or unexpressed need to respond to an issue of health. According to Newman's definition (1986, 2008), health encompasses all the potentialities of function and dysfunction, comfort and pain, brokenness and healing, strength and weakness, connection and isolation, or hope and fear for a person who is whole in the moment. Patterns of persons or communities reveal the aspects of their wholeness. The nurse is also whole in the moment and reveals aspects of that wholeness through pattern. All persons (not only nurses and patients) relate in their wholeness, so how does the nursing encounter differ from an encounter that might happen between any two people?

Reconceptualizing Nursing Decision Making

Nursing is a profession that is granted by society access to the intimate spaces of other persons' lives for the purpose of accompanying them on journeys of wholeness, health, and healing: "Nursing does not exist to identify and solve problems; nursing exists to support human beings as they encounter human processes such as growing, developing, healing, recover[ing] and dying" (Chase, 1998, p. 63). The new view of nursing process is as a circle of (1) coming to know the wholeness of person and pattern in their complexity over time; (2) determining the meaning, intention, or directionality of the patient's wholeness; (3) choosing goals or outcomes as new directions; (4) designing activities and explorations for both nurse and patient that support chosen outcomes; and (5) coming to know the new state of being for nurse and nursed, which is a new first stage for the process to continue.

This circle of meaning making and decision making is repeated over and over again in cycles that are determined by the journey of the patient (see Figure 13.1). In a critical situation, the cycle might be repeated more than hourly; in acute care daily, and in a community setting, it might be a cycle of months between encounters. One of the decisions the nurse makes is how frequently to reenter the circle. Each step in the cycle requires meaning making and decision making.

13.1

Circle of meaning making in nursing © S. Chase, 2008

An ideal model that allows for this new way of understanding practice is a complexity science model. The complexity model recognizes that complex adaptive systems (which may be individuals or groups) relate in their wholeness, that they are open to influences from outside themselves, that they have self-correcting capacities, and that small changes in one part of the complex system can have unpredictable and large effects in the overall system. Complex systems are adaptive. They are engaged in movement and change, and they thrive because of their diversity (Lindberg, Nash, & Lindberg, 2008).

The nurse is unique in that he or she may be the only health care professional who systematically assesses the wholeness of the health care experience and takes into account the complex systems that characterize the patient's life process. Physicians use an empirical or problem-solving approach

to planning and delivering services. The·
system or cellular level of the person, a.
increasingly specialized in how they view
Therapists work to support a patient in regain.
strength and skill, and counselors work with pat.
meaning of life stress and to assist in pattern change
nurse takes into account the physiological, the function.
the meaning of a patient's journey simultaneously.

Working in nursing in the new way presented in th.
book requires a new view of decision-making processes and
a new commitment to understanding and supporting the
thinking of nurses. There are similarities, however, between
the old and the new processes, and complexity science is
large enough to hold multiple processes and realities. In the
new process, information is gathered and considered, actions
are taken, and new states of being evolve and can then come
to be known. The difference for this new view of process is
that it respects the wholeness and complexity of person and
context over time. It supports self-determining actions by
patients, be they individuals or communities, and it provides
for care that is focused on wholeness and wellness and not
on deficit or disease. The nurse is not the paternalistic, all-
knowing, powerful person who carries out activities against
the wishes of the patient, albeit "for the patient's own good."

The traditional nursing process begins with an assessment of the patient's condition (Yura & Walsh, 1967). Too often
this view focused on the identification of deficits or needs. In
contrast, Tanner, Benner, Chesla, and Gordon (1993) identified in a study designed to understand expertise in critical
care nursing that knowing the patient was a central idea.
They found that knowing involved both the pattern of the
patient's responses to the challenge of critical illness and the
pattern of knowing them as persons.

The knowing that provides for the new kind of nursing
exists not in the nurse but between the nurse and the patient.
So, on the surface, the nurse may appear to be collecting data,
choosing actions, and performing professional nursing activities with and for the patient, and documenting their effects;
but in reality a very different process is occurring. The nurse
comes to know the person in wholeness and complexity; the
nurse considers pattern and direction of events, considers
and offers options in redirecting pattern, and accompanies
the patient in taking steps to evolving pattern. The nurse

attentively adjusts care and support to the responses of the patient and is faithful to the patient, not abandoning the patient even if he or she does not choose options that lead to the nurse's preferred view of what is a healthy pattern. The new model allows for and extends caring theory to explicate not only the essence of nursing, but also its process. In this model, the nurse is present and invested in engaging actively in assisting patients to recover from illness events or to develop new patterns of health.

It is the underlying models of the old and new processes which differ. In the old model, the nurse identifies problems, makes decisions, and takes action to solve them. This has been the focus of the nursing process for decades. The focus is on the nurse's activities and presumes a linear causality. In the new model, the nurse still engages actively in responding to patient health concerns and patterns, but the nurse understands that the patient and the patient's life are continuing on their own path. There is power in the human encounter to recognize and change pattern, to form new meanings and purpose, and to emerge into a new state of health (Newman, 1986). The nurse is not solving problems but accompanying the patient and respecting the human capacity to grow and develop and to transcend loss and challenges in the evolution of life. The model is one not of linear causality but of complexity and change. The patient, the nurse, and the system in which they meet are all self-correcting systems. They are each open to the energy of the other and are constantly growing and changing.

Knowing and Meaning

For a nurse to respond to a patient in the patient's wholeness, the nurse must come to know the patient as a person and as a complex system. The nurse needs to consider simultaneously all the knowledge he or she has about the patient, which may include physiological data, knowledge of treatments and medications (including the individual patient's life/health story), and the knowledge the nurse has about the range of ways that humans respond to situations similar to those this particular patient is experiencing. For example, for a male patient who has experienced a cerebral vascular accident, the nurse needs to consider the path that the patient and his partner are taking to recovery or to redefining his life, taking into account changes in his physiological functioning. What will this mean for his partner, given their culture and values? What decisions must they make for rehabilitation and support? Attending to these questions as a central part of care will then assist the nurse in gathering or providing the support that the patient and partner need to move forward.

The level of knowing that we describe here is much deeper than a quick scan of a medical history. The illness or disability of a person is not the person's wholeness. The person may have an illness, but the knowing of wholeness requires knowing much more. This knowing that nursing requires involves attentiveness, persistence, sensitivity, and reflective understanding. It requires the use of the wholeness of the nurse. Nurses convey their understanding of who patients are in ways that are unique to each of their complex systems. The thinking process used is one of discernment, sorting possible meanings, thinking analogically, or using metaphor to characterize pattern.

Nurses know their patients directly. They know them from the wholeness of their own being. Nursing is physical. The feel of a person's skin becomes one element of pattern. If a nurse never touches the skin of a person and relies on data collection by delegated ancillary people, then the nurse does not know as much about that person as he or she might. In this time of nursing-unit complexity, the nurse may have to decide which of his or her patients requires direct knowing and for which the nurse can rely on secondary data. Physical touch and the capacity to provide physical comfort are important elements of nursing. The nurse who is overseeing a team of ancillary caregivers can still engage in knowing patients though touch, even while making surveillance visits to a bedside.

Nursing is intellectual. It requires understanding complex mechanisms of physiology, pathophysiology, pharmacology, psychology, anthropology, and sociology, and how those principles are working in the moment for a particular person. It requires the capacity to evaluate data and their meaning as a picture of the wholeness of the person emerges. Experienced nurses describe seeing how all the pieces fit together. Nurses are curious. Their commitment to nursing and to patients is fueled by deeper questions. What will this new treatment mean for the recovery of this kind of patient? What new nursing research illuminates ways of responding to health concerns? What is really going on with this patient? What kind of information will team members need in order to develop a good treatment plan?

Nursing is spiritual. Spirituality is concerned with the questions of life and its ultimate meaning. Nursing is ultimately concerned with the meaning of the human condition. What does this illness mean in the course of the patient's life? What will assist this person in engaging in health behaviors that will change the direction of his or her life? How are these health events related to earlier life events? What are the patient's hopes and deepest fears? By considering these questions, all nursing may be considered spiritual caring.

Meaning is developed with regard to patients' health on a continuous basis by attentive nurses. There are variations in the level of engagement that a nurse can choose. Patients who are progressing well in their recovery from an acute event will have energy to engage in progressive activity, will begin to make choices for themselves regarding care, will relate to staff and family members with strength and not with fragility, and will be open to asking for help when they need it. Patients who are focused on details of comfort and discomfort, who are fearful of participating in care, and who resist activities that will increase their strength reflect a different pattern of wholeness that indicates the need for the nurse to determine the meaning of their experience. Is the patient in pain? Is this only the most recent in a long series of health care system encounters that have progressively resulted in lost capacity to live as the patient would wish? Is the hospital setting the only place where humans offer care and support for this person, and therefore moving toward discharge is not the patient's goal? Or is the patient experiencing a physiological change that threatens his life? The nurse only knows what the patterns of data mean in the situation by pursuing a process of coming to know the patient and uncovering the meaning of the situation for all relevant parties. Without understanding the meaning of the moment, the nurse cannot decide how to proceed. Meaning is essential to decision making.

Nurses and patients together determine the meaning of the moment. A study designed to uncover processes of judgment in three different practice settings found common features of "the nurses' connection with the patient that contribute to nursing judgment" (Doona, Chase, & Haggerty, 1999, p. 55). The analysis revealed "that something more than how a nurse processed information was occurring. This gestalt was tentatively labeled *presence*" (p. 55). Elements of presence identified in this study included recognizing uniqueness, connecting with the patient's experience, sensing, going beyond the scientific data, knowing what will work, knowing when to act, and being with the patient.

This discussion of meaning making as an activity of the nurse, perhaps the central activity of the nurse, will serve as background for a more detailed examination of how this meaning making offers a new perspective on nurse decision making.

Processes of Decision Making

Simultaneous processes are difficult to describe in writing, which is by nature linear. This section will provide an overview of a new process of decision making that directs nursing activities—a process in which the actual processes may occur in a different order or even simultaneously. This model is reflective of Benner's view of expert practice (1984), and by intentionally focusing on its features, it may be possible to support students and practicing nurses to move to this level of expertise more efficiently than simply by waiting until the nurse has multiple years of experience.

Coming to Know the Wholeness of Person and Pattern in Their Complexity Over Time

The first moments of the nurse-patient encounter reveal the beginning elements of pattern. Ideas emerge as to what the pattern might entail. Based on knowledge and experience, the nurse simultaneously looks for expected patterns of responses and comes to know the patient as an individual. A hospitalized patient who had surgery will likely have pain-management concerns. Pain is a likely experience or fear of the patient, and it can affect the entire experience of healing. If the nurse learns that a patient's husband is under treatment for cancer, then the meaning of the patient's current illness might include fear, anticipatory grieving, or motivation to get back to full strength in order to be available to her husband. A picture of wholeness or what is happening starts to emerge.

When a nurse encounters a patient, the patient usually has some previously identified health issue, even if the current appointment is for a routine health screening. In most cases, something of the health issues of the person are identified based on admitting medical diagnoses, procedures, or statements of complaint. These initial ideas regarding health are not the end point in the nursing process; they are the beginning. The nurse must actively determine the pattern of response that the patient is exhibiting to the stated complaint or the identified medical diagnosis. The nurse must also determine if there are other, seemingly unrelated issues of concern to the patient that might affect healing and wholeness. Patients decide which providers they will trust and reveal themselves to. Patients are attentive to nurses, too. If a nurse keeps promises, is fully present, respects dignity, and is competent to provide comfort and solve problems, then the patient may choose to trust the nurse with more openness. Patients may have an intuitive sense of whom to trust, but demonstrable commitment to the whole person, on the part of the nurse, will support this openness. How does the nurse become trustworthy in this sense? The nurse is present, shares aspects of wholeness, and extends beyond routine tasks to meet the patient on the patient's health journey.

Data Elements

A systematic approach to data collection is useful in that it becomes a routine. On the surface, that might seem to be a return to the old model that we have been describing in coming to know individuals, but a systematic approach serves as a safety net so that important data elements are not recalled individually, placing a cognitive load on the nurse. By using a routine, one can transcend the process of data collection itself and reflect on the meaning of data that are being generated. Necessary data elements have been proposed by a number of sources. It is the professional nurse's responsibility to determine what elements are necessary for groups of patients under her care who have common experiences. Determining screening or monitoring data collection for nursing is not limited to physician orders on frequency of vital signs. In the new view of nursing process, the group of nurses decides together how to approach and record data regarding patients on a unit or in a practice. Appropriate data collection for an oncology unit would differ from that in an orthopedic unit or for a clinic in the community. Organization of data collection does not violate knowing and nursing the individual. The nurse is part of a complex system and needs to coordinate, direct, and participate in care activities that collaborate with other people. A unit staff might benefit from thoughtful reflection on what data each person finds important to track as they all come to know patients as people and to determine their progress in healing. Thoughtful systems that nurses are empowered to create provide a context in a complex system that supports growth in nurse knowing and caring.

One classic system of data collection for nursing is the Functional Health Pattern Assessment (Gordon, 1994). This system focuses on elements of human function and provides for collection of data that reflect patterns of the whole (see Table 13.1).

13.1 Data Elements for Nursing Judgment

Functional Health Patterns (Gordon, 1994)	Related Data Elements
Health Perception/Health Management	What do you do to stay healthy? Do you see yourself as healthy?
Nutrition/Metabolic	What is your usual dietary pattern?
Elimination	Any problems with urination or bowel function?
Activity/Exercise	What is your usual activity pattern? Any limitations? What are your preferences?
Sleep/Rest	Is your sleep restful? Are you easily tired?
Cognitive/Perceptual	How do you learn new things? Are you in any discomfort?
Self-Perception/Self-Concept	How would you describe yourself?
Role/Relationships	Who are the important people in your life? How about your pets?
Sexuality/Reproductive	Do you have any concerns about your sexuality?
Coping/Stress Tolerance	How do you relieve your stress?
Value/Belief	What is most important to you? What is the source of your strength? Do you have preferences for your care?

These data elements are not collected in order to determine specific deficits. This framework allows the nurse to come to know things about the persons that will help the nurse respond to the whole person under his or her care. It is possible that using such a data-collection tool can uncover health issues early in their process. For example, waiting until the patient complains of constipation as a problem before establishing a plan for bowel function support is not engaging in recognizing patterns as they are emerging. The patient may be surprised to see how much information the nurse collects because it extends beyond expectations. The patient who feels known in the otherwise impersonal health care system will benefit from the human connection made with the nurse. The nurse must seek out data to accurately characterize wholeness. What data are significant will depend upon the practice setting and the nature of the relationship. A basic decision that a nurse must make is the range and depth of data to collect in order to come to know the patient.

For clinical judgment to occur, data must be sought out, attended to, collected, processed, and recorded. The nurse is active in this search for data. Research into human decision making in general and nursing and medical diagnostic processes in particular has shown that the most efficient way to gather and process clinical data is through a hypothetico-deductive process. This process does not guarantee responsiveness to whole-person concerns. It can be used in a mechanical, objectifying way, but it does not need to be used that way. If the nurse is attentive to a wide range of data and considers a range of ways to come to know the person, then the hypotheses about the patient's situation contain elements that are reflective of wholeness.

The hypothetico-deductive model is useful because it allows nurses to consider how they are making meaning of the wide range of data that are presented to them in a nursing encounter. The model makes the assumption that human information processing has limits related to processing and memory. If data are considered as discrete elements with no relationships among them, then short-term memory of humans is limited to approximately seven items. If, however, humans cluster data, sometimes known as *chunking*, then vastly more data can be organized and considered (Chase, 2004). The very process of chunking requires meaning. There must be a reason that urine output and heart rate are considered together to determine a physiological pattern. The reason is both of the data bits' relationships to the concept of cardiac output. Nurse educators and leaders can review information-processing concepts with nurses in practice and encourage them to reflect on their decision-making processes.

The hypothetico-deductive model involves the systematic evaluation of data as they confirm or disconfirm specific hypotheses. The nurse might have "grieving" on a mental list of possible concerns for a female patient. As the nurse comes to know the patient, asking about the recent death of the patient's husband, its suddenness, its meaning to the patient, the nurse may find that the loss, while felt, has been accepted as part of the person's meaning of life. The patient may describe how she is reaching out to others for support and how her memories sustain her. The nurse no longer considers grieving a likely possibility for the patient. If, on the other hand, the patient cannot discuss her loss, appears disengaged, and is unable to participate in care, then it is more likely that exploring the meaning of her life now in her new circumstance would be an appropriate response.

The nurse looks for the "soft spots" not as deficits or problems, but as ways of coming to know the wholeness of person. A person who is absorbed in grief needs different kinds of support than a person who is proceeding in hope. Nurses risk errors in two different ways: first by not coming to know sufficiently even to recognize pattern, and second by failing to engage courageously in being present in human suffering. Naming a pattern of response such as grieving does not objectify or judge the patient. It provides a focus for caring.

Seeing wholeness of pattern is close to the model of intuition described by Benner (1984). Intuition is a way of seeing the whole of a situation. An intuitive model does not preclude a model that uses information processing. There are two ways in which these models connect. In the first, it is the expertise of the nurse that allows the processes of data collection and analysis to be transcended so that patterns of data being presented are matched with patterns of data that the expert has seen before. This pattern matching happens in a moment, and the expert nurse is unaware of the processes that occurred. The data evaluation and assembly is speeded though the use of heuristics, or rules of thumb, and the expert sees the wholeness of the situation in a moment.

Another view is that different kids of situations or problems require different kinds of processes. Evaluating a wound that has redness and pus does not require an existential analysis. What that wound infection means to the patient, however, requires deeper analysis. It might mean the necessity for more surgery or fear that the wound will never heal. Responding to the meaning for the patient will require deeper engagement by the nurse, but the care of the wound itself may proceed based on wound-care guidelines.

Determining the Meaning, Intention, or Directionality of the Patient's Wholeness

How the nurse assembles a picture of wholeness will vary by setting and nurse, but essential elements are maintaining openness to possible meanings of data patterns, a curious attitude, and a view of wholeness. Aside from evaluation of the meaning and pattern of specific data elements, the nurse attends to larger questions: Is this patient experiencing expected responses to the first course of chemotherapy, or are there subtle signs that things are not gong well? Does this patient look better today or worse? Does the patient have increasing strength and resilience, or is the patient drawing inward? Nurses need time to reflect on how data elements interact with each other to form patterns. The data collection and documentation system must allow them to see the data simultaneously so that possible elements can be compared and integrated. In critical care, the flow sheet serves this function, but nurses in every setting are assembling complicated sets of data, and understanding wholeness requires seeing how the pieces fit together.

Determining the meaning of a situation is an outcome of a process that occurs between the patient and nurse. Patients who are unconscious respond in their wholeness with changed physiological responses to the challenges of care, even of being turned in the bed, and meaning is made from the pattern of their responses to treatment and challenge. The nurse attends actively to determine the meaning of the health experience for the patient and develops a meaning of his or her own of the overall encounter. This meaning includes considering what is going on here and now and also what the likely possibilities are if this pattern continues. This list may include possible eventualities of which the patient may not be aware. Some of these eventualities might be valued by the patient, but others may be potentialities the patient would choose to avoid.

Directionality. Directionality is a concept that can be addressed using this new model of nursing process. The patient assessment is not an event that happens when the patient is admitted to a unit or a practice. Data elements from one point in time are not sufficient to know the patient's status and progress. What does one blood pressure reading mean by itself? Very little. The trend in the blood pressure readings, how stable or changeable they are, and what the direction of these changes might mean are essential to nursing practice using the new model. Critical care flow sheets allow for monitoring trends. Outside of critical care, electronic health records may make it possible to track trends in data. Expert nurses pay attention to trends in data because they reflect the direction of patient progress. This attention to change's speed and direction is characteristic of the expert thinker. It is a kind of calculus of care. Novice nurses will likely not automatically see these relationships, but experts who are teaching, mentoring, or leading neophyte practitioners can invite them to reflect on meaning in this way.

Goal Setting

Once a pattern of health state and direction begins to emerge, the next question that must be addressed is whether this direction is what the patient and/or nurse would choose. At this point, goals or outcomes can be identified. The health care system is moving to a deeper commitment to delivering specific outcomes of care. This is part of the complexity of the health care system in which the nurse works. For example, one of the goals determined for a patient with limited mobility is that she will not develop a pressure ulcer. Another goal might be that a patient will not develop a deep vein thrombosis. In a complexity model, there is room for these considerations simultaneously with a consideration of hope for recovery. The seemingly small thing of discussing a patient's best hopes for a future life might change the patient's interest and motivation for mobility, which in turn will result in better outcomes even for skin integrity or vascular function. The nurse using a complexity model understands these relationships.

The patient is involved in goal and outcome setting, which is a kind of mutual decision making between the nurse and the patient and family or community. In fact, the patient is the most important person in determining outcome. It does no good to push people who choose not to move. What the expert nurse does is determine what is at stake for the patient. A patient who is unconscious does not seem to participate directly in determining goals. Family members and loved ones can assist the nurse in knowing what the patient might have chosen for himself or herself.

These questions are particularly important when end-of-life considerations are involved (Hiltunen, Medich, Chase, Peterson, & Forrow, 1999). In a study of end-of-life decision making, nurses assisted family members in making decisions about life support and other issues for their loved ones. The nurses in the study described how they accompanied the families in a lengthy process of reviewing who their loved one was and what he or she valued. Not all decisions are of the same ultimacy, but nurses participate with patients and family members as they make choices for their health, even if that choice includes withholding life-sustaining treatment.

Examining the idea that nursing decision making occurs as a circle brings out a difference between the old nursing process and this new view. In the old method, data are collected, a diagnosis named, and interventions selected to correct something. Then the patient is reassessed. In the new process, a consideration of outcome is central to the practice. A possible outcome is the pattern that the patient and nurse together choose. In this way, the outcome state is a direct evolution of the pattern identified by the nurse and patient in their coming to know each other. Outcomes will be an extension of initial pattern. This view of outcomes was developed for teaching nursing students in acute care nursing settings and focuses on overall patterns of function (Chase, 1998). In this case study, the students learned to base their projections of what was possible for their acutely ill patients on their initial knowledge of and collaboration with the patient using a general set of parameters (see Table 13.2).

Over the course of a semester, students were able to determine achievement of outcomes and develop language to reflect goal attainment (Chase, 1998).

13.2	Outcomes to Nursing

Outcomes of Nursing (Chase, 1998)	Data Elements
Control	What aspects of life does the patient choose to control?
Comfort	Is the patient comfortable in body, mind, and spirit?
Communication	Does the patient need assistance in communicating preferences for care, or in communicating with loved ones?
Mobility	What mobility status is the patient's preference? What activities will improve the patient's strength?
Exchange	Is the patient receiving adequate nutrition, fluid, and oxygen? Is the patient able to eliminate wastes? Is the patient giving and receiving energy?
Safety	What are the specific issues that will support this patient's safety?

Organizing frameworks do not violate the wholeness of persons if they do not become an end unto themselves. If these frameworks support a broad understanding of the person, then they serve to assist the nurse and patient in seeing wholeness. The Iowa Outcomes Project has systematically collected and refined a list of outcomes to nursing care that could be chosen for individual patients (Moorhead, Johnson, & Maas, 2004). These outcomes are organized into seven domains with associated classes of outcome statements (see Table 13.3). Each of these classes has specific, identified outcome statements with scales that indicate the level of outcome attainment. Just as with the hypothetico-deductive model, there is a potential that the use of such integrated systems can lead to a focus more on the labels chosen than on the patient. However, if the nurse is clear on the model of practice that he or she is choosing to use,

13.3   Iowa Outcomes Project Domains and Representative Classes of Outcomes

Domains	Representative Classes
Functional Health	Energy Maintenance
	Growth and Development
	Mobility
	Self-Care
Physiological Health	Cardiopulmonary
	Elimination
	Fluid and Electrolytes
	Immune Response
	Metabolic Regulation
	Neurocognitive
	Nutritional
	Tissue Integrity
	Sensory Function
Psychosocial Health	Psychosocial Well-Being
	Psychosocial Adaptation
	Self-Control
	Social Interaction
Health Knowledge and Behavior	Health Behavior
	Health Beliefs
	Health Knowledge
	Risk Control and Safety
Perceived Health	Health and Quality of Life
	Symptom Status
	Satisfaction with Care
Family Health	Family Caregiver Performance
	Family Member Health Status
	Family Well-Being
	Parenting
Community Health	Community Well-Being
	Community Health Protection

then categories become concepts that reflect patterns of wholeness. "Diabetes Self Management" (Moorhead et al., 2004, p. 256) may be a chosen goal for both patient and nurse, and to reflect this directly in plan development does not violate wholeness. It focuses on a way of measuring progress and celebrating success that will empower the patient for care. It reflects the meaning of the care.

One of the ways in which the new nursing process is radically different from the former one is that it sets goal or outcome determination at its core. It is not focused on problems or diagnoses; it is organized from the beginning of the cycle around determining movement of the pattern of the whole and around making choices about new direction. In this new view, even critical care nursing is about assisting patients to move to new levels of stability and independence with decreasing reliance on technology. The problem is not the focus. In fact, it need not even be named. The goal is the entire focus, and it leads to decisions about how the patient can be assisted in meeting chosen goals. This use of goals is different from King's theory of goal attainment, which uses outcomes as "data to evaluate quality nursing care" (2008, p. 110), and which bases the nursing process in the traditional model.

The view of outcomes described here also differs from the Outcome-Present-State Test (OPT) view of nurses and patients selecting goals, as described by Pesut and Herman (1999). This view claims a link with complexity science (Pesut, 2008) but remains rooted in a problem-based framework with a consideration of the interrelationship of specific problems. The new view described in this chapter includes very directly the meanings and goals of the patient and from a complexity model, the patient's family and the system of care with other professionals. The new process includes nursing attention to possible health problems that patients can encounter on a health journey as an accompaniment to goal attainment. Failing to take action to prevent deep vein thrombosis for a patient who is not aware of his or her risk is a failure to prevent harm to the patient. Problems and potential problems are a part of the new view of nursing process. They are simply not the focus. The patient's goal is the process, and the problems are dealt with as they prevent the ultimate goal attainment of the patient.

Designing Activities or Explorations for Both Nurse and Patient That Support Chosen Outcomes

Once goals are determined and shared, the nurse next makes another set of decisions. The nurse decides what needs to be in place or to occur in order to bring the patient to the desired outcome. Expert nurses frequently speak in terms of movement. Where are we going here? Where do I want this patient to be (in health status) by the end of my time with the patient? When will the patient be ready to move to the next level of care? Complex health care systems are very much about movement of patients through systems. This depersonalized movement can violate human wholeness and meaning, but if the nurse engages with the patient and family in determining direction and choosing actions to assist preparation for movement to the next level of care, then care has meaning for the nurse and for the patient.

The nurse makes decisions about such aspects of care as what the patient might need in order to recover strength or capacity for self-care as well as knowing what roadblocks commonly are encountered along the path to recovery. This outcome setting and planning for support requires a kind of future thinking that is frequently not taught to nurses in school. This is a kind of decision making used by artists and craftsmen. Using concept as a goal, artists arrange material, shape objects, or assemble elements to create something new that makes a new statement. Artists often say that the story creates itself or the marble holds the shape within it. When working with humans, nurses as artists cannot objectify the patient or treat him or her as plastic to be molded. Humans, as open systems, do respond to the influence of artful attention of the nurse. The thinking of the nurse is directed to meeting a goal and making decisions along the way to accomplish a goal. Documentation systems that focus more on problems than on goals also work against this future thinking. Providing reflective space and time even at change of shift rounds can be an investment in developing nursing skill in decision making, and it can also focus care activities on what matters, which may result in more efficient care. Each care activity must be directed to meeting goals that patients and caregivers are committed to achieve.

Decisions in choosing activities appropriate to the nursing care of patients include knowing all that the nurse can know about the individual patient's preferences, joys, and values, along with all the knowledge the nurse has about specific health problems and healing, social and cultural meanings, and resources that are available. In a classic article by Eisenhauer (1994), the concept of nursing therapeutics was analyzed: "Nursing therapeutics can be described as singular or multiple interventions (actions) by the nurse to alter life processes, life patterns, functional health patterns and responses in order to alter the health–illness trajectory of a person" (p. 261). The typology she presents reflects that not all nursing actions are directed at the same level of issue. Some actions are chosen to respond to simple symptoms or cues, and that is sufficient. An ingrained pattern of symptoms may reflect altered health patterns that require responses at a deeper level. Focusing full attention on the symptom will not help the patient develop new patterns that may be leading to the symptom.

Going even deeper, life patterns and life processes may be addressed. The nurse must discern through analytic and imaginative thinking how the elements of behavior, relationships, and habits come together for the patient in the moment. Nursing interventions need not be seen as mechanical or objectifying. An intervention comes between and influences events. In this way, the nurse's decision as to how to influence the health path of the patient is an intervention. The codified Nursing Intervention Classification is an organized list of validated activities engaged in by nurses in caring for patients. It can be used as a source document to describe nursing activities. The assembly and refinement of this list is an open process that invites dialogue and contribution to its evolution (Dochterman & Bulechek, 2004).

Nursing at this level is creative, personal, and efficient. Nursing activities include care of the body—its comfort, its protection, its strengthening and balance. They include providing the patient with knowledge and skill in self-care so that after the nursing encounter, the patient is empowered to choose activities that will support the patient's goals and health. They also include understanding of the family and its culture, and the community context of the patient's life. Supporting the patient in choosing self-care activities will involve the entire family and may also include community agencies and contexts such as faith communities, social organizations, and support mechanisms. These are all decisions that nurses make that come not from a mechanistic, fix-the-problem mentality but from knowing the person, what matters to him or her and what will have meaning for him or her.

Prevention. This new model includes clear support for preventive care. Mobilizing patients to prevent deep vein thrombosis, engaging in mouth care for patients with mechanical ventilation, or changing a moist dressing are all activities that prevent complications that will delay recovery. One way to focus these activities is to determine what issues the patient is at risk for that may not yet exist. By identifying risks, the nurse can communicate and coordinate care activities with the entire care team. Preventive care activities are increasingly important in the increasing complexity of the health care system, which will be reporting and reimbursing for care based on rates of adverse outcomes to care.

The nurse is expert in small things. Adjusting body position for comfort, arranging the environment of care to support order and peace, communicating concern with a touch, offering fluids between meals, and updating family or other care providers on patient status all convey caring and offer the nurse an opportunity to attend to wholeness and directionality. In a complexity model, small things are recognized for the power they have to affect directionality of large systems. Nurses may use humor or distraction to assist the patient to see beyond current difficulties. Humor or irony only work when people understand each other and share a perspective. The nurse who knows the wholeness of person designs unique and creative responses to patient status that assist in recovery and health.

Uncertainty

At times, the picture of patient stability or direction is not entirely clear. The old, linear process does not account for uncertainty. In real practice, however, nurses and other clinicians make decisions based on hypotheses to establish care systems. In these cases, patient response to treatment can confirm or disconfirm the view of the patient pattern. For example, a postoperative patient may have reduced urine output. This could be due to a number of reasons, but two likely ones are fluid deficit and reduced cardiac output. If the patient had good cardiac function prior to surgery, a pattern that would have been assessed before the surgery, then increasing fluid delivery is a reasonable approach to improve fluid balance. If urine output increases, then the original hypothesis of fluid deficit is confirmed. If the output does not increase, then the team must consider other patterns, which might include decreased cardiac output. An openness to pattern and its probabilistic nature are consistent with the complexity model.

Coming to Know the New State of Being for Nurse and Nursed

The circle of meaning making continues as the nurse attends to how the patient responds to challenges. As the circle continues, the nurse comes to know the patient on deeper levels. The patient builds trust in the nurse and in the care of the team that the nurse directs. Patterns of healing are reinforced, and new direction is attained. Patients can report their own progress in maintaining health and in meeting identified goals. In fact, in many cases, patients are the best source of data in recording progress. Patients can also participate in resetting goals as care or recovery proceeds.

The new nursing process sees making meaning as its core process (Newman, 2008). In the old view, the assessment is the judgment as it is formed about the problems of the patient. In the new form, the assessment is the overall statement describing the pattern of the whole person's health. It includes possibilities for growth, healing, and evolving meaning. Being present with people at this level reminds the nurse daily of the reason for being a nurse. It promises patients that they will not be alone in their health/illness journey. As the nurse accompanies the patient, there are times when health problems progress, when cancers reoccur, when cardiac function declines, or when meaning making for the individual is destroyed by dementia. The nurse has not failed the patient even if the medical treatment plan cannot offer any new treatments. The nurse accompanies, offers support, and witnesses to suffering, attending always to the wholeness of the person.

Documentation. Documentation of nursing practice has had a long history. From the days of "nurses' notes" that recorded patient activity and physician visits but were discarded on patient discharge, to the use of nursing diagnoses to record focused attention of care activities, to electronic health care records, the changes to nursing documentation have resulted in mixed responses from nurses. Some nurses believe that lengthy documentation takes time from patient care, many do not take time to read the documentation recorded by other nurses, and some believe that using nursing diagnosis language objectifies the patient and fails to reflect wholeness.

Despite all this resistance, documentation continues to have general purposes that are important to the patient and to the profession. These include providing a written record of patient data, which supports the understanding of patterns of health at various stages of the patient encounter with the health care system. This data recording can assist other nursing and other professionals to detect the meaning of the data pattern so that care can be individualized and effective. Documentation records decision-making activities by nurses and reflects the basis for actions taken. This is useful as a communication device for the health care team and can support and defend nursing actions should questions or lawsuits challenge the quality of care delivered. Documentation also supports quality improvement activities in the complex systems in which nursing is delivered. Have multiple patients had difficulties with a new system of parenteral feeding? Have multiple patients had to return to the hospital for care shortly after discharge? What was different about their care?

For all these reasons, documentation must be accurate in recording the events of care and must be complete, which may include adding elements outside standardized data-collection instruments because the patient's unique situation cannot by captured within those parameters and the situation must be clearly communicated to a range of potential audiences. Deciding what to communicate is another major area of nurse decision making.

Nursing is different from many professions, and the intimacy of the nurse-patient encounter may seem to be violated by the use of language. Nursing is frequently conducted in a social framework (Chase, 1995). Other professionals, such as physicians or therapists of various types, engage with the same patients that nurses do. Acute care nursing usually involves a team of nurses who provide care. Communication about the uniqueness of an individual patient's wholeness is necessary to prevent fragmented and impersonal care. It is true that a patient may find one nurse to be the one he chooses to be open with, but the entire staff needs to know the situation in order to be sensitive to the patient's needs for care. Communication that is sensitive to describing overall issues and goals of the patient without revealing confidences requires a deft use of language. One principle that serves the nurse well is to write in such a way that if the patient read the record, he or she would agree and feel that the story had been represented well.

The level of communication required by this new model of caring cannot be captured in systems of documentation that rely completely on check boxes or charting by exception. Charting by exception is a way of reducing routine and repetitive language that reveals nothing about the uniqueness of the patient situation. Care activities that need routine documentation, such as turning, ambulating, or dressing changes, might be sufficiently recorded with a check. The nature of the patient's wound, the patient's response to the challenge of walking, and the condition of skin visible when the patient turns, however, may not be well captured in check boxes unless the system is very sophisticated. Nurses can contribute to the development of individualized documentation elements that are important to their patients' concerns (Chase, 1997).

An ideal system of documentation would

1. Capture the essence of the patient's story of health care, perhaps by using a broad range of data elements such as the functional health pattern assessment. At very minimum, the living situation of the patient and his or her stated goals and concerns must be recorded.
2. Specify patient goals for health. These goals could be elements of the Nursing Outcomes Classification (Moorhead et al., 2004) or could be creatively determined between the nurse and patient. Depending upon the setting, midrange goals for the day can be declared, and progress in meeting these goals can be recorded in summary statements that reflect the direction of the patient's progress.

3. Specific actions taken to assist the patient in meeting goals are recorded along with their effects. These might be specific nursing interventions (Dochterman & Bulechek, 2004) or actions at the system level that coordinate activities of other elements of the health care system that will support the patient. These might be referrals or consultations. Activities chosen to reduce the development of problems can be recorded along with data that reflect that the potential problem has been assessed and has not developed.
4. Comments on the effectiveness of activities chosen will assist the team in coordinating care.

Data elements not directly related to goals could be recorded on flow sheets or checklists. Deciding which data elements to record in detail because of their salience to patient goal attainment is another decision that nurses make.

Systems of documentation that are designed around the use of nursing diagnoses can be adapted for use with this new model for nursing process. When considering what matters most to patients, or the meaning of the health situation to the patient, certain concepts tend to reoccur. Using a concept label that reflects the wholeness of patient pattern does not violate the nurse-patient encounter. It can be a way of reflecting the pattern of the person. The North American Nursing Diagnosis Association (NANDA), now NANDA International (NANDA-I), began using an inductive method to identify health concerns or problems for which the nurse was independent in care in order to differentiate nursing practice from following doctor's orders. The early days of NANDA coincided with a problem-solving view of the nursing process, and the early language reflected that view. Currently the NANDA labels are conceptual and can reflect actual problems that patients may experience, but they can also reflect potential issues or areas for growth that the patient might choose through the use of axes that allow for more flexible use of the concept labels. These concepts can be applied to the new view of nursing process by taking time to reflect on the essence of that patient's health pattern. Are there concepts that can put words to those patterns? For example, a patient facing rehabilitation following stroke who has a goal of returning home with minimal assistance may have focused care activities related to physical mobility, health maintenance, and verbal communication (NANDA-I, 2007). Using these concepts to focus the attention of the multidisciplinary team and to prepare the patient for the goal of returning home does not violate the new nursing process. What is different is that it is not a "problem" label that drives nurse decision making. It is the goal statement of the patient-documented attention on aspects of care that maintain respect for the wholeness of person. Whole persons need specific care individualized to their pattern.

Sadly, using the old, problem-solving model and routine documentation, the patient record never records nursing's best contribution to the health of the patient. By focusing on meaning and direction, the most exquisite contributions that nurses make can be recorded in a way that honors the process and the persons. It is nursing's obligation to represent the patient encounter and activities in such a way that the health care system can recognize the contributions of nursing. If a surgery is seen as successful because of the surgeons' skills and not the nurses' then the story of care has not been accurately recorded. If nurses do not record their decisions so that the quality of those decisions can be evaluated, then nurses will not learn to improve their decision making. Recording what nurses really do as they are present with their patients, coming to know them, and assisting them in making choices about their health allows for knowledge development in ways not yet realized.

Summary

Nurses make decisions regarding the care of their patients in a continuing process of coming to know them, recognizing patterns of health and movement to new levels of health, assisting patients in setting goals for their health, choosing activities that assist patients in meeting goals, and then in coming to know the person as he or she continues to evolve. The thinking of the nurse is an important part of the wholeness of what he or she brings to the encounter. Responding to patients comes from knowing the patient and having access to growing nursing knowledge. When these come together, then nursing truly happens and individuals, families, and communities are assisted in attaining new levels of health. As students learn to use the thinking skills that professional nursing requires, faculty can guide them in thinking in creative ways about assembling patient information, coming to know patients in their wholeness, and discovering the meaning of patterns of living. Research into how nursing promotes health and healing requires retrievable records that reflect the most powerful aspects of nursing. With further research, nursing's contribution to the health of society will be more understood and more highly valued.

References

American Nurses Association. (2003). *Nursing's social policy statement* (2nd ed.) Silver Spring, MD: Author.

Benner, P. (1984). *From novice to expert: Excellence and power in clinical nursing practice*. Menlo Park, CA: Addison-Wesley.

Chase, S. K. (1995). The social context of critical care clinical judgment. *Heart & Lung, 24,* 154–162.

Chase, S. K. (1997). Charting critical thinking: Nursing judgments and patient outcomes. *Dimensions of Critical Care Nursing, 16,* 102–111.

Chase, S. K. (1998). Teaching baccalaureate nursing students to project outcomes to nursing interventions. *Nursing Diagnosis, 9*(2), 62–70.

Chase, S. K. (2001). Response to "The concept of nursing presence: State of the science." *Scholarly Inquiry for Nursing Practice: An International Journal, 15,* 323–327.

Chase, S. K. (2004). *Clinical judgment and communication in nurse practitioner practice*. Philadelphia: F.A. Davis.

Dochterman, J. M., & Bulechek, G. M. (2004). *Nursing interventions classification (NIC)* (4th ed.). St. Louis: Mosby.

Doona, M. E., Chase, S. K., & Haggerty, L. A. (1999). Nursing presence: As real as a Milky Way. *Journal of Holistic Nursing, 17*(1), 54–70.

Eisenhauer, L. A. (1994). A typology of nursing therapeutics. *Image: Journal of Nursing Scholarship, 26,* 261–264.

Gordon, M. (1994). *Nursing diagnosis: Process and application* (4th ed.). St. Louis: Mosby.

Hiltunen, E., Medich, C., Chase, S., Peterson, L., & Forrow, L. (1999). Family decision making for end of life treatment: The SUPPORT nurse narratives. *Journal of Clinical Ethics, 10,* 126–134.

King, I. M. (2008). King's conceptual system: Theory of goal attainment, and transaction process in the 21st century. *Nursing Science Quarterly, 20,* 109–116.

Lindberg, C., Nash, S., & Lindberg, C. (2008). *On the edge: Nursing in the age of complexity*. Bordentown, NJ: Plexus Press.

Moorhead, S., Johnson, M., & Maas, M. (2004). *Nursing Outcomes Classification (NOC)* (3rd ed.). St. Louis: Mosby.

NANDA-I. (2007). *Nursing diagnoses: Definitions and classification 2007–2008*. Philadelphia: Author.

Newman, M. A. (1986). *Health as expanding consciousness*. St. Louis: Mosby.

Newman, M. A. (2008). *Transforming presence: The difference that nursing makes*. Philadelphia: F. A. Davis.

Pesut, D. J. (2008). Thoughts on thinking with complexity in mind. In. C. Lindberg, S. Nash, & C. Lindberg (Eds.), *On the edge: Nursing in the age of complexity* (pp. 211–238). Bordentown, NJ: Plexus Press.

Pesut, D. J., & Herman, J. (1999). *Clinical reasoning: The art and science of critical and creative thinking*. New York: Delmar Press.

Tanner, C. A., Benner, P., Chesla, C., & Gordon, D. R. (1993). The phenomenology of knowing the patient. *Image: Journal of Nursing Scholarship, 25,* 273–280.

Yura, H., & Walsh, M. (1967). *The nursing process*. Norwalk, CT: Appleton, Century Crofts.

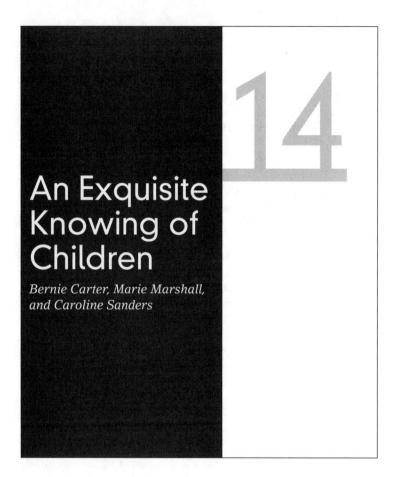

An Exquisite Knowing of Children

*Bernie Carter, Marie Marshall,
and Caroline Sanders*

Chapter Overview

Knowing children reflects a particular sense and aesthetic about the way in which nurses approach every element of their care. Knowing children becomes possible if nursing practice is characterised by being reciprocal, attuned, relational, dialogic, dynamic, still, nonjudgmental, reflexive, and committed to understanding the child. This involves understanding how the child is making sense of his or her illness, how the child is generating a sense of what is happening to him or her and their family, trying to determine how his or her life world is being changed, and what these changes will mean. An exquisite knowing might best be described as an almost perfect knowing, when all the elements of knowing are in place and where the nurse and child have a meaningful, genuine, empathic, and engaged relationship that sustains and supports the child, and which mediates the consequences, effects, and disruptions of the child's illness. Knowing is a point of mutual recognition.

A World That Is Too Small?

Knowing children is a rich, compelling, and complex aspect of nursing children. Knowing the children we nurse is more than just knowing their names, their diagnoses, and what their treatment sheet says they need in terms of medication. It means knowing something about whom they are as special, important, and unique individuals. It means knowing about their hopes, concerns, and joys. Rather than just knowing their names, it may mean knowing what is special to them about their names. Rather than just knowing what their diagnoses are, it means knowing what they understand about their illness, what concerns them—if anything—about their symptoms and why they think they are in hospital. Rather than us just knowing about the drugs they are prescribed and potential side effects, it means knowing what the children think and understand about their treatment. It means knowing how they see their illness, their treatment, and our nursing care fitting into their lives.

Knowing the child who is sick is important, but it is equally important to know about what the child is like when they are well as much of this aspect of their life, personality, hopes and aspirations may be muted or masked by their sickness. So we need to understand something about the children's life worlds. We need to understand about their beliefs, their toys and imaginary companions, their pets, and the games they like to play. We need to know whether they are serious or silly, shy or bold. We need to know about their previous illnesses and how they managed these, what they like and dislike, what frightens them and what reassures them. In brief, it seems we need to know a lot.

Knowing children involves finding out about them and they, rather than anyone else, are best placed to tell us about themselves even though children's nurses can benefit immeasurably from the expertise, sensitivity, and insights of parents and caregivers. Children can be excellent first-person reporters of their own health and illness experiences (see Olsen et al., 2007; Riley, 2004), although health professionals need to give them time, space, and opportunity to do this. Even very young children can tell us about themselves, providing we ask simple questions. For infants and children, where verbal communication is not possible, we can come to a powerful and engaged knowledge of a child through touch, space, silence, and caring.

However, despite the rhetoric of inclusion, studies suggest that in most health care encounters, children are silenced or contribute in constrained ways. Many of the studies that have focused on this area have looked at doctor-child or doctor-parent-child communication rather than at nurse-child communication, perhaps reflecting the almost universal assumption that nurses communicate well with children. Wassmer et al.'s (2004) study of clinical encounters in an outpatient clinic showed fairly typical findings. Doctors were involved in 61% of conversation, parents in 35%, and children in only 4% of conversation. The consultations were directive, communication was primarily instrumental, and children's contribution was small. A small study by Shin and White-Traut (2005) of the interaction patterns between eight triads of nurses, hospitalized children, and their parents found that the total amount of interaction was limited. The average interaction in the 8 hour period was only 4–24 minutes long, and these interactions were triggered by other nursing activities such as monitoring or providing technical care. The children were generally passive participants. Opportunities for knowing the children may well be missed in such scenarios.

Determining how to present a chapter on knowing children was, in itself, challenging. Indeed it is pertinent, at the start of this chapter, to question whether adults can ever really know children. The fact that this question is raised is, in itself, important as it reflects a position of humility about children. It questions the typical arrogance of adults that they know and that children are knowable. In his beautiful and evocative poem "Children's Song," R. S. Thomas wrote of the impossibility of adults, despite or maybe because of their sophistication, cleverness, and world-weariness, to enter the world of children which he described as:

A world that is too small
For you to stoop and enter
Even on hands and knees, the adult subterfuge. (1986)

Thomas evoked the preposterousness and absurdity of adults being able to physically, emotionally, and socially reenter the world(s) of children. The poem is a place to start thinking about the world of children and the limits to how we can know them.

The chapter could have adopted a strongly philosophical, psychological, pedagogical, or theoretical perspective; but, although these perspectives are valuable, they could miss some of the points that we want to make. They also shift the emphasis and focus away from the children and their families who should, we believe, have center stage in a chapter on knowing children. Indeed, it is ironic in many ways that we—as adults, professionals, academics—far removed from being children, should be writing a chapter on knowing children. Children writing this chapter or answering this question would write from their own frames of reference and their response would likely be constructed very differently from the way in which we have chosen to respond.

However, we have tried to create a chapter that resonates with a sense of childhood and children—a chapter grounded in children's experiences, in which a polyphony of children's voices helps to actively co-construct and co-constitute the text. We have acknowledged and respected children, childhood, and their worlds. We have woven their worlds, words, stories, and experiences, as well as literature on children and childhood, into our writing and thinking. In doing so, we are presenting our perspective—shaped from our years in practice and research, from years of reading as children and adults. It is informed by the children who have led us into their worlds, shared parts of their stories and their lives, and taught us much of what we now know is fundamental to children's nursing practice.

Children and Their Knowing About Illness

Illness is part of children's everyday world. They bump and bruise themselves, catch colds and coughs, go down with vomiting and diarrhoea, develop fevers and rashes, and suffer from aches and pains. All of these experiences are par for the course of childhood. For most children, these episodes of acute illness are over and done with relatively quickly and do not require medical intervention (Bruijnzeels, Foets, van der Wouden, van den Heuvel, & Prins, 1998) and the illness is contained within the family (Neill, 2000).

These minor episodes may seem inconsequential, especially to nurses involved in caring for children presenting with more significant symptoms and illnesses. These minor illnesses are, nonetheless, important—not least because they provide the context to subsequent illness. They become the backdrop to the dramas where nurses may become involved. These minor illnesses not only challenge the child's immune system, but they also challenge the child's sense of self, the child's sense of his or her body and its boundaries. Usually when illness disrupts the child's sense of self, this disruption is managed by their parents and, as Neill (2000) noted, within the boundaries of their family and their home.

Children learn from adult responses to illness. They learn about how they are expected to respond, behave, and react, and the degree of seriousness (or not) attributed to different illnesses or injuries. They also learn how their siblings, friends, and relatives react, and they in turn learn from these reactions. They start to create an understanding of illness and health. This understanding is created through their own personal experiences of illness within the family. They also learn through family stories and fairy tales, nursery rhymes and poems, books, and other media. These vicarious experiences of illness also shape their behavior, expectations, and attitudes. Despite their actual illness experiences, children's imagination may project an illusion about illness that is a long way from the truth of real illness. Imagined illness may be perceived as being something dramatic, an adventurous opportunity to be relished, in which the child becomes the hero or heroine, drama king or queen. Within children's literature the romance of illness can be played out. In Ransome's *Swallows and Amazons*, a story set in England in the early 1930s, a group of children are getting their stores prepared for a voyage of discovery. They are packing their small sailing boat for a camping trip to an island in the middle of a lake. Having sorted out the frying pan and food, their thoughts turn to medical supplies and the potential need for doctoring. Susan, the oldest girl, says,

"I ought to take some bandages and medicines and things."
"Oh no," said Titty. "On desert islands they cure everything with herbs. We'll have all sorts of diseases, plagues, fevers and things that no medicine is any good for and we'll cure them with herbs that the natives show us."

> *At this point mother came in and settled the question.*
> *"No medicines," she said. "Anyone who wants doctoring is*
> *invalided home."*
>
> *"If it's really serious," said Titty, "but we can have a*
> *plague or a fever or two by ourselves." (Ransome, 1930)*

The interplay between Titty, Susan, and their mother provides a neat little vignette. Susan is being practical and sen-
sible about the need for doctoring. Titty (a child who lives in
her imagination) is being romantic about illness and is rather
looking forward to something deliciously desperate happening in the way of plague, fever, and disease. Meanwhile,
their mother is decisive, places clear limits, and is not at all
wrapped up in the notion of illness being fun. The excerpt is
full of lessons for children: the notion that medicine might
not be good for everything, the concept of gradation of seriousness in illness, and the practicality of Susan being prepared (as a mother would be) with "bandages and medicines
and things" that can remedy illness and injury.

Interestingly, apart from the possibility of "plagues and
fevers," the worst illness experienced by the children in any
of Ransome's novels is mumps. In *Winter Holiday,* Ransome
(1933) provided an insight into an everyday, routine sort of
childhood illness. He touched upon the ways in which adults
react, the importance of doctors who treat children well, and
the longing of Nancy, the child who is ill, to be well and to be
fully part of the world of other children again. He also demonstrated quite brilliantly how illness changes the dynamics
and relationships of the children who remain well.

A more contemporary hero would be J. K. Rowling's Harry
Potter, whose adventures bring their fair share of glory and
suffering (see Rowling, 1997). Interestingly, not all episodes
of illness and injury are speedily rectified by the application
of magic; they often involve periods of time spent in bed,
being looked after by a nurse and being separated from
everyday (wizarding) life. In nearly all of the books, Harry
and his friends experience illness, injury, and pain, and the
children reading the books start to understand that medicine
(and magic) have limits.

Children can and do learn from literature. We feel that it
is a real shame and a missed opportunity that, for the most
part, nurses do not study children's literature. It should perhaps be an integral part of nursing curricula because it has

the potential to help nurses question what they know about children, illness, and nursing. Humanities are embedded within some narrative curricula (Charon, 2007).

"Play illness" is important because it allows children to act out their fears, concerns, and potential strategies for dealing with illness; but it is not the same as being ill. As children grow older, their understanding about illness changes, shifting from magical thinking (such as coughing up frogs) to a more concrete appreciation of causes, effects, and consequences (such as a spitty cough because of a pseudomonas bug). This is aligned to their shift from being oriented to the present moment to being more future oriented, although even children as young as 4 or 5 years old have a sense of how physical and emotional reactions to illness or injury can unfold over time. They are also relatively sophisticated in their ability to link biological causes with common illnesses (Raman & Gelman, 2007).

Children grow up learning about the rules and social mores that guide illness behaviors in their own family and within wider society. Through their previous experiences of ill health, they accumulate a repository of knowledge that they bring with them to subsequent illness. They link the use of plasters (band-aids) to helping heal the hurt of a grazed knee, the cuddle from their mother or father with the comfort it brings to a sore tummy, and the stroking of their head with the calming feeling after they have been sick. They know that banana-flavored medicine sorts out "green coughs" and that pink medicine is pretty much good for everything.

In some senses, their knowledge may not be terribly sophisticated. They will not necessarily know why the pink medicine helps them when they are sore or have a fever or feel ill, but they trust in it. Children become wise about treatment and interventions, picking up their knowledge pragmatically—two teaspoons of pink medicine *does* work—and even being able to recommend treatment to their siblings and friends. Children pick up information about illness from those around them, and they piece this knowledge together, although sometimes the connections they make are not accurate. Although sometimes these misconnections can be amusing for adults, they can be bemusing and confusing for children, creating moments of anxiety, misunderstanding, and distress.

One of the authors has a clear memory from her own childhood: I was angry and upset when the doctor dismissed my concerns about the eczema cream I was prescribed. I wanted to know why it bleached my skin. My mother did not know why and the doctor brusquely told me, "Don't be silly; it's not bleaching your skin." However, as far as I was concerned—and I was concerned—the cream I was applying was creating pale patches on my arms, at the back of my legs, and near my ears. What I failed to recognize and what the doctor was too busy or dismissive to bother to explain to me was that something different but equally real was happening. Rather than the cream bleaching my skin, the skin was always so new that it never got the chance to tan the same as the surrounding skin and so it appeared to be lighter. The explanation was not complicated; it would have taken the doctor less than a minute to explain, and it would have helped me to make sense of what was happening and would have made me feel I was being taken seriously.

Years later, I was caring for a very distressed little girl who had eczema that was far worse than mine had ever been. It would have been easy enough to have just explained that she had to have cream if she wanted to get better and gloss over her stubborn refusal to apply the cream. Her distress took me back to my own experience and we talked about why she was so unhappy. She explained that her friend had told her that the cream would make her invisible and no one would be her friend anymore. Rather than repeat the patronizing response I had received, we talked about how I had believed my cream had been bleaching me and she giggled. Then, using almost the same words as my doctor, she told me that it was a silly idea; we went on to talk about invisibility cream, how much fun it could be, and that unfortunately eczema cream did not make you invisible.

Children's understanding of health and ill health is facilitated and guided, initially, by their parents, who provide the first line of care for everyday illness. Just as children learn about illness and injury, parents learn about how each of their children reacts and responds to the challenges that illness creates. Parental knowing and knowledge builds over time, reflecting each individual child's sources of strength and resilience and repertoire of skills and capacities. Rubovits and Wolynn (1999) have clearly shown that mothers are "able to reflect their children's conceptual strength and weakness" (p. 103) in terms of their children's understanding of illness, etiology, treatment, and prevention. Parents develop a repository of knowledge about their children and use this knowing to determine the seriousness of any changes they notice their children presenting with. In a study of parents and children living with the child's diabetes in the months and years after formal diagnosis, Marshall, Carter, and Rose (2006) and Marshall in her ongoing doctoral study (Marshall, ongoing) found that parental knowing of their children was crucial. This was particularly clear in the pre-diagnostic stage, where the parents gradually developed a sense of unease or dis-ease as their children started to display behavioral and other differences. Initially, the changes were subtle or could be relatively easily dismissed as these mothers explained,

> "She [Sonia] had lost a lot of weight but I never thought of anything else," or "She [Polly] put her tongue out and there was froth on it and I thought, 'bit weird,' but it was a hot day and everything."

As the integrity of their knowing was progressively breached, parents came to recognize the changes as threatening. For example, as John's mother explained,

> "It [diabetes] wasn't something that came on all at once. It started with drinking lots. Obviously, he would be going to the toilet more. It was like pieces of a jigsaw putting them together.")

(Please note that in the above examples and the ones following, pseudonyms have been used to protect the identity of the children and their parents.

Sensing that something is physically amiss is difficult enough, regardless of how well a parent knows a child, and it is even more difficult to sense emotional distress. Even a very close knowing does not mean that it is sufficient to reach across to the child who is sick or worried about an aspect of their illness. Knowing a child is not the answer to everything; knowing does not necessarily create solutions. In fact, knowing a child well can reveal difficulties that are not readily resolved, and this can often cause parents distress. In Sanders' doctoral study (Sanders, under examination; see also Sanders, Carter, & Goodacre, 2008), one of her interviews with a parent of a child with ambiguous genitalia portrayed the mother's anguish about the sense of knowing that her daughter wanted to talk and her concern that her child did not know how:

> She's sensible and she does listen and she doesn't know why, and it's all confusing inside her. She won't talk about it, especially in front of anyone else. And when she talks to me about it, it's not childish. In a heartbreaking way, you know you sort of go, it's all right, talk to me about it if you want to; but she doesn't know what she wants to say.

A skilled nursing response to such a scenario would be to consider how best to help the child and her family. This might be through working directly with the parents rather than the child. Another mother in Sanders' study talked of the isolation she was experiencing. She was clearly desperately in need of an informed professional to reach out and make contact with her, to provide a safe place for her to talk through the things affecting her child. This mother was clearly making a plea from her heart when she said,

> I have to say it's a lonely condition to be around; it is lonely. 'Cause sometimes you know when you want somebody to talk to that you think might understand what you've heard and what you're doing and what you're talking about really, but they don't.

Often parents welcome guidance and support from trusted professionals who know them well and who build their esteem and confidence. However, it is important to acknowledge that although parents have expertise about their child, they are not infallible. Sometimes their expertise can be clouded and their insight only partial. Worry and concern about their child and competing demands on their time can affect parental knowing. Sometimes parents can fail to recognize an aspect of their child's response to illness because the child is trying to protect the parents. Regardless of how attuned parents are to their child, there will inevitably be differences between what the child knows, thinks, and feels about his or her illness and what the parents perceive that their child knows, thinks, and feels.

An example from Marshall's study (Marshall, ongoing) clearly reflects the dissonance between the child's views and those held by her mother. When Zoe's mother was asked about Zoe's thoughts about having diabetes, she talked of how she did not think that Zoe was bothered by her diabetes but that she sometimes used her diabetes to gain sympathy or get "a packet of crisps." She went on to say,

> *I reckon she is proud of it sometimes, being a diabetic as well, because she is quite happy talking to strangers about it ... So it is not—I don't see, like, when you see some teenagers, and they hide it—I'm normal; she will quite openly say, "I am a diabetic," and she will explain it to you if you want to know, but I don't think she knows any difference.*

Whereas her mother's immediate response was that she did not think that Zoe was bothered by her diabetes, Zoe's response was that having diabetes was "bad." Her stark, almost diametrically opposed, response reflects Zoe's lived experience of *being* diabetic, whereas her mother is looking in to that experience from outside. Zoe's reason for saying why diabetes is "bad" related to being teased, as she explained:

> *When we went to the youth club, everybody teases me with sweets. I got upset, everybody always goes, "Ah, Zoe, look— do you like a bit of it? Oh no, I forgot; you're not allowed it, are you? Right." But if they are buying stuff from the shop, they go, "Ah, look, Zoe," and they walk away, and people tease me, saying that I am not allowed it.*

The fact that dissonance exists does not represent a failure on Zoe's or her mother's part, but it is important that their nurse know both of them well enough to acknowledge their different positions and to help weave a path between both views without judging or finding fault. The aim of nursing care may not be to bring these views into perfect alignment but to help resolve the tensions that may arise from the situation. Zoe clearly is bothered by her diabetes, and if her mother is aware of this, she may be able to provide additional support to Zoe. If Zoe knows that her mother is unaware of how much the teasing is bothering her rather not caring, she may seek advice from her mother about how to deal with it.

Knowing a child is complex. It is challenging for a child's parents and even more so for nurses who become uniquely positioned in relation to a sick child. Nurses are positioned outside of the family but undertake some aspects of the caring role for the sick child. Knowing the sick child can mediate the child's experience of illness through mitigating suffering and reducing distress. However, knowing a child is rarely simple and, for nurses, knowing a child means coming to know the child's family as well. Knowing a child who is ill, injured, or facing an operation, for example, requires nurses to somehow tap into the child's experiences, to understand something of the ways in which the family deals with illness/ill health, to appreciate what the illness means or may mean to that child, and to be prepared to help the child make sense of *their* illness.

The Adult Hegemony in Retreat

In order to come to know children, nurses need to have some sort of sense of what is meant when we talk of children and childhood. The terms *child, children,* and *childhood* are often used relatively carelessly, assuming "a monolithic social category" (Matthews, 2001, p. 154) that simply does not exist in reality. However, the assumptions that are inherent in the discourses (e.g., in the media, government policy and reports, academic research, curricula) surrounding children and childhood, position children as 'Other' than adults. These discourses frame children negatively, defining them "by not what the child is ... but is subsequently going to be"(Alanen, 1999, p. 16). Children are described in terms of lower linguistic skills and being pre-social, incomplete, and less rational than adults. They are beings requiring socialization into the world of adults. In this portrayal of children, a core purpose of socialization is to render them "same," not 'Other'. The hegemony of adulthood encompasses and can overwhelm children and their childhoods. However, childhood is a pluralistic concept. As Matthews and Limb (1999) noted, there is

> Neither such a thing as "the child" nor a uniform social category which can be called "children" ... Children come in all shapes and sizes and may be distinguished along various axes of gender, race, ethnicity, ability, health, and age. Such differences will have an important bearing on their geographies and should not be overlooked in any discourse. We emphasize the need to recognize the importance of "multiple childhoods" and the sterility of the concept of the "universal child." (p. 65)

Greene and Hogan (2005) would support the notion of the individuality and uniqueness of each child's childhood because each has been exposed to different "historical and cultural influences" (p. xi).

Acknowledging that the adult hegemony exists is important because it influences, to a greater or lesser extent, the ways in which adults think about children, the spaces that children are able to occupy within our society, and the contribution they can make. This in turn influences us as nurses and our professional knowing of children. If we see the life worlds of children in the way that some writers suggest (as being fundamentally different and inaccessible to adults/nurses), then any attempts at knowing children will be constrained by that perception. Jones (2001) noted that "children's worlds are irretrievably alien to adults: bizarre (to us) 'other' worlds, closed off by the 'dark reason' that limits adult gaze" (p. 174). Horton (2001) talked of children's geographies as being "horrible to 'adult' sensibilities" (p. 162). If we fully or even partially accept the notion that children's life worlds and the spaces children occupy are alien territory for adults, then this suggests that we will never be able to come close to knowing children. Their world would be, as Thomas (1986) suggested in his poem, "too small" for us as adults to enter. However, alternative views on children, childhoods, and life worlds exist that provide a different set of possibilities for understanding, engaging with, and knowing children.

A social constructionist view of children and childhood rejects the notion of children as being passive "adults-in-waiting" but frames them as "embodied health care actors" (Mayall, 1998). James and Prout (1997) see children not as "human becomings" but as "human beings"—agents who are "actively involved in the construction of their own social lives, the lives around them and of the societies in which they live" (p. 4). Children "both construct their worlds and are constructed by their worlds' (Kincheloe, 2004, p. xii). Accepting that children are "meaning-producing beings," as proposed by Young and Barrett (2001), demands that nurses engage with children in a meaningful way. We embrace the notion that children are meaning-producing and sense-making beings; evidence of this can be seen in the way in which they approach the world with curiosity and insight, questioning how things work, why things happen, and why things are.

Children often outstrip adults in their quest to make sense of the world they live in. In their hunger to understand and make meaning, children are reaching out to be known. Thomas implies that "adult subterfuges" cannot take us to the centre of a child's world. We would agree (in part) with this as adults will always be "a very definite and readily identifiable other" (Graue & Walsh, 1998, p. xiv). Knowing a child and basing our nursing care on that knowledge requires a nurse neither to know the absolute centre of the child nor to lose his or her identity as an adult/nurse.

Nursing and Knowing Children

Philosophically, children's nursing practice is underpinned by a commitment to nursing and knowing the child *within* the context of his or her family. This, in itself, is complex. It requires nurses to know the child and his or her family and to understand the way in which the child fits into the relational web of family ties. As Stein (2003) noted, "We know—and should remember anew *that* we know—with all our senses" (p. 29); knowing comes through a synthesis of senses.

Knowing children is essential if we are to nurse children well. It reflects a particular sense and aesthetic about the way in which nurses approach every element of care. Knowing children becomes possible if nursing practice is characterised by being reciprocal, attuned, relational, dialogic, dynamic, still, nonjudgmental, reflexive, and committed to understanding the child. This involves understanding how the child is making sense of the illness, how the child is generating a sense of what is happening to him or her and his or her family, and trying to determine how the child's life world is being changed and what these changes will mean for the child. An exquisite knowing might best be described as an almost perfect knowing, when all the elements of knowing are in place, and where the nurse and child have a meaningful, genuine, empathic, and engaged relationship that sustains and supports the child and that mediates the consequences, effects, and disruptions of their illness.

Knowing is a point of mutual recognition.

Although we would argue that knowing is an essential element of nursing care, it lacks visibility. It is not measured and it is rarely documented. However, knowing children allows nurses to create therapeutic spaces, landscapes, and possibilities for children and their families that respect their individuality as children and their own specific childhoods.

Knowing a child is powerful.

It is powerful in the way it can support a child who is ill and help him or her flourish despite the challenges and disruptions to their life world that illness presents. Knowing a child is powerful for nurses who see the boundaries of their care extend beyond mechanical competence, beyond caring for symptoms to caring for the child experiencing the sense of desolation, desperation, fear, isolation, and anxiety that symptoms can engender. Although Schmidt et al. (2007) did not specifically report on knowing within their study, it is clear that the type of nursing engagement that they are advocating is closely aligned with what we would call *knowing*.

Knowing a child means we can truly nurse the child. It requires us to acknowledge an "ethic of caring" (Noddings, 1984) where fidelity (an acting in faith with the children's own life worlds) is a central quality of our relationships with children. Fidelity suggests devotion and acting faithfully or in faith with the children's own life worlds. Knowing can be accomplished through a sense of mindfulness.

Knowing requires us to nurse differently, to move away from professional monologues where we (nurses)—the so-called experts—"colonize" (Porter, 1998) the life worlds of children and parents. It forces us to understand that nursing by numbers, algorithms, and formulae can never fulfill the needs of children who are ill or nurses who want to make a genuinely human difference to those children. Knowing a child means that our interactions with the child cannot be unidirectional; knowing means we are involved. Knowing a child is not something we do to them; it is something we do with them. Knowing is co-constructed and co-constituted. Knowing a sick child through entering the child's life world can create a sense of closeness, a sense of (professional) companionship between the child/family and the nurse.

Our knowing has to be a humble knowing; we need to be aware that, despite our professional knowledge and expertise, we know very little in comparison to the child's/parents' experiences of being ill and living with illness. However, by adopting a dialogic approach—whereby we attend to a child's stories about illness, respect the concerns the child raises, listen to the silences and pauses between the child's words, and try to hear the things that the child does not say—then we can start to know a child.

By being reflexive and dialogic practitioners, we can enter into what Christensen (2004) called children's "cultures of communication" (p. 166). Stories are often the currency of communication used by children; their stories illustrate their desire to be involved, to understand more about their illness, their treatment, and what is happening to them (Carter, 2009). Although stories are quintessentially part of knowing children, stories can reveal difficult things for nurses to attend to. Stories are not benign—they have the potential for good and bad, and nurses are morally bound to act/to nurse in a way that honors their knowing of the child and the child's story (Carter, 2008). Knowing the children we are nursing can transform the way that we nurse; we can align our communication with their needs. Knowing a child may mean that we give ourselves permission not to be active, to choose to be still and to share their silence. Choosing to be still can be a significant act that is respectful and necessary if the relationship is to have balance.

Children are perceptive and can see the difference between professionals who remain distanced from them and those professionals who are willing to get to know them through reciprocal dialogue. As Ben, one of the children who talked to me during a study on children's pain, explained:

> There are some [doctors] better than others. There are some [the better ones] who like talk to you about your illness and everything and about your social life ... They'll ask you what you're doing ... Whilst others, like, ask you, "OK, so how are you feeling? What's wrong with you?" ... And then they'll tell you about your illness ... But the better ones chat to you ... and treat you like a person, not just someone who's ill, and let you tell them.

Although nurses undoubtedly can develop expertise in knowing children and can develop a sense of knowing about groups of children within their care, they should never become complacent and assume that knowing many children with a particular diagnosis or symptom means that they know all children. Experienced and expert nurses also need to be humble in their knowing and try to recover what Suzuki (1986) called a "beginner's mind." This means that we do not base our practice on assumptions and suppositions but try to approach every child open to their individual possibilities.

Ways of Getting to Know

Stein's (2003) reminder that "we know—with all our senses" (p. 29) provides a useful starting place for a consideration of some of the ways in which we might approach getting to know children. Nurses who are open to knowing children will not require a recipe book or a toolbox of how to come to know children; they will follow the lead that the individual child gives and align their approach with things that the child feels comfortable with and which have resonance with the child.

The temptation is to use the terms *tools* or *methods* as handy labels for some of the things that we may use to engage children. The temptation is strong, not least because it is difficult to think of other terms that fit the bill; but the problem with condensing child-centered approaches to engagement to words like *tool* or *method* is that it makes them seem mechanistic, reductionist, and directive. However, there are approaches—such as drawing, writing stories, making scrapbooks, taking photographs, or using existing family photographs alongside some of the more everyday nursing practices such as playing, observing, talking, touching, holding, explaining, listening, and involving—that can help nurses come to know the children in their care. These additional approaches do not have to be time-consuming or difficult, but they can provide imaginative and non-medically focused ways of deepening a relationship with a child and the child's family. They can be integrated into play activities if that is appropriate for the child. Play is core to children's lives, and as Buchbinder (2008) emphasizes, play does not necessarily "privilege discursive skills" (p. 154) and therefore simply observing (or becoming involved in) children's play—even when the children are being strongly dialogic—can help illuminate issues that are preoccupying them.

Some approaches such as drawing and doing other artwork have a long-established history as a means of expression for children and are part and parcel of most play activities. More recently they have been utilized in research as a means of trying to understand children's perspectives, and there is enormous potential for nurses to utilize drawing and artwork as a way of establishing and sustaining a close relationship.

Rollins (2005b) discussed the value that drawings can have in transferring the "focus from the child to the drawing," which seems "to relax the child by relieving the pressure of being the object of direct communication" (p. 215), describing this as the "camp fire" effect.

There are many creative ways of bringing art to the bedside and humanizing the way in which nurses (and other health professionals) engage with children (Rollins, 2005a). Rollins, Bolig, and Mahan's work also showed that hospitalization and illness can be triggers for growth (2005). Carter (2005) used scrapbooks as a means of triggering stories and engagement with children with complex needs and with their siblings. The scrapbooks that the children freely created consisted of a mélange of stories, poems, pictures, photographs, and collages. Each page represented something of importance to the child and provided a focus for child-centered discussion. All of the discussions added depth to Carter's knowing of the children, and many reflected the depth and sophistication that the children had in relation to the sick child's illness and its effect on family life. Some of the children chose to protect their parents by containing their worries about whether the respite nurse who was coming to their home for the first time would be "as good as Mum" and could be "trusted." Amy and Sophie said,

> We didn't tell her [we were worried], we just wanted her [Mum] to get out the house ... We wanted her to have a nice time ... I was a bit worried 'cause I didn't know who they were, but when [nurse] came, she was dead nice and I knew everyone else would be nice ... so, no worries!

Conclusion

Knowing children means moving into more ambiguous, uncertain, and very human ground in our practice. Despite the ambiguity, it is intensely rewarding. Children might be smaller than we are, but their worlds are not. Their worlds can often be immense, unlimited by the boundaries that constrain adult thinking. Billy Collins' poem "On Turning Ten" summed up some of the magic of the way a 4-year-old thinks:

> At four I was an Arabian wizard.
> I could make myself invisible
> by drinking a glass of milk a certain way

Children navigate their worlds with remarkable skill and dexterity, but illness and injury can challenge them, making territory in which they usually feel secure feel unfamiliar and frightening. One of our roles as children's nurses is to act as pilots for the child, offering guidance and support through that unfamiliar territory.

Coming to know a child does not require grand plans. It requires commitment to take the opportunities that arise in the micro-moments of practice. In some senses it is simple. All we need to do is to prioritize getting to know the child—to see it as equally as important as 'doing the obs',(i.e., observations or vital signs), There is already a drive to have pain as the fifth vital sign; maybe the sixth vital sign should be knowing the child. We need to attend to children when they are talking to us, to provide spaces in our nursing talk for child talk to come through, and to engage meaningfully with children when we are checking their infusion lines.

We need to be the nurses we want to be—to be the nurses that we know we can be.

An Epilogue: Knowing James

James is a beautiful child moving toward being a gracious, handsome, and disarming young man. It is early February and late at night; James can't sleep and he wants to talk. He chooses me. As he talks to me, we move from the mundane, superficial chart-talk exchanges about his temperature to a more hesitant, beginning exploration about him, his feelings, and what he tells me is the "important stuff." Quietly and tentatively, he starts to talk about his family; not in the joking way he has talked about them before, but as if talking about them to me was starting to reveal them to himself. As I listen to James, he becomes less hesitant, more certain that he wants to talk; stories pour out of him. They need to be told.

James talked of lots of things—his friends and friendship, his parents and his older brother. Sometimes he talked directly, but often his stories were more indirect—circuitous but purposive and talking to and for himself as much as to and with me. What James talked most about was his "big trip." James's trip was partly an homage to a holiday his brother had done the year before, when he and his girlfriend had hitched to Greece and eaten octopus. James's brother had come back with beads in his hair. James saw this trip as a good starting point, although he explained that he was more ambitious, definitely better looking, and was not going to stop at Greece. He was going to have more beads in his hair. His trip was going to continue on beyond Greece, through to India, Nepal, China, and then back via the Americas. Although his motto for the trip was going to be "no worries," he did have some aspects planned down to the last detail. The girlfriend he had yet to meet was going to be perfect, although during the course of the several nights he talked about the trip, his notion of the perfect girl friend changed somewhat. She turned from blonde to brunette, from a punk (to upset his mum) to someone who was great at sports and who'd be as good as he was at running. The trip got bigger and bigger and his story projected farther and farther into the future. We talked about the places he wanted to visit (definitely no museums!) and the places that were on my list—he mostly approved of my choices. He promised that he would "almost definitely but then again probably not" send me postcards.

Through parts of five or six nights in between me checking his observations, regulating his oxygen, recording his fluid balance, giving his medication, and making him comfortable, I listened with his story and travelled with him.

James was 14, bald, and beautiful, and full of stories.

Through his stories, I came to know him; and through my listening to his stories, he came to know me and something about nursing and nurses. I finished my week of night duty, but I promised I'd pop back to see him the following day to listen to the next instalment of what we were now calling his "fantastic voyage." But it was not to be. James had died. It was expected and inevitable. It was unexpected and profoundly shocking.

I went over to talk with his family, to offer something to them. His mother squeezed my hand and gave me an envelope saying James had been insistent that she give it to me. Inside the envelope was a Valentine's Day card signed by James and saying that he would have to "make do" with me as his first valentine. The valentine was, in many ways, the last—albeit poignant—installment of his "fantastic voyage." The stories he spun and shared with me helped me to reach across to him, to help care for those parts of him that could not be recorded on intake/output, medication, and vital signs charts. His stories allowed him to explore and express his hopes and fears and to be the child/young man he wanted to be and to become. James was bald but longed for a future in which he had long, blonde, beaded hair. He was trapped in a cubicle yet able to travel to lands farther flung than his brother had ever aspired to. He knew he had limited time, but that did not constrain him.

The time that James and I shared during what I look back on as a defining set of night duty was not an unbroken therapeutic period. Some of the parts of the stories were related during snatched moments of time; others were told when I was able to create longer periods of space for him. As rewarding as it was for me to come to know James, I believe that James gained from being known and from knowing that someone cared.

James was then and always will be for me a special child who taught me about the fragility and the resilience of life. James was one of my first teachers—one of the first children who helped me to fully realize how vital knowing can be.

Knowing James became an exquisite knowing.

References

Alanen, L. (1999). Rethinking socialization, the family and childhood. *Sociological Studies of Child Development, 3,* 13–28.

Bruijnzeels, M. A., Foets, M., van der Wouden, J. C., van den Heuvel, W. J., & Prins, A. (1998). Everyday symptoms in childhood: Occurrence and general practitioner consultation rates. *British Journal of General Practice, 48,* 880–884.

Buchbinder, M. L. (2008). 'You're still sick!' Framing, footing, and participation in children's medical play. *Discourse Studies, 10,* 139–159.

Carter, B. (2005). "They've got to be as good as mum and dad": Children with complex health care needs and their siblings' perceptions of a Diana community nursing service. *Clinical Effectiveness in Nursing, 9,* 49–61.

Carter, B. (2009 – in press). Nursing amidst stories (and knowing what to do with them). *Journal of Clinical Nursing, 18,* 477–484.

Carter, B. (2008). "Good" and "bad" stories: Decisive moments, "shock and awe" and being moral. *Journal of Clinical Nursing, 17,* 1063–1070.

Charon, R. (2007). What to do with stories: The sciences of narrative medicine. *Canadian Family Physician, 53,* 1265–1267.

Christensen, P. H. (2004). Children's participation in ethnographic research: Issues of power and representation. *Children and Society, 18,* 165–176.

Graue, M. E., & Walsh, D. (1998). *Studying children in context: Theories, methods and ethics.* Thousand Oaks, CA: Sage.

Greene, S., & Hogan, D. (2005). Preface. In S. Greene & D. Hogan (Eds.), *Researching children's experience* (pp. xi–xiii). London: Sage.

Horton, J. (2001). Do you get some funny looks when you tell people what you do? Muddling through some angsts and ethics of (being a male). Researching with children. *Ethics, Place and Environment, 4*, 159–166.

James, A., & Prout, A. (1997). Re-presenting childhood: Time and transition in the study of childhood. In A. James & A. Prout (Eds.), *Constructing and reconstructing childhood: Contemporary issues in the sociological study of childhood* (pp. 230–250). London: Falmer Press.

Jones, O. (2001). Before the dark of reason: Some ethical and epistemological considerations on the otherness of children. *Ethics, Place and Environment, 4*, 173–178.

Kincheloe, J. L. (2004). Foreword. In L. D. Soto & B. B. Swadener (Eds.), *Power and voice in research with children* (pp. xi–xiv). New York: Peter Lang.

Marshall, M., Carter, B., & Rose, K. (2006). Adolescents living with diabetes: Self-care and parental relationships. *Journal of Diabetes Nursing, 10*, 421–429.

Marshall, M. (ongoing) Normal but Different, Different but Normal: Children's and their Parents' Perceptions of Living with Diabetes. PhD thesis. University of Central Lancashire.

Matthews, H. (2001). Participatory structures and the youth of today: Engaging those who are hardest to reach. *Ethics, Place and Environment, 4*, 153–159.

Matthews, H., & Limb, M. (1999). Defining an agenda for the geography of children: Review and prospect. *Progress in Human Geography, 23*, 61–90.

Mayall, B. (1998). Towards a sociology of child health. *Sociology of Health & Illness, 20*, 269–288.

Neill, S. J. (2000). Acute childhood illness at home: The parents' perspective. *Journal of Advanced Nursing, 31*, 821–832.

Noddings, N. (1984). *Caring, a feminine approach to ethics & moral education.* Berkeley, CA: University of California Press.

Olson, L. M., Radecki, L., Frintner, M. P., Weiss, K. B., Korfmacher, J., & Siegel, R. M. (2007). At what age can children report dependably on their asthma health status? *Pediatrics, 119*, e93–102.

Porter, S. (1998). *Social theory and nursing practice.* Basingstoke, United Kingdom: Macmillan.

Raman, L., & Gelman, S. A. (2007). Children's recognition of time in the causes and cures of physical and emotional reactions to illnesses and injuries. *British Journal of Psychology, 98*, 389–410.

Ransome, A. (1930). *Swallows and Amazons.* London: Jonathan Cape.

Ransome, A. (1933). *Winter holiday.* London: Jonathan Cape.

Riley, A. W. (2004). Evidence that school-age children can self-report on their health. *Ambulatory Pediatrics, 4*, 371–376.

Rollins, J. (2005a). *Art activities for children at bedside.* Washington, DC: WVSA, Arts Connection.

Rollins, J., Bolig, R., & Mahan, C. (2005). *Meeting children's psychosocial needs across the healthcare continuum.* ProEd Austin, Texas.

Rollins, J. A. (2005b). Tell me about it: Drawing as a communication tool for children with cancer. *Journal of Pediatric Oncology Nursing, 22*, 203–221.

Rowling, J. K. (1997). *Harry Potter and the philosopher's stone.* London: Bloomsbury.

Rubovits, D. S., & Wolynn, T. H. (1999). Children's illness cognition: What mothers think. *Clinical Pediatrics, 38,* 99–105.

Sanders, C., Carter, B., & Goodacre, L. (2008). Parents' narratives about their experiences of their child's reconstructive genital surgeries for ambiguous genitalia. *Journal of Clinical Nursing. 17,* 23, 3187–3195.

Sanders, C. (under examination) Parents of children with ambiguous genitalia: Stories of experiences of reconstructive genital surgeries and finding harmony. Unpublished 2007 PhD thesis. University of Central Lancashire.

Schmidt, C., Bernaix, L., Koski, A., Weese, J., Chiappetta, M., & Sandrik, K. (2007). Hospitalized children's perceptions of nurses and nurse behaviors. *MCN, The American Journal of Maternal/Child Nursing, 32,* 336–342.

Shin, H., & White-Traut, R. (2005). Nurse-child interaction on an inpatient paediatric unit. *Journal of Advanced Nursing, 52,* 56–62.

Stein, H. F. (2003). Ways of knowing in medicine: Seeing and beyond. *Families, Systems & Health: The Journal of Collaborative Family HealthCare, 21,* 29.

Suzuki, S. (1986). *Zen mind, beginner's mind.* New York: Weatherhill.

Thomas, R. S. (1986). Children's song. In *Selected Poems 1946–1968* (p. 34). Newcastle: Bloodaxe Books.

Wassmer, E., Minnaar, G., Aal, N. A., Atkinson, M., Gupta, E., Yuen, S., & Rylance, G. (2004). How do paediatricians communicate with children and parents? *Acta Paediatrica, 93,* 1501–1506.

Young, L. & Barrett, H. (2001). Ethics and participation: Reflections on research with street children. *Ethics, Place & Environment, 4,* 130–134.

Knowing Persons With Disabilities: Nurses Illuminate Difference in a Natural Light

15

Donna Carol Maheady

Chapter Overview

Many of us recognize that we will experience some form of disability, either permanent or temporary, at some point in our lives. Still others would say that we are all disabled in some way. Given this reality, why do we struggle so hard to cure, name, and/or explain disability?

Who are these persons who include all or most of us? How can we humbly gain deeper understanding of and insight into the issues persons with disabilities face, and come to know and celebrate them as whole—just as they are?

If disabilities were more commonly recognized and anticipated in the way that we designed our environments or our systems, would they be seen as abnormal? If environments became more accessible and more universal design concepts were implemented, wouldn't all persons in society enjoy such benefits?

For answers to these questions and more, we turn to nurses with disabilities for discussion of issues and controversies. Through their stories, the reader will be challenged to reflect on old and new perspectives about disability—in a natural light.

Introduction

Black bodies, white bodies; male bodies, female bodies; young bodies, old bodies; tall bodies, short bodies; beautiful bodies, unattractive bodies, broken bodies; right bodies and wrong bodies. Our bodies have framed our futures and explained our pasts; our bodies write our stories. But it is not our bodies, per se, that write the story; rather it is the way in which we, as a society, construct our bodies that shapes our history and our future (Clapton & Fitzgerald, 1997, p. 20).

Bodily difference has for centuries determined social structures by defining certain bodies as the norm and defining those that fall outside the norm as "other." The degree of otherness has been defined by the degree of variation from the norm. In doing this, we have created an artificial "paradigm of humanity" into which some of us fit neatly and others fit very badly (Clapton & Fitzgerald, 1997, p. 20), particularly those with "normality" differences—for example, in human physiological functions, anatomical features, or physiognomy.

For persons with disabilities, the body is also the center of political struggle. In the 1800s, people with disabilities were considered unfortunate, tragic, sick, useless, pitiful individuals unfit and unable to contribute to society, except to serve as ridiculed objects of entertainment in circuses and exhibitions (Anti-Defamation League, 2005). They were assumed to be abnormal and feeble-minded and were often forced to undergo sterilization and live in institutions and asylums. As society's definitions of *bodies* have been challenged by people with disabilities, a new group of people with disabilities has emerged with a focus on positive self-image and self-determination. A movement has grown as persons have refused to be warehoused in institutions, restricted from public places, and discriminated against in employment (Eiesland, 1994). They often live a difficult life ordinarily.

Reflection on the Past

Table 15.1 chronicles events and dates significant to our understanding of the evolution of societal attitudes toward persons with disabilities. The time line documents the struggle persons with disabilities have had to move toward equality and full participation in the mainstream of life. The events speak for themselves and provide the background to this chapter for thought and reflection.

15.1	Time line of Significant Events Affecting Persons With Disabilities

Date	Description of Event
3500 BCE	The Rig-Veda, an ancient sacred poem of India, includes what is said to be the first written record of prosthesis.
355 BCE	Aristotle said those "born deaf become senseless and incapable of reason."
1500 CE	Girolamo Cardano was the first physician to recognize the ability of the deaf to reason.
1784	Abba Silvestri opened the first school for the deaf in Rome, Italy.
1790	In Paris, Philippe Pinel unshackled people with mental illnesses.
1815	Thomas H. Gallaudet departed America for Europe to seek methods to teach the deaf.
1817	Connecticut Asylum for the Education of Deaf and Dumb Persons opened in Hartford.
1829	Louis Braille invented the raised point alphabet now known as Braille.
1872	Alexander G. Bell opened a speech school for teachers of the deaf in Boston.
1887	Women were admitted to the National Deaf-Mute College (now Gallaudet University).
1921	The American Foundation for the Blind was founded.
1935	The League for the Physically Handicapped protested discrimination by the Works Progress Administration (WPA).
1939	Hitler ordered widespread "mercy killing." The Nazi euthanasia program was code-named Aktion T4 and was instituted to eliminate "life unworthy of life."

(continued)

15.1	Time line of Significant Events Affecting Persons With Disabilities (continued)

Date	Description of Event
1974	The Disabled Women's Coalition was founded at UC Berkeley by Susan Sygall and Deborah Kaplan.
1976	The Federal Communications Commission authorized reserving line 21 on television sets for closed captions.
1977	A group of people with disabilities took over the San Francisco offices of the Health, Education, and Welfare Department to protest Secretary Joseph Califano's refusal to sign regulations for Section 504 of the Rehabilitation Act.
1980–1983	National Disabled Women's Educational Equity Project was established. National Disabled Women's Educational Equity Project put on the first national Conference on Disabled Women's Educational Equity in Bethesda, MD.
1988	"Deaf President Now" protest occurred at Gallaudet University in Washington, DC. ADAPT took on the inaccessible Greyhound buses.
1990	Americans with Disabilities Act (ADA) signing ceremony occurred at the White House.
1990	The Secretary of Transportation issued regulations mandating lifts on buses.
1995	Two women disability leaders were elected to parliament in South Africa and Zimbabwe. The First International Symposium on Issues of Women with Disabilities was held in Beijing, China. The organization of people with disabilities in Cuba held their first international conference on disability rights.

Source: Disability Social History Project (n.d.)

Coming to Terms
The difference between the almost right word & the right word is really a large matter—it's the difference between the lightning bug and the lightning. (Twain, 1890)

There is no universally agreed-upon definition of disability. A definition of disability or a descriptor may become a sociopolitical passport to services or legal status. Beyond that, definitions

are up for debate, and much depends on which service system is used—for example, Social Security disability benefits,
special education services in schools, transportation services,
state vocational/rehabilitation programs, Medicaid/Medicare,
or workers compensation programs (Snow, 2008).

Some argue that we need to go beyond conceptions of
constructed disability to a notion of universalism in which
disability is actually seen as a fluid and continuous condition that has no boundaries but that is, in fact, the essence
of the human condition (Bickenbach, Chatterji, Badley, &
Ustun, 1999). As a condition that is experienced by us all at
some stage in our lives, disability is actually normal (Clapton
& Fitzgerald, 1997).

The politically correct language surrounding disability
issues has changed over time. According to Disabled People's
International (1993), disability is the functional limitation
within the individual caused by physical, mental, or sensory
impairment. Handicap is the loss or limitation of opportunities to take part in the normal life of the community on an
equal level with others.

Disability is currently the most generally accepted term.
Referring to persons with disabilities using person-first language remains most important. Persons with disabilities are,
for example, mothers and fathers who are bipolar, sons and
daughters who are autistic, friends and neighbors with multiple sclerosis, physicians who are blind, nurses who are deaf,
and presidents who use wheelchairs. They are not a homo-
geneous group called "the handicapped" or "the disabled"
(Snow, 2008).

Models of Disability. Socially constructed models of disability came about as a way to define or explain disability. Some
of the models have evolved into tools that serve to provide a
basis upon which a government or society meets the needs
of people with disabilities. Persons with disabilities often
view models with skepticism, and some resist categorization
because they feel that the resources and needs of individuals with the same diagnosis can differ greatly. People who
experience disability do not always conceptualize their lives
in terms of a neat model (Smart, 2006–2007).

The religious model. The religious model views disability
as something inflicted upon an individual or family by an

external force. From some religious perspectives, it can be related to actions committed by the person, someone in the family or community group, or even forbears.

According to Eiesland (1994), "The Christian interpretation of disability has run the gamut from symbolizing sin to representing an occasion for supererogation. The persistent thread has been that a person with a disability is either divinely blessed or damned" (p. 70). Eiesland (1994) offered as an example a story in the New Testament gospel of John. In this account, a man who was unable to walk was sitting by the pool of Bethesda. After healing this man, Jesus said, "Do not sin anymore, so that nothing worse happens to you (p. 71)." Eisland (1994) stated that passages like this have been cited as proof that disability is a sign of moral imperfection or retribution for sin. She also offered a contrasting passage from the same gospel. In this passage, Jesus had a different reply when questioned about a blind man. When his disciples asked him, "Rabbi, who sinned, this man or his parents, that he was born blind?" Jesus answered, surprisingly, "Neither this man nor his parents sinned; he was born blind so that God's works might be revealed in him" (Eiesland, 1994, pp. 71–72).

The obligation to engage in charitable giving is fundamental to many faiths. This charity focus has resulted in establishment of hospitals and clinics for people with disabilities. These efforts have contributed to medical advances that have benefited persons with disabilities.

An unintentional outcome of some faith-based efforts has been the environmental and social segregation of people with disabilities from the religious community. Often people with disabilities are denied full social and religious participation within the life of the church, synagogue, or mosque through practices, attitudes, and structural barriers that limit rather than empower and segregate rather than include.

When disability is addressed in terms of themes of sin-disability confabulation, virtuous suffering, or charitable action, it will be seen as a fate to be avoided or pitied, a tragedy, or a cause to be championed rather than an ordinary life to be lived (Eiesland, 1994, p. 75).

The biomedical model. The biomedical model of disability is a lens through which the person is viewed as the problem in need of cure or rehabilitation—the person needs to be fixed. The disability exists solely within the individual, privatizing it in ways that absolve society from responsibility of dealing with disability issues such as civil rights and accommodations. The person has to adjust and adapt. Disability is dysfunction, abnormality, inferiority, pathology, or defect. It is simply "better not to have a disability" (Smart, 2006–2007, p. 42).

This view has been challenged by some persons who are deaf and refuse to be considered disabled. They see themselves as members of a cultural group, with a shared language (e.g., American Sign Language).

Whereas many medical professionals see disability as a personal tragedy, many persons with disabilities feel that the disability is a valued part of their identity. Many people with disabilities feel that "difficulty does not automatically translate to tragic" (Smart, 2006–2007, p. 42). The greatest difficulties or challenges may have nothing to do with the disability but may be the result of social isolation, prejudice, discrimination, and poverty (Guernsey, Nicoli, & Ninio, 2007). Societies make people with disabilities foreigners in their own countries (Higgins, 1992).

The biomedical model divides persons into groups based on diagnostic categories or functional traits, effectively fragmenting persons with disabilities into groups competing for resources and services (Smart, 2006–2007). The person is viewed as an object or collection of body parts that lacks wholeness. The body machine is viewed as broken, a view that is endemic to contemporary health care.

American President Franklin Delano Roosevelt is well-known to have disguised and minimized his disability in his role as a political leader. Less well-known is the remarkable nature of the colony he established for people with disabilities from polio in Warm Springs, Georgia, in 1927. The colony at Warm Springs represents a unique historical community in which disability was not stigmatized, where people with disabilities controlled their own resources and their own lives, and where the medical model of disability was repudiated (Holland, 2006).

The social model. The quest to find medically based cures distracts people from looking at the causes of the impairment or disability. In a worldwide sense, most disabilities are created by war, poverty, hunger, malnutrition, medical advances that prolong life, population growth, HIV/AIDS, lack of clean water, exploitation of workers, land mines, lack of safety, and child abuse (UN Chronicle, 2004). People need to address these issues more robustly, rather than just responding to the injuries and impairments that result from them.

The social model addresses these issues and also recognizes that it is society that is disabling people with disabilities. Disability is a social state and not a medical condition (Harris & Enfield, 2003; Oliver, 1990, 2004). The problem rests squarely with society. The social model, although not rejecting medical intervention, recognizes that some people have physical or psychological challenges that may affect the means by which they function. In this model, people are disabled primarily due to the barriers that exist for them in a society, such as stairs without lifts or elevators, information that is not available in large print, or negative societal attitudes. How we react to difference is a social and policy choice. For example, a person with a disability is not disabled by spina bifida or multiple sclerosis, but rather is disabled by structural barriers to offices, bathrooms, and restaurants, and by discriminatory attitudes held by society.

Disability, when viewed as a long-term social state, is not treatable or curable. This view is in direct conflict with traditional views of medicine and rehabilitation, which are founded on an ideology of normality. The goal of medicine and rehabilitation is to restore the person to normality or to a state that is as near normal as possible; whatever the costs in term of pain or suffering, the ideology of normality rules (Oliver, 1990).

The human rights model. The human rights model moves beyond the social model by focusing on the rights of people with disabilities. Disability continues to be seen as a socially created problem and not an attribute of a person, but dignity as a value has been added as a crucial factor. Often invisible, people with disabilities have been treated as objects to be protected or pitied, and as recipients of charity. A crucial change occurred when persons with disabilities saw themselves and were seen by others as subjects and not as objects (Quinn & Degener, 2002). This social perspective is reflected in the WHO International Classification of Functioning, Disability, and Health (ICF), which defines disability as a universal human experience and not the concern of a minority; every human being can suffer from a health loss and thus experience some disability (World Health Organization, 2001; UN Chronicle, 2004).

The changing nature of disability and the realization that it is an inevitable part of the life of any individual or society required that the concept of disability be related to the issue of human dignity (UN Chronicle, 2004). Every human being is to be valued and respected. In a recent study on human rights and disability conducted for the Office of the United Nations High Commissioner for Human Rights, human dignity was identified as one of the four most essential values. The other three identified were autonomy, equality, and solidarity (Quinn & Degener, 2002).

The growth of the international disability movement, "Nothing About Us Without Us" encapsulates this shift in perspective towards a principle of participation and the integration of persons with disabilities in every aspect of political, social, economic, and cultural life (Charlton, 2000). The process of ensuring that persons with disabilities enjoy their human rights is inspired by the values that underpin human rights: the dignity of every person, self-determination that demands that the person be placed at the center of all decisions affecting him/her, equality of all regardless of difference, and solidarity that requires society to sustain the freedom of the person with appropriate social supports (Quinn & Degener, 2002). This is profoundly encapsulated in the following:

> Human dignity is the anchor norm of human rights. Each individual is deemed to be of inestimable value and nobody is insignificant. People are to be valued not just because they are economically or otherwise useful but because of their inherent self-worth. People with disabilities have a stake in and claim on society that must be honored quite apart from any considerations of social or economic utility. (Quinn & Degener, 2002, p. 14).

Commemorating the 2004 International Day of Disabled Persons, "Nothing about Us, Without Us," Secretary-General Kofi Annan stressed that "no society can claim to be based on justice and equality without persons with disabilities making decisions as full-fledged members" (United Nations Enable, 2004).

Pause for Reflection. Can One Model Fit All? If a model as a lens for knowing is too general and covers everything, it becomes useless. A model may also retain a name even when it has become something different because the context society has changed (Finkelstein, 2007).

Which model of disability influences your practice as a nurse? Do you use one or a combination? Is the influence of the model conscious or unconscious? How do you come to know a person?

Example: A child is born with a hearing loss.

Religious Model:	"She is a gift from God... here to teach us."
Medical Model:	"If she gets a cochlear implant, she will be able to hear so much better."
Social Model:	"We should all learn sign language so that we can communicate with this child and other persons with hearing loss."
Human Rights Model:	"When she grows up, she will be able to attend a university if she wants to."

Example: A child is born with Down syndrome and a cardiac condition.

Religious Model:	"This is God's will."
Medical Model:	"Surgery will be able to fix his heart."
Social Model:	"He should attend the neighborhood school so he is surrounded by persons without disabilities."
Human Rights Model:	"Where does he want to go to school? Let's ask him!"

Legal Protections. Many countries still do not have laws that address disability issues. According to the Inter-Parliamentary Union, only one third of countries have antidiscrimination and other disability-specific laws (United Nations, 2008). For example, national disability nondiscrimination laws have been passed in the following countries: Colombia, 1997; Costa Rica, 1996; Ghana, 1993; Israel, 1998; Jordan, 1993; United Kingdom, 1995, 2005; United States of America, 1990;

and Zambia, 1996 (Disability Rights Education and Defense Fund, 2008).

Passage of legislation does not instantly change hearts and minds with the stroke of a pen. Deep-rooted assumptions and stereotypical biases can be difficult to change, and enforcement of laws may be weak or lacking. People with disabilities continue to face prejudice and bias in the stereotypical portrayal of people with disabilities in movies (British Film Institute n.d.); in the media; in physical barriers to schools, housing and voting stations; and in lack of affordable health care (Anti-Defamation League, 2005). The consequences of disability are particularly serious for women because they are discriminated against on the double grounds of gender and disability (UN Chronicle, 2004).

Pause for Reflection. Is Disability Natural? If adolescents with disabilities were asked about their daily lives and well-being, how do you think they would respond? Do you think they would see their disability as a natural part of life?

In a research study, adolescents with disabilities reported the desire to be allowed to prepare for living a normal life integrated in society. They reported needing a feeling of support, personal growth, and acceptance of their illness/disability as a natural part of life (Berntsson, Berg, Brydolf, & Hellström, 2007, p. 419).

Coming to Know Persons with Disabilities—Vignettes

Nurses born with disabilities and those who acquire disabilities later in life offer a unique perspective on those nursed. Lived experiences illuminate disability in deeply personal ways that serve to guide our path to a deeper understanding of being whole—a notion that transcends body parts and functional abilities. When the tables are turned, the lens of caring clears the view and frees the nurse to look beyond standardized plans of care and see the whole person in a new light. Sowers and Smith (2002) reported that nurses with disabilities believed their disability actually helped humanize them in their patients' eyes—it helped to ameliorate the "myth of perfection" (p. 332) of the health care profession.

The following stories invite us to examine our views of disability in a new, more natural light. Each story is followed by a series of questions that provoke and encourage further thought and deeper reflection, while encouraging us to identify the issues and challenges of coming to know the person as whole.

Storytelling has been successful in teaching many topics in nursing (Diekelmann & Diekelmann, 2000; Cangelosi & Whitt, 2006). Stories can inspire us, challenge us to think in new ways, and bring us back to the core values of our work (Drake, 2002). Exemplar stories can describe scenarios that are unusual as well as those that are ordinary (Benner, 1984). Each person who hears the story begins to cocreate new stories and to think about solutions (Denning, 2000).

A wheelchair? A nurse who suffered a spinal cord injury following an automobile accident spoke about her experiences and responses from patients in her care:

> *"Oh my gosh. She's in a wheelchair!" some would say. My being in a wheelchair seems to project to people that I'm not as smart as someone who doesn't use a wheelchair... They question my ability as though my having a physical disability has affected my mind... If I were a smart nurse, in other words, I wouldn't be in a wheelchair.*
>
> *Coworkers will say, "fix your ankle," or comment about my chair, "You're kind of... slouchy." They frequently make me feel like a child again. (Maheady, 2003, p. 112)*
>
> *I have incredible insight into my patients and they with me... People with a disability seem to understand each other. As a nurse I like to show people how to lose focus on their problems and to believe they can do more than they expect. Children are interesting to work with also. They immediately want to know, "Can you walk? How did you get that injury? Hey, lady, how do you get that chair in the car? Do you sleep in that chair?" (Maheady, 2003, pp. 113–115)*
>
> *I'm Catholic and... I have grown even closer to God now. I had a few problems with religion when I was injured, and I didn't want to talk to the priest. I had all of the "why me" questions... My faith is very important to me, and I know my beliefs. My injury solidified them; they did not break them.*

Years later, I interviewed at two graduate schools. I didn't like the Catholic university because of their attitude. They treated me as though I was inadequate. The administrator said, "Come through the back door, because the office isn't accessible for a wheelchair. You're going to have to come through the back, because I have to find another room for us." It was a dreadful experience. (Maheady, 2003, p. 114)

Following her injury, the nurse graduated from nursing school and worked as a head nurse of a spinal cord injury unit. She now works as a legal nurse consultant in Florida and loves sailing in the Atlantic Ocean.

Is this a self-care deficit? What influences our perceptions of intelligence?

Why would coworkers feel the need to comment about her chair or ankle?

Do children react differently than adults to a person with a disability?

How could you come to know this person using the religious/medical/human rights/social model?

Would she be welcomed by faith-based organizations (churches, synagogues, mosques)?

Wheel power! A nurse who has multiple sclerosis works as a legal nurse consultant in Ohio. She shares her adjustment to using a wheelchair:

Nothing is as easy when you're doing it from a wheelchair, but I took figuring out ways to do things differently as a challenge. To this day, the creative problem solving that goes with adapting to life on wheels is something I enjoy... I love kids; and now that I'm on their level, I find they love dealing with an adult who always looks at them eye-to-eye. I never have to worry about ironing the back of my shirt or jacket. I frequently get to sit at the head of the table in business settings... and I must admit, I love the feeling of power. (Maheady, 2006, pp. 12–13)
I know some of that may sound silly, but it reflects an attitude change that was essential for my survival. I couldn't change my circumstances, but I knew I could keep from letting them change me for the worse. I look at

> *my adaptive equipment as no more or less than the tools*
> *I need to remain active and independent; it's no different*
> *from the glasses I've been wearing since I was 8 years old.*
> *(Maheady, 2006, p. 13)*

This nurse is married and has three children. With the help of her state Vocational Rehabilitation program, she received the financial support necessary to complete a legal nurse certificate program and adapt her van with hand controls; she went off disability payments and returned to work.

How could you come to know her using the human rights/social model?

Is this an alteration in mobility? Survival?

How could you come to know this nurse better as a person?

Would ramps, bi-parting doors, and accessible bathrooms help her as well as others?

You didn't ask. Another nurse who was born missing her left hand recounts,

> *"I came home after the first day of school and said to my*
> *mother, "I was the only one in my class missing a hand.*
> *Why didn't you tell me?" Her mother replied, "You didn't*
> *ask" (Maheady, 2006, p. 26).*
>
> *Another day, she was watching a television commercial*
> *that featured several children with sorrow on their faces—*
> *all with various handicaps. Her mind began to wander. Is*
> *this my destiny?*
>
> *She recalls, "I remember children actually getting nau-*
> *seated when they saw my hand. During school dances, when*
> *other children held hands on the dance floor, I knew my*
> *place was next to the teacher. However discouraging these*
> *experiences, I gained strength" (Maheady, 2006, p. 27).*
>
> *Another day she asked her mother, "Am I handicapped?"*
> *Her clever mother replied, "Only if you want to be" (Fleming*
> *& Maheady, 2005, p. 535).*

She also shares perspective on dating and married life:

> *When I was young and dating, some young men could*
> *not accept my hand. However, my husband was differ-*
> *ent. After 20 years, he has shown love and acceptance...*

My missing hand acted as a 'meter' of sorts, keeping me single long enough to meet the right man. (Maheady, 2006, p. 30)

This nurse is married and the mother of four children. She teaches nursing at a university in Washington state. She and her husband often participate in medical missions to South America.

How could you come to know this nurse using the human rights or social model?

Does she have a musculoskeletal alteration, freedom of choice, or courage?

The Gift. A nurse who is HIV-positive states,

When you live with a chronic disease day in and day out, you become familiar with what is changing in your body. Over time, people learn to see you in a different light—not as a person with a chronic illness, but a person who takes life and runs with it into their dreams... I go to work every day; and by going to work, I'm contributing to the nursing profession and to the reputation of all people with disabilities. I'm an example of that if you decide to take charge of your life and health, you can do anything, no matter what type of disability you may have. (Maheady, 2006, p. 83)

When you are given this gift, you can either choose to keep it wrapped up or open it up and learn to use it to help others. By choosing to open your gift... you begin the process of education, ending discrimination against persons with disabilities and becoming a role model. It's easy to sit on the sidelines, do nothing, and watch the world go by. It's hard to get on the court with a disability and play. When I question, "Why am I here, God?" I know the answer. I am here to share my positive gift with everyone. (Maheady, 2006, p. 84)

This nurse received the 2005 Nurse of the Year Award from the neuroscience unit at his place of employment. He and his partner live in Florida.

Is this an immunologic alteration or a gift to share?

How could you come to know his gift?

How could you come to know him using the human rights or social model?

Giving 150% A nurse who has experienced progressive vision loss since childhood due to retinitis pigmentosa describes the situation when she was hired for a position:

> *There was palpable resentment among the nurses. They had been forewarned that I was visually impaired. They feared that they would have to "carry" a handicapped nurse. I had to prove myself. I had to give 150% to receive credit for 50%. Patients and visitors have made disparaging comments at times that I have tried to attribute to ignorance. But they hurt no less. (Maheady, 2006, p. 43–45)*
>
> *Lighting in our hospital rooms has changed. We now have energy-saving fixtures and wall switches located in the center of the room's back walls, requiring one to stumble through the dark to find the switch. More forms with increasing items requiring documentation have been added to nurses' daily tasks, and the print has shrunk. I didn't like having to ask others to do my job for me... I became determined to work my way into the educational aspect of nursing. (Maheady, 2006, p. 45)*
>
> *With the help of a large computer monitor and Zoomtext, I received my master's in nursing education with a 4.0 GPA. I don't know whose smile is bigger in the graduation picture—my guide dog's or mine. (Maheady, 2006, p. 46)*
>
> *I learned from my patients that life is a precious gift... I live my life by a creed... I am only one, but I am one. I cannot do everything, but I can do something. What I can do, I ought to do. And what I ought to do, by the grace of God, I will do. (Maheady, 2006, p. 47)*

This nurse has a master's degree in nursing and works as a diabetic nurse educator at a hospital. She and her husband live in Florida.

Does she have a visual alteration?

Do persons with disabilities have to work harder than others in order to prove themselves?

How could you come to know this person using the human rights or social model?

Would brighter lights, large-print documents, and audio book recordings help her as well as others?

Cool wheels. A nurse born with spina bifida states, "My family raised me with a 'can do' attitude, and I was never treated any differently than the other kids in my family" (Maheady, 2006, p. 75). Today, she has a BSN and is a registered nurse on the pediatric unit of a rehabilitation hospital.

She recounts,

> *I was raised to focus on what I could do. Becoming a nurse was the ultimate goal for me, and from day one, I was not going to let anyone or anything stand in my way. It was my calling. As strange as it may sound, a part of me always felt like I belonged in the hospital, even as a patient. I didn't enjoy the pain I endured during my many hospital stays, but I still felt that I belonged there. (Maheady, 2006, p. 75)*
>
> *One of my professors suggested that I meet the assistant dean of the nursing college. I was a little afraid that she was going to tell me that nursing wasn't for me. Instead, she vowed to help me in any way she could. We knew that we were going to have to pick apart each clinical experience and assess whether or not I absolutely had to perform every skill. If it was not an essential function, then we discussed delegating the task to someone else. If I knew there was a lift or transfer that I could not perform, I asked a classmate to do it for me, promising to lend my help when he or she needed it. (Maheady, 2006, p. 76)*
>
> *After graduation … I interviewed constantly, but I got turned down for every job. I met with the people from the disability services office and the assistant dean of the nursing college. We agreed to team up to help the next person with a wheelchair who decides to go through the nursing program (Maheady, 2006, p. 78).*
>
> *Soon after, "I flew out to an interview… I knew it had gone well… I wasn't even out of the airport parking garage when I got a phone call requesting a second interview" (Maheady, 2006, p. 78).*
>
> *I now work as a full-time registered nurse on the pediatric unit. The biggest lesson I learned from the experience is to never let go of a dream. My younger patients think it is cool that their nurse has a wheelchair just like them. (Maheady, 2006, p. 79)*

Does she have an alteration in mobility, or did she fulfill her destiny?

How could you come to know her using the human rights or social model?

How has the medical model influenced her life?

Hope. It is nearly impossible to find a nurse who has a serious mental illness who isn't terrified to talk about it. A nurse recounted being unable to shower, being too afraid to get her mail, and having her husband dress and undress her. Another nurse shared being in a dark, suicidal hell and being unable to get out of bed. She wanted to die, but she still got up to go to work. She did her shift with her supervisor aware of her condition:

> *"It wasn't easy to walk with legs made of lead, or breathe when the air weighs you down. A professional leaves their depression at home. No one would have guessed how low I was."(personal communication, September, 2007)*

This nurse stated,

> *"I begged for help. I was nearly hospitalized again. Then I spoke to my psychiatrist about a medication change. A medication change gave me a reason to have hope that I could escape the despair. Hope is a powerful antidote."(personal communication, September, 2007)*

Out of the shadows. The journey of a nurse with bipolar disorder who now has a master's degree in nursing and lives and works in San Francisco, CA, includes the following:

> *At two years of age, she would sit by herself for hours, obsessively sorting her toys by colors, size and shapes. When she attended school, she was often the scapegoat who was picked on, bullied and abused by other children because she did not participate and respond socially the way other children did. As an adult, she had manic episodes characterized by grandiosity: excessive spending on shopping for clothes, rushing into relationships, and being irritable and unkind when angry. During one episode, depression robbed her of her business, house, and a nine-year relationship. This nurse openly shares her journey in an effort to help others move out from the shadow of their illnesses into the light. (Vo, 2008)*

Does she have an alteration in thought process?
Could she or others like her be scared silent?

How could you come to know this person using the human rights or social model?

Why do issues concerning mental health continue in greater measure than other health concerns?

How can nurses help to move persons with mental illness into the light?

Putting others at ease. At four years of age, a nurse learned that she was different. She was hospitalized to repair a congenital heart defect and recalls that the other children in the room didn't have to look at each other to talk and play: "It was the first time that I felt left out of the world around me" (Maheady, 2006, p. 58).

> *In nursing school, I learned quickly during my clinical rotations not to use the word "Deaf" when identifying myself. Doing so often triggered an automatic pathological reaction from the patient that someone defective could not be an effective caregiver. I found that the label "hearing impaired" put the patients at ease more than the term "Deaf."*
>
> *"Hearing impaired" is a generic and sometimes confusing term. It covers all kinds and degrees of hearing loss. It can be used as a safety net or to hide how grave the hearing loss is. Now, it is a relief not to have to identify myself as "hearing impaired," since I work for Deaf and Hard of Hearing Services. Now, I do not have to give up my self-identify as a Deaf nurse to reassure my patients of my competence as a caregiver. (Maheady, 2006, p. 60)*
>
> *When I was in my early 20s, I was offered the opportunity to get a cochlear implant. I declined the offer due to the invasiveness of the procedure and failure rates. (Maheady, 2006, p. 62)*

This nurse has a master's degree in nursing. She lives with her husband, who played on the water polo team at the Deaf Olympics, and their two "profoundly hearing" children in Connecticut. She works as a clinical case manager with clients who are deaf at a mental health center in Connecticut.

Is this a communication impairment?

Is this a demonstration of the need to soften the impact of a hearing loss on people without hearing loss?

Who is comforting whom?

Do you consider her disabled?

How could you come to know her using the medical, human rights, or social model?

What technology could assist her as well as others with hearing loss?

Live, chuckle, and smile. A nurse with dystonia, a movement disorder, works in an ICU in New York City. She founded a nonprofit organization and wrote two books. In addition, she underwent deep brain stimulation and chronicled her experiences in a photo journal.

She writes,

> *Working as a nurse while having a movement disorder is difficult. I don't think most people realize how difficult it is to work with a "visible" disease. One can hide diabetes and a glucometer, but one can't hide tremors, pain, abnormal twitching and posturing... Personally, I am more embarrassed on the street, because a social stigma exists when one looks different. Some people are so afraid of others with a disability that they make every attempt to avoid you. (Maheady, 2006, p. 87)*
>
> *I would not be able to work as a nurse without the support of my colleagues—nursing, medical staff and others. There are high rates of depression, isolation, unemployment and loss associated with having dystonia.*
>
> *Being a patient and a caregiver—being on two sides of the coin— has brought me other opportunities: writing books, working as a patient advocate and as a consultant for pharmaceutical companies. (Maheady, 2006, p. 88)*

In her book, this nurse writes,

> *My patients are asking me "how I do it?"*
> *Do what?*
> *LIVE??*
> *Work with dystonia?*
> *I don't know.*
> *I amaze myself.*
> *I amaze everyone.*
> *I chuckle and smile.*
> *(Serdans, 2000, p. 30)*

Is this an alteration in comfort, social isolation, or joyful living?

How does a visible disability differ from an invisible disability?

How could you come to know her using the medical, human rights, or social model of disability?

Coming to Know the Person as Person. The aforementioned vignettes express situations and conditions affirming the need to know persons with disabilities more fully as persons. These vignettes show us that persons experience disability in a variety of ways at different points in their lives. Experiences range from feeling childlike, hurt, isolated, and fearful to having freedom to make choices; feeling a sense of belonging, humor, smiles, and chuckles; having hopes and dreams; and being the recipient of a gift. They also demonstrate determination, resourcefulness, and resilience.

Traditionally, nurses have made assessments in a habitual approach based on functional abilities and stereotypical labels. A more inclusive approach would be to invite the person to the assessment table and allow the person to lead the way to *our* understanding. Questions might include these:

> *Tell me about your thoughts, joy, pain, plans, goals, and expectations.*
> *Tell me about your life and your view of health. Describe feeling well.*
> *Tell me about your daily activities, mobility, and recreation.*
> *How do others help you? How can you be helped? How can I help you?*
> *How should I describe you to others?*

Discussions may be facilitated by parents, caregivers, sign language interpreters, or technology.

Do We Need to Label Persons? People with disabilities, like people without disabilities, do not speak with one voice on many issues that uniquely affect their quality of life. Pathologizing differences may be unnecessary or counterproductive if we presume that all are whole—just as they are.

If we recognize that disability is part of life, a human experience that impacts most persons at one time or another, should we consider disability to be normal? Part of the whole? Part of all of our imperfections or perfection? Do we need models or labels? And if the labels are needed, who should decide who is the mental, physical, and emotional norm against which others should be judged? Should the government decide? Society? Insurance companies? Physician? Nurse? Should nondisabled persons decide? Or should the person whose life is affected ultimately make the decision?

After reflection on persons with disabilities in this light, do we need a monolithic model in order to come to know them? Or, is it as simple or complicated as coming to know ourselves?

Reflective Exercise. Record your health status today.

Now, imagine becoming disabled tomorrow. If you are currently disabled, imagine having another disability or complication tomorrow:

- Describe the disability and your strengths and limitations.
- What challenges would you anticipate?
- How would your family and coworkers respond?
- How would you like society to see you?
- What environmental, structural, or attitudinal barriers would influence your full participation in life? What supports would you need?
- What would you tell people about who you are as a person?
- How could society and health care come to know you as a whole person?

References

Anti-Defamation League. (2005). A brief history of the disability rights movement. Retrieved on May 30, 2008, from http://www.adl.org/education/curriculumconnections/fall2005/fall2005lesson5history.asp

Benner, P. (1984). *From novice to expert.* Menlo Park, CA: Addison-Wesley.

Berntsson, L., Berg, M., Brydolf, M., & Hellström, A. (2007). Adolescents' experiences of well-being when living with a long-term illness or disability. *Scandinavian Journal of Caring Sciences, 21*(4), 419–425.

Bickenbach, J., Chatterji, S., Badley, E., & Ustun, T. (1999). Models of disablement, universalism, and the international classification of impairments, disabilities and handicaps. *Social Science and Medicine, 48*, 1173–1187.

British Film Institute. *Medical model vs. social model.* Retrieved on June 27, 2008, from http://www.bfi.org.uk/education/teaching/disability/thinking/medical.html

Cangelosi, P. R., & Whitt, K. J. (2006). Teaching through storytelling: An exemplar. *International Journal of Nursing Education Scholarship, 3*(1), Article 2, 1–7..

Charlton, J. (2000*). Nothing about us without us: Disability oppression and empowerment.* Berkeley, CA: University of California Press.

Clapton, J., & Fitzgerald, J. (1997). The history of disability: A history of "otherness." *New Renaissance, 7*(1), 20–21.

Denning, S. (2000). *The springboard: How storytelling ignites action in knowledge-era organizations.* Boston: Butterworth-Heinemann.

Diekelmann, N., & Diekelmann, J. (2000). Learning ethics in nursing and genetics: Narrative pedagogy and the grounding of values. *Journal of Pediatric Nursing, 15*, 226–231.

Disability Rights Education and Defense Fund. *Directory of national disability non-discrimination laws.* Retrieved on June 22, 2008, from http://www.dredf.org/international/lawindex.shtml

Disability Social History Project. *Disability history timeline.* Retrieved on June 24, 2008 from http://www.disabilityhistory.org/timeline_new.html

Disabled Peoples' International (1995). *Constitution of disabled peoples' international preamble.* Retrieved on June 10, 2008, from http://v1.dpi.org/langen/index?page=4

Drake, E. (2002). The power of story. *The Journal of Perinatal Education, 11*(2), ix–xi.

Eiesland, N. (1994). *The disabled God: Toward a liberatory theology of disability.* Nashville: Abingdon Press.

Finkelstein, V. (2007). *The social model of disability and the disability movement.* Retrieved on July 4, 2008, from http://www.leeds.ac.uk/disability-studies/archiveuk/archframe.htm

Fleming S., & Maheady, D. (2005). Empowering persons with disabilities. *WHONN Lifelines, 8*(6) 534–537.

Guernsey, K., Nicoli, M., & Ninio, A. (2007). Convention on the rights of persons with disabilities: Its implementation and relevance for the World Bank. Retrieved on July 8, 2008, from http://siteresources.worldbank.org/SOCIALPROTECTION/Resources/SP-Discussion-papers/Disability-DP/0712.pdf

Harris, A., & Enfield, S. (2003). *Disability, equality and human rights: A training manual for development and humanitarian organisations.* Oxford: Oxfam Publishing.

Higgins, P. C. (1992). *Making disability: Exploring the social transformation of human variation.* Springfield, IL: Charles C. Thomas.

Holland, D. (2006). Franklin D. Roosevelt's Shangri-La: Foreshadowing the independent living movement in Warm Springs, Georgia, 1926–1945. *Disability & Society, 21*(5), 513–535.

Maheady, D. (2003). *Nursing students with disabilities change the course.* River Edge, NJ: Exceptional Parent Press.

Maheady, D. (2006). *Leave no nurse behind: Nurses working with dis-Abilities.* Lincoln, NE: iUniverse.

Oliver, M. (1990). *The politics of disablement.* London: Macmillan.

Oliver, M. (2004). The social model in action: If I had a hammer. In C. Barnes (Ed.), *Implementing the social model of disability: Theory and research* (pp. 18–31). Leeds: The Disability Press.

Quinn, G, & Degener, T. (2002). *Human rights and disability: The current use and future potential of United Nations human rights instruments in the context of disability.* Office of the High Commissioner for Human Rights. Retrieved on June 22, 2008, from http://www.unhchr.ch/html/menu6/2/disability.doc

Serdans, B. (2000). *I'm moving two: A poetic journey with dystonia.* Philadelphia: Xlibris.

Smart, J. (2006–2007). Challenges to the biomedical model of disability. *Advances in Medical Psychotherapy & Psychodiagnosis, 12,* 41–44.

Snow, K. (2008). *People first language.* Retrieved May 29, 2008, from http://ftp.disabilityisnatural.com/documents/PFL8.pdf

Sowers J., & Smith, M. (2002). Disability as difference. *Journal of Nursing Education, 41*(8), 331–332.

Twain, M. (1890). Letter to George Bainton, 10/15/1888. In G. Bainton, (Ed.), *The Art of Authorship: Literary reminiscences, methods of work and advice to young beginners* (pp. 85–88). New York: D. Appleton.

UN Chronicle. (2004). Nothing about us without us: Recognizing the rights of people with disabilities. United Nations, vol. XLI (4). Retrieved May 29, 2008, from http://www.un.org/Pubs/chronicle/2004/issue4/0404p10.html

United Nations. (2008). *Backgrounder: Disability treaty closes a gap in protecting human rights.* Retrieved June 6, 2008, from http://www.un.org/disabilities/documents/toolaction/backgroundermay2008.doc

United Nations Enable. (2004). *Nothing about us, without us.* Retrieved on June 22, 2008, from http://www.un.org/esa/socdev/enable/iddp2004.htm

Vo, B. (2008, December 22). UCSF professor a *Student* nd student share struggles with mental illness. *Synapse: The UCSF Newspaper, 51,* 6. Retrieved on May 29, 2008, from http://www.ucsf.edu/synapse/content/2006/10/12/mental.html

World Health Organization. (2001). *International classification of functioning, disability and health.* Retrieved on June 10, 2008 from http://www.who.int/classifications/icf/site/onlinebrowser/icf.cfm

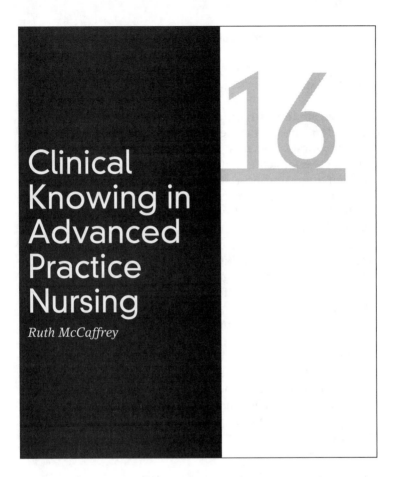

16

Clinical Knowing in Advanced Practice Nursing

Ruth McCaffrey

Chapter Overview

Nurses, as expert professional practitioners, are charged with caring for the whole person. As a professional practice grounded in a succinct body of disciplinary knowledge, nursing is charged with safe and competent care through the use of clinical knowing. Research on clinical judgment in nursing practice strongly supports clinical knowing as an essential core element in the process of decision making. This chapter describes clinical knowing across dimensions of advanced nursing practice, including nursing theory as a guide for clinical knowing; the role of evidence; collaboration; and use of the intuitive, reflective self.

Prelude

In a large southeast Florida health care institution, an educational program was developed to foster collaboration
between nurses and new medical residents. This endeavor
focused on enhancing mutual understanding of disciplinary
knowledge grounding their respective practices. Findings
from this endeavor showed that physicians (both residents
and their teachers) had very little idea about professional
nursing. Their focus was on being able to complete technical
procedures and diagnose disease, rather than on seeing the
patient and understanding the situation from the patient's
point of view. In this program, by fostering communication
skills and a new appreciation of membership in a health care
team, there ensued a new appreciation for the complexity of
the practice of professional nursing. It was clearly evident
that both the practice of medicine and the practice of nursing,
although distinct and separate, are integral to the health and
welfare of all persons in their care. Mutual clinical knowing is
imperative, leading all concerned to a deeper understanding
of the nature of persons through nursing and its practice, and
through medicine and its practice. Collegial collaboration is
essential in the practice of health care.

Introduction to Clinical Knowing

Nurses, as expert professional practitioners, are charged
with caring for the whole person. As a professional practice grounded in a succinct body of disciplinary knowledge,
nursing as a profession is charged with safe and competent
care through the use of clinical knowing. Clinical knowing is
evidenced in the day-to-day practice of nursing and is the
underlying foundation for the profession. Florence Nightingale wrote, "I think one's feelings waste themselves in words;
they ought all to be distilled into actions which bring results
(Nightingale, 1860, p 36)." Clinical knowing is the distillation
of knowing put into action on behalf of patients. Society grants
the foundations of existence to all professions, and in most
societies throughout the world today, nurses are considered
to be important providers of care. Clinical knowing allows
nurses to continue to earn the public trust and advance the
discipline and practice of professional nursing.

In this chapter, the many aspects and co˙
clinical knowing are examined including histʳ
clinical competence as knowing, the role of evideͺ
cal knowing, and the role of collaboration, reflection, ͺͺ
and the senses. Each of the components of clinical kͺͺ
ing is an aspect of larger concepts of holism. Contemporarʏ
advanced practice nursing literature supports the fact that
clinical knowing improves patient health and safety while
creating increased job satisfaction among nurses.

Clinical knowing is advanced as nurses offer direct care
and advocate for patients in navigating through complex
health care systems. To accomplish this task, nurses use
clinical knowing that advocates collection of data during the
assessment phase, and from these data they develop a diagnosis and plan of care. Within this process is consistent evaluation and adjustment of the plan of care within the nursing
situation. Sometimes this process is formal and documented,
and sometimes it is informal—when more immediate decisions must be made at the bedside. Whether undertaken as
a formal or informal process, clinical knowing and the ability to care for the patient are the cornerstones of clinical
nursing practice. However, what professional nursing activities are used in the practice of clinical knowing by advanced
practice nurses?

Coming to know the patient from a clinical perspective
is a fast-paced, ever-changing challenge that is built upon
a foundation of many different aspects of knowing. Clinical
knowing is identified, described, explained, and modeled to
beginning practitioners in undergraduate programs. Profi-
ciency with clinical knowing is expected as the nurse assumes
the role of novice to expert, modeled from Benner's (1984)
view of competency in nursing practice. In nursing school,
students are taught to care for patients in a safe manner. This
is an outstanding feature of beginning clinical knowing. As
clinical knowing skills continue to be developed throughout
a lifetime of nursing, through formal education, and experience, novice nurses usually take more time to express their
clinical knowing in a plan of care, whereas more experienced and expert nurses often develop and practice clinical
knowing skills more efficiently and effectively, using these
skills routinely for planning care. Oftentimes, the practice of
clinical knowing of expert nurses occurs almost without any
conscious effort.

Nurses use clinical knowing when they interact with patients, families, physicians, and other ancillary persons, for the purpose of providing evidence as required to obtain insurance coverage. Clinical knowing is important when educating patients about health promotion and disease prevention, as well as when discussing current health problems and management. Nurses must possess a vast array of knowledge concerning medical, pharmacological, social, financial, emotional, cultural, and spiritual aspects of care. Nurses are the professionals whose clinical knowing encompasses a vast amount of information that makes each person unique and identifies the person as whole and complete. This means that nurses must integrate different types of knowledge when creating a care plan. Clinical knowing therefore requires the nurse to use many different skills and thinking processes to care for patients.

Exceptional clinical knowing exhibits competence, compassion, intuition, self-awareness, and a high level of consciousness. This type of knowing uses theory-based planning, the knowledge of research, a genuine presence with patients, and expert clinical competence to promote health and well-being among patients.

Example 1.

SS, a new nurse on the unit, has compiled an assessment of Mr. T, who was admitted yesterday for a gastrointestinal bleed. She knows that his vital signs are within normal limits, and today's blood work shows only a slight anemia, which can be attributed to the bleed. SS proceeds to plan her care for Mr. T based on the fact that he seems stable and is getting better. BC, the charge nurse on the unit, who has years of experience as a nurse, comes to see Mr. T on rounds. She notices that Mr. T is pale and somewhat withdrawn; he is also not as alert as he was when he came in. When talking to Mr. T, BC notices that he seems tired and lethargic. BC is concerned and notifies the physician, who orders further testing and finds that the bleeding has not stopped. Mr. T needs surgery. What aspects of clinical knowing were more advanced in BC's assessment of Mr. T? How did BC's advanced clinical knowing improve patient care for Mr. T?

In her original article about the ways of knowing in nursing, Carper (1978) states that the ways of knowing influence nursing knowledge, including how that knowledge is gathered, tested, and applied. One way nursing knowledge can be actualized and tested is through clinical knowing. In the clinical setting data are gathered, plans of action are applied to assist the patient with health and well-being, and testing is applied to determine the success of the action plan. Each of these steps requires clinical knowing. Therefore, we might say clinical knowing is the result of many different types of knowing and that it formulates the basis for all nursing.

Nursing Theory as a Guide for Clinical Knowing

Nursing theory is integral to all aspects of nursing care (Meleis, 2007, p. 31). In the clinical setting, theory may be compared to the assessment nurses undertake with each patient because theory provides a way of looking at a situation which is specialized and concept driven. This means that theory presents the basis from which knowledge grows, including clinical knowledge and clinical knowing.

Theory-guided clinical knowing can assist the nurse to decide what actions are needed and what interventions would work best in the present situation. Theory helps to prioritize patient needs and then evaluate the nurse's success in meeting those needs.

The development of theory begins with an examination of the paradigm from which the theory is founded. A paradigm may be defined as a pattern or model which includes a collection of assumptions, concepts, practices, and values that constitutes a way of viewing reality. The metaparadigm elements within which nursing exists are that of person, environment, nursing, caring and health. Any clinical action or series of actions taken by nurses that cannot be designated as advancing one of the elements of the paradigm is outside the scope of clinical knowing. Meleis (2007) states, "Nursing theory is then defined as a conceptualization of some aspect of reality (invented or discovered) that pertains to nursing. The conceptualization is articulated for the purpose of describing, explaining, predicting, or prescribing nursing care" (p. 41). Using theory as part of clinical knowing requires that assumptions be defined and concepts of the phenomenon of clinical knowing be described.

Clinical knowing can be described using theory as a biopsychological and cultural way of understanding the human condition in both health and illness.

Clinical nursing in some theories focuses on providing self-care needs and providing interactions between nurse and patient that are efficient, functional, and productive while sensing, perceiving, and concaving. Using theory to shape clinical practice provides the nurse with a framework around which to plan care and judge the effectiveness of that care. Therefore, clinical knowing in the context of theory means that the nurse bases his or her knowing on a definite set of concepts and definitions.

Theory is a tool that can be used to increase efficiency and effectiveness in clinical knowing. Theory-guided clinical knowing develops expertise in the nurse, prepares the nurse for all eventualities based on the nursing paradigm, and validates clinical nursing work as important and meaningful.

Finally, basing clinical knowing on nursing theory builds professional autonomy and accountability in practice. Theory allows the nurse to articulate responses and nursing plans for patient care based on an identifiable model of practice. Clinical knowing that is based on theoretical knowing provides a focus and creates goals for nursing practice.

Example 2.

Using Martha Rogers's theory—the science of unitary human beings—the nurse realizes that human beings exhibit patterns that guide the nurse to know what is happening. These patterns are constantly influenced by the environment in which the patient resides. The environment and the human being are constantly interacting in a way that moves the human being forward. The nurse in this case uses this theory to enable the patient to change his or her pattern of pain perception through manipulation of the environment. To do this, the nurse adds music to the environment. This is a nursing intervention that is easily accomplished, inexpensive, and safe. In doing this, the nurse changes the pattern of pain perception for the patient. The nurse then measures the change in pain perception and evaluates the usefulness of this theoretical intervention to changing the pattern of pain perception. When reporting the positive effect of the intervention to other nurses, the physician, the family, and the hospital, the nurse is able share the reason for his or her decision to change the environment as having a theoretical basis and being focused on the paradigm of nursing (human, environment, caring, and health).

The Role of Evidence in Clinical Knowing

Evidence-based clinical knowing may be defined as the ability of the nurse to obtain and use evidence that specifies the best therapeutic choices for a given circumstance in accordance with the nurse's experience and the patient's wishes. This type of knowing links research to practice. For example, nurses use evidence-based clinical knowing when they explain to a post-heart attack patient the reason for taking a beta-blocking medication—because it has been shown to decrease the chance of a second heart attack. Using evidence in decision making is an essential skill the nurse must possess in order to know the best clinical options for a given patient.

In order to effectively use evidence-based knowing as part of clinical knowing, the nurse must have the ability to access relevant information, read it critically, and finally adapt information from the evidence in clinical knowing. Evidence-based knowing integrates clinical knowing and patient preference with the best external clinical evidence (Melnyk & Fineout-Overholt, 2004).

Nurses should be guided by the evidence to structure decision making that is accurate and timely. Applying evidence in the practice setting enables the nursing profession to communicate with other health care providers in a way that has meaning for both professions and establishes the value of nursing in the health care setting. The use of evidence-based knowing provides a systematic approach to rational decision making that facilitates achievement of best practices in clinical knowing and thus demonstrates accountability. "The odds of doing the right thing at the right time for the right patient are potentially improved when the strongest available evidence is systematically appreciated" (Melnyk & Finehout-Overholt, 2004, p. 28).

There are several misconceptions about evidence-based knowing. The first misconception is that using evidence as a guide for practice ignores patient preference and both patient and nursing values. Patient preference, values, and nursing experience are all part of evidence-based knowing. Combining evidence-based knowing with other types of knowing (such as personal knowing or aesthetic knowing) to complete the plan of care provides the best opportunity for the health and well-being of the patient.

Another misconception is that evidence is too complicated and hard to understand, and therefore it is better to stick to the way things have always been done rather than trying new ways of knowing patients based on the findings of research. Clara Barton is quoted as saying, "I have an almost complete disregard of precedent, and a faith in the possibility of something better. It irritates me to be told how things have always been done. I defy the tyranny of precedent. I go for anything new that might improve the past" (Oates, 1994 p. 247)". Not being familiar with the current research regarding patient care is disregarding an important tool that has demonstrated ability to improve outcomes. Professional nurses must be aware of advances in patient care that have proven to be effective and use those advances to promote accountability. Continuing to base clinical knowing only on past experience creates a situation where patients are not receiving the best possible care. Studies have shown that using evidence-based knowing for patient care has improved patient safety and outcomes as well as nurse satisfaction (Ciliska, Pinelli, DiCenso, & Cullum, 2001; Retsas, 2000).

The skills necessary for the effective use of evidence as part of clinical knowing include the ability to complete a literature search using a computer database on a given topic to find the available research, ability to critically evaluate the research to determine the quality and generalizability of findings, and the ability to use the information to produce a protocol for practice. Finding the appropriate research literature is accomplished by defining the topic of interest and then either searching or approaching the librarian at the health care or academic institution to assist in performing a search for relevant research literature. Research studies are often obtainable online as well. Assistance from a nurse in an academic position is also possible.

Reading and evaluating the literature can be done by those with a general knowledge of research. Many times nursing faculty are willing to assist in this type of work. Finally, from what has been read, a protocol for practice using evidence-based knowing can be developed. This process does not have to be done by one nurse, but rather can be undertaken by a group of nurses who work together to formulate the practice protocol and share it with other nurses to improve the clinical knowing of a larger group, thereby improving patient care.

Example 3.

A number of nurses in a hospital are frustrated because they seem to be unable to identify patients at risk for venothrombotic events (VTE). They also feel that physicians would be more willing to use preventive treatments in patients at risk if the nursing staff could clearly identify who was at risk and why. The nurses go to the hospital librarian and ask her to do a computer search for them regarding patients at risk for VTE. They receive many research studies as well as guidelines based on a meta-analysis of the research. One thing they learn from the literature is that over 300,000 patients die each year from VTE in hospitals. Therefore, they know that their concern was justified and that the work that they are undertaking will probably save patients' lives and improve patient outcomes.

The nurses describe the magnitude and seriousness of the problem to hospital administrators and ask for help to read and understand the research. Hospital administrators hire a research consultant to work with the nurses on this project. From the information obtained through the computer search and the evaluation of the research studies found, the nurses are able to design a VTE assessment tool to be used on every patient admitted to the hospital to evaluate the patient's risk for VTE. This tool is then connected to a treatment option sheet presented to physicians so that they can choose the most appropriate treatment for their patients. This is an example of nurses using evidence as clinical knowing to improve patient care. Can you think of other examples of clinical issues or questions that could be answered using evidence-based clinical knowing?

Historical Knowing

Historical knowing is an important part of clinical knowing. Understanding the patient's history and coming to know the patient as a unique individual that cannot be separated from the effects of history is imperative to the development of a successful nursing plan of care. Historical knowing requires authentic presence with the patient and listening skills, to discern which parts of the history affect the health problem being presented. To adequately use historical knowing in planning care, the nurse must put aside judgmental thinking about such things as appearance, gender, age, and other preconceptions that could influence coming to know the patient's history. This is not to say that appearance and other features do not factor into the nursing care plan. If a patient appears dirty and unclean, a plan must be made to remedy the situation; however, preconceived judgment about the meaning of being dirty might decrease the nurses' ability to truly know the person by labeling the person.

As part of historical knowing, the nurse comes to know each person as a unique and completely whole individual. This includes coming to know the person's culture, ethnicity, spiritual beliefs, and family history, and the areas of life that bring joy and sadness. This not only assists the nurse to establish a plan of care, but also engenders the trust and confidence required to establish a therapeutic relationship between the nurse and the patient nursed.

After coming to know the history of the patient, the nurse can make adjustments to the medical, nursing, or other plans to fit the needs of the patient. When a patient is labeled noncompliant in health care, it is often only that health care providers have not come to know the patient and his or her history. When health care providers use historical knowing, the necessary steps to increase compliance will be evident.

Example 4.

FM is a 42-year-old, obese male who has diabetes, hypertension, and high cholesterol. He says he does not like medical offices or hospitals, and does not feel as though they would ever do him any good no matter what was wrong. After listening to FM's history, the nurse learns that FM has been overweight since he was a child and that his pediatrician told him at age 16 that he was a fat slob and that if he did not loose weight, everyone in society would be laughing at him. FM's family has a tendency to be overweight, and no one ever told him how to diet or that exercise was good for him. No one in his family played sports or spent much time at anything except watching television, reading, and eating. FM states that he is sure that all health care providers are just laughing at him and thinking he is fat, lazy, and stupid.

How does FM's history and the nurse's historic knowing play a role in his compliance with a plan to assist him to lose weight and get his blood pressure and diabetes under control?

Clinical Competence as Knowing

Clinical competence is defined as the practice of acquiring and using scientific knowledge and skill in the application of therapeutic interventions in the clinical setting. Competence in nursing is reflected in the cognitive and technical performance that constitutes calls for nursing and answering those calls in an efficient and effective manner to improve patient outcomes.

Nursing is a science-based profession that uses the art and science of the discipline in serving the health care needs of society. While nurses are responsible for decision making and education, they are equally responsible for skill-based tasks that are essential when caring for patients. As health care evolves, technological skills become increasingly complex and specialized. Therefore, clinical and technological competence is essential in providing the best care at the appropriate time in a manner accepted by the patient and family.

Rapid changes in science and technology, coupled with reduced time for personal connection with patients, have increased the importance of competence among nurses providing care and have become the cornerstone of nursing practice. Competence in growing areas of health-related science such as genomics, assistive devices, telemedicine, and complementary and alternative therapies requires nurses to investigate and continue learning in order to maintain competence. With the advent of the Internet, patients have the ability to learn about therapies and treatments for medical problems and are likely to ask knowledgeable questions about information gained on the Web. Nurses must be competent in answering these questions so that patients can make informed decisions about care and treatments.

Professional nurses are increasingly concerned about patient safety and quality of care as well as about nurse safety and quality of career (Knapp, 2004). Competence is connected with each of these concepts. Competence is a form of knowing that provides a level of comfort to the patient and the nurse. Competence as knowing means that both the patient and the nurse have a certain level of confidence that the patient will receive the care required to promote health and well-being.

Sr. Simone Roach has written of competence as one of the C's of caring. She defined competence as "having the knowledge, judgment, skills, experience, and motivation required to respond adequately to the demands of one's professional responsibility" (1987, p. 61). Competence as knowing then means that the nurse knows what is appropriate to promote health and well-being for patients and uses that competence to provide the best care possible.

Competence as knowing also includes the ability of the nurse to modify care based on coming to know the person as a whole and complete person in the moment. This is the opposite of using competent knowing as a source of power. If a patient is resistant to a treatment or therapy, competent knowing uses education, open discussion, and inclusion of ideas in order to help the patient make the best choice about treatment. Competent knowing allows for deviation from the norm in order to accommodate patient desires and needs.

Critical thinking is part of competent knowing. Critical thinking consists of using the processes of discernment, analysis, and evaluation. It includes processes of reflection and judgment that coincide with scientific evidence and common sense. Critical thinking clearly involves synthesis, evaluation, and reconstruction of thinking in addition to analysis and is therefore an essential component of competent knowing. The nurse cannot analyze, synthesize, and evaluate without knowing.

Competent knowing is essential to the development of a nursing plan that is scientifically appropriate and meets the needs of both the patient and the nurse. In this way, nursing competence requires many levels of skill. It is not enough to be competent in diagnosis and technological treatments. Competent knowing includes technological knowing; understanding the body and diseases; being able to share knowledge with patients and families; and identifying patient emotional, spiritual, and cultural issues regarding care. If any of these components of competent knowing is missing, the goal of responding adequately to meet the demands of the nursing profession will not be realized.

Competent knowing as a subcategory of clinical knowing can be divided into four sections (Taylor, 1995). Interpersonal competent knowing is the ability to know how to establish and maintain relationships that are able to achieve health care goals. This type of knowing increases the ability of nurses to elicit patient strengths, identify knowledge deficits, establish a collaborative setting between providers and recipients of health care, and identify patient goals and objectives.

Intellectual competent knowing is the ability to reason out the nature of what is happening to the patient and what should be done about it to facilitate good health outcomes. This type of knowing encompasses scientific knowledge, a command of nursing interventions and their outcome goals, and the ability to solve problems creatively.

Technical competent knowing enables the nurse to manipulate equipment skillfully to achieve a desired physical goal. This includes manual dexterity, eye-hand coordination, and the ability to troubleshoot equipment. This type of competent knowing enables the nurse to use creativity to master equipment technique in the patient-care setting.

The final type of competent knowing is moral competent knowing. This type of knowing allows the nurse to have a consistent, professional moral code and responsibility. This type of knowing establishes a sense of accountability in the nurse to patients, the caregiving team, and society. Moral competent caring enables nurses to provide care in a manner that is faithful to the nurse's code of ethics.

Using the idea of competence as a way of knowing, how would you answer the following?

- Do I know my patients well enough to promote anything more than the well-being of their bodies?
- If asked to describe a patient, would I be able to report on anything other than the patient's physical condition?

- Is the care I provide prioritized according to the patient's interests as well as according to medical need?
- What are my strengths and deficiencies in creating caring relationships?
- When being competent with machines, do I still see the patient as part of the equation?

Example 5.

Mr. F is a 68-year-old, complex patient who is in the hospital for heart failure. Mr. F is married and has three children who live out of state. Mr. F has an ejection fraction of 13 and is often short of breath. He is unable to complete most of the activities of daily living such as bathing and dressing. In addition to this problem, Mr. F is overweight and has diabetes and hypertension. Mr. F is on a fixed income and finds it difficult to afford all of his medications even with the insurance plan from Medicare. He also finds it hard to diet because he feels he can only afford a limited amount of money on his food budget, and that money goes farther with carbohydrates and inexpensive, processed foods that are often high in salt or fat content.

Mr. F's doctors are very frustrated with him and have labeled him noncompliant with his medical plan. Mr. F is admitted to the hospital at least four times a year and stabilized, but then he leaves the hospital and seems unable financially and physically to stay on the course prescribed.

- How can your competent knowing help Mr. F? Is Mr. F truly noncompliant, or are there reasons he cannot follow the medical plan laid out for him in the hospital?
- Are there ways of getting him financial assistance for his medications so he can be more compliant?
- How could the nurse facilitate assistance from Mr. F's family in his medical plan? Do you think a family conference might be useful to assess the children's knowledge of Mr. and Mrs. F's situation and how they might help?
- How can the nurse share thoughts with the physician so they can work together to help Mr. and Mrs. F?

The Role of Collaboration in Clinical Knowing

Working together with other health care professionals is a skill necessary for the development of clinical knowing. Collaboration as part of clinical knowing improves patient care, reduces morbidity and mortality, reduces length of hospital stays, and provides for improved patient satisfaction (Nelson, King, & Brodine, 2008). Dimensions of nurse-physician collaborative communication are leadership, communication, coordination, problem solving/conflict management, and team culture. Health care must develop a culture of collaboration that includes shared norms, values, beliefs, and expectations.

Researchers have found significant associations between higher nurse-physician communication and the positive patient outcomes of lower risk-adjusted mortality and higher satisfaction (Boyer & Kochinda, 2004). Professional communication has been described as a complex process involving education, vigilance, and evaluation. There is evidence that interprofessional collaboration between physicians, other medical professionals, and nurses is important to ensure quality clinical outcomes. Traditionally, the physician-nurse relationship has been seen as adversarial, based on viewing the roles of physicians and nurses as contradictory rather than complementary and positive. Conversely, appropriate and successful communication and collaboration skills among health care professionals has been shown to improve the quality of patient care and enhance positive patient outcomes. Communication and collaboration are essential to providing a healthy work environment. Poor communications have been linked to medication errors, patient injuries, and death.

Several studies have found that more medical errors are set in motion by poor communication than by any other cause. Data from the Joint Commission on the Accreditation of Healthcare Organizations Sentinel Event Program have demonstrated that communication problems are the most common root cause of serious medical errors. The inability to communicate factual knowledge and problem solving has been shown to be a barrier to collaboration between professionals. The United States Department of Health and Human Services compares hospitals throughout the United States for quality and publishes this data on the Internet. Out of the 34 areas rated, 10 areas have to do with communication skills. Positive communication and collaboration begin with mutual respect, openness, honesty, and trust.

The Role of Reflection in Clinical Knowing

Reflection is a part of many types of knowing or coming to know. It is the ability to stop and think, to use contemplation and introspection in order to know what is appropriate for any given patient clinically. The nurse can use reflection as a method of clinical knowing, becoming a detached observer and using logic and observation as tools to make clinical judgments. Therefore, the use of reflection within the practice of clinical knowing and nursing care has a constructivist epistemology, based on learning from experience. Although this seems the antithesis of basing practice on the evidence, reflection can be used alongside evidence in order to come to the best understanding of the patient and the situation, and to make clinical knowing possible.

Thoughtful practice can be mistaken for reflective practice, but reflective practice can only exist when practice is deliberate and not taken for granted. Reflective practice is learning from experience and using reflection to cement that learning in memory and in the foundation of practice. Reflective practice often can result in unexpected but important new knowledge (Kilpatrick & Purden, 2007).

Atkins and Murphy (1993) have defined the steps in reflective nursing practice that affect clinical knowing. In these steps, the nurse moves from an uncomfortable thought or feeling that the knowledge being applied to the situation is not sufficient in itself to explain what is happening in that unique situation to a critical analysis of the situation, in which new knowledge is generated, and then finally to the development of a new perspective where all three stages are integrated. Reflection as part of clinical knowing occurs while practicing and influences decisions made and care given (Atkins & Murphy, 1993).

Using reflection as an aspect of clinical knowing helps the nurse make sense of what is happening in any given situation. Experience and reflection are often the most important components of clinical knowing. Reflective thinking is a highly adaptive and individualized response to a gap-producing situation and involves a range of cognitive activities in which the individual deliberately and purposely engages in discourse with self in an attempt to make sense of the current situation or phenomenon, in order to act. Reflective thinking contributes to better contextual understandings and therefore may influence future behavior. Reflecting on one's own practice is self-empowering because it adds to personal understanding and control. The individual is thus both shaped by, and the shaper of, his/her world (Teekman, 2000).

The nurse may use reflection as an aspect of clinical knowing every day. In the clinical setting, there are many opportunities that require "sense making" and therefore make reflection a useful tool. As the nurse becomes more adept at reflection, critical thinking and judgment will be improved, decision making will have a new depth, and the nurse will develop a sense of trust in his or her own understanding of a situation, leading to feelings of autonomy and professionalism.

Example 6.

Sally had been a nurse in her unit for about 4 years. She had started at this job immediately after nursing school. Sally was caring for Mr. T, who was just admitted to her unit today, and noticed that he was very anxious. His diagnosis was gastroesophageal bleeding, and the physicians were sure that the bleeding had stopped but wanted to keep Mr. T for a few more hours of observation. Mr. T kept telling Sally that he was fine and did not know why he couldn't go home.

Sally reflected on several other patients she has had that were as anxious as Mr. T. These patients all had a problem with alcohol or drug addiction and wanted to be discharged because they were feeling the need for alcohol or drugs. Sally also reflected that these patients were very furtive, just the way Mr. T was being, not really stating why they were so anxious to leave. Sally reflected that with all of the prior patients, she was able to talk to them about their problem and get them some help, although she was not sure how well they followed up after discharge.

Sally sat down in Mr. T's room and started the conversation by saying, "You know, I have had other patients who were as anxious to leave as you are, Mr. T. They wanted to leave because they wanted a drink or a hit of a drug. You remind me of those patients. If you tell me about what is going on, I might be able to help you." Mr. T stated that it had been a day since he had a drink and he was used to drinking about a quart of whiskey every day. He told Sally he was feeling a little jittery about not having a drink and would appreciate any help she might be able to provide.

Sally called Mr. T's doctor, who was unaware of his drinking habits. He prescribed an anxiolytic medication for Mr. T to avoid any problems with not getting a drink. He also asked Sally to talk to Mr. T about his drinking and how that might be the underlying cause of his gastrointestinal bleeding. In a nonjudgmental way, Sally discussed these issues with Mr. T. Mr. T said he knew that the drinking was not good for him and would like to stop but he just didn't know where to start. Sally gave Mr. T information about alcohol addiction and ways it could be treated. She told Mr. T that a meeting of alcoholics anonymous met right at the hospital every evening and he could go whenever he felt better. Mr. T told Sally that she was very kind to care about him and that he was grateful for the information and concern. Sally stored away her understanding of patients who had hidden alcohol or drug addictions and knew that she would use this information when another patient with similar problems appeared on the unit.

The Role of Intuition in Clinical Knowing

Nurses have traditionally used intuition when caring for patients and making clinical decisions about their care. *Intuition* can be defined as instinctive knowing, or an immediate cognition without the use of conscious or rational processes. Intuition is a perceptive insight making available an immediate form of knowledge in which the knower is directly acquainted with the object of knowledge. Intuition differs from other ways of knowing because it does not use rational or analytical thought processes to come to conclusions but rather simply knows something to be true.

Intuitive knowing is antithetical to the positivistic domains of medicine and other sciences. Science requires truths to be proven in ways that are replicable. Intuition simply knows that something is true without any proof; it relies on past experience, the development of relationships, and the simple act of being with. Scientist Albert Einstein is quoted as saying, "The only real valuable thing is intuition. The intellect has little to do on the road to discover. There has to come a leap in consciousness, call it intuition or what ever you will, but the solution comes to you and you don't know how and you don't know why. The intuitive mind is a sacred gift and the rational mind a faithful servant. We have created a society that worships the faithful servant and has forgotten the gift (Physics: Discovery and Intuition, 2007). Nurses often have a moment when they know something about a patient in their care that cannot be explained through measurable means either physiological or psychological. This type of clinical knowing should be honored and encouraged among nurses. The use of intuition as part of clinical knowing provides an added layer of knowledge that benefits the patient and the nurse.

Recognition of the use of intuition in clinical nursing practice has risen in prominence over the last 20 years. Research evidence would suggest that intuition occurs in response to knowledge and is an important component of clinical decision making. Intuition in nursing practice involves the recognition of previously experienced patterns and the detection of subtle clinical changes (Benner & Tanner, 1996). Intuition in practice has been linked to enhanced clinical judgment, effective decision making (McCutcheon & Pincombe, 2001), and crisis aversion (Cioffi, 1997).

In a study on the use of intuition as clinical knowing, researchers found that intuition was able to facilitate the depth of nurse-client relationships, lead to a deeper understanding and connection with client patterns, and contribute to excellence in nursing care (Lerners, 1992). When the nurse has an intuition about a patient and uses that feeling to aid in clinical decisions, intuition becomes integral to clinical knowing. Nurses should trust their intuition and document the outcomes of intuition as part of clinical knowing so that an understanding of the importance of intuition can be appreciated. In addition, nurses should not be afraid to discuss their intuitions with other health care providers so that the idea of intuition as an aspect of clinical knowing can become more mainstream.

Example 7.

Mr. U is an 86-year-old man who comes to the nursing unit for treatment of his heart failure. He is a very sweet, older gentleman, and the nurses love talking to him and hearing his stories of growing up in Germany. He is always polite and shares with the nurses his gratitude for their care.

Today, Mr. U tells his nurse that he feels more tired than usual and wants to stay in bed and rest instead of taking his usual stroll around the unit. He says that he feels his age today. He tells the nurse a story about when he and his wife first came to the United States and how they were so in love. He tells the nurse that he is a lucky man to have had such a wonderful wife and two incredible children. He tells the nurse that when he dies, he will be reunited with his wife and with his son who died in Vietnam.

The nurse does a regular assessment on Mr. U. His blood pressure is stable at 140/84, and all of his other vital signs are stable. His lungs are clear and his skin color is good. The nurse, however, has an uneasy feeling about the tone of Mr. U's voice and general demeanor. She holds his hand and asks him if he feels all right. He squeezes her hand and says he feels fine and just wants to rest today. His daughter is coming to see him this afternoon and he wants to be strong when she comes. Later that day, Mr. U's daughter comes to visit, and they have a long and happy time together. The nurse checks on Mr. U at about 5 p.m. and he tells her, "You know, I am a lucky man; life has been good to me. I have no complaints."

Because of the nurse's intuition, she checks on Mr. U frequently. At change of shift the nurse shares her intuition with the night nurse and tells her that Mr. U seems fine, but something is just not the same. At 10 p.m., Mr. U becomes obtunded and the night nurse is unable to rouse him. The nurse calls Mr. U's physician and the physician orders tests, X-rays, and a transfer to the ICU. The night nurse goes into Mr. U's room to get started and as she approaches the bed, Mr. U opens his eyes, tells her he is tired, and stops breathing.

The night nurse reflects on the intuition of the day nurse as well as her own intuition. Because of Mr. U's wishes were not to be resuscitated and the physician had orders to that affect on the chart, the night nurse simply stays with Mr. U a few minutes and then calls the physician. Looking back, both the day and night nurse feel positive about Mr. U's death. They know that their intuition was telling them he was ready to die and that he was peaceful and did not want extraordinary measures to keep him alive. Both nurses know that Mr. U died the way he wanted and that their intuition supported him and his decision.

Have you ever had an intuition about a patient? Have you listened to that intuition or feeling? How has it played out? What can nurses do to validate intuition as a method for clinical knowing?

The Role of the Senses in Clinical Knowing

When we describe the senses that humans use to perceive their world, we think in terms of five senses: sight, hearing, touch, taste, and smell. In other cultures there are other senses that are considered of importance. One is the sense of proprioreception or the exact position a person has in space. Another sense is the sense of connection to the earth or the feeling a person has that his or her feet are firmly planted on the earth and that the person is connected with all others on the planet. Nurses use all of these senses in their clinical knowing. It is one of the aspects of nursing knowledge that sets the expert nurse apart from the novice. Using sensory information to make clinical decisions is a fundamental aspect of clinical knowing.

Clinical knowing requires a heightening of the senses. What appears to be a casual observation when the nurse enters the patient's room is often a very detailed use of the senses to size up the patient's condition and problems. The expert nurse is always aware of sensory information coming into his or her mental database and uses this information along with other assessments to develop a plan of care for the patient. This makes the nursing assessment different from medical assessments in that the medical assessment is completed in a very short time period, usually without a thorough observation of the patient and the notice of sensory information. The medical assessment is focused only on the system identified in the diagnosis rather than on the whole person.

The sense of sight is essential in making clinical decisions. The nurse watches the patient move to determine the patient's functional status. Is the patient able to stand straight and walk, or is he or she bent and unsteady? Does the patient have a look of pain on his or her face even though the patient denies being in pain? Does the patient appear anxious? What is the patient's skin tone? Is there any skin breakdown? These are only some examples of the ways that nurses use the sense of seeing to clinically know their patients. Those nurses who are not discerning in their sense of seeing often miss subtle clues in the patient's appearance that lead to missing critical knowledge.

Other aspects of seeing include these: Does the patient have visitors? Is the patient smiling? Does the patient read books? Does the patient watch TV? What shows does he or she watch? These types of information gathered by seeing can tell the nurse something about the psychosocial and spiritual aspects of the patient's condition.

The second sense, hearing, is able to provide the nurse with clues to the patient's understanding of directions, cognitive abilities, and interactions between the patient and family or friends. As the nurse listens to and speaks with the patient, assessment can be made. Is the patient able to verbalize and repeat directions about medications, treatments, and diets? Does the patient seem forgetful, unaware of his or her surroundings? Does the patient ask the same questions over and over? Does the patient have questions that need answering? Does the patient have fears and worries that he or she would like to discuss?

Hearing can also provide the nurse with information about how well the patient is coping in the current situation and how he or she will cope once discharged. If the family does not seem to be able to communicate or is not caring with one another, then the nurse may determine that the home environment may not be conducive to recuperation. Being authentically present with the patient requires the nurse to use the sense of hearing as well. Truly hearing what the patient says and responding in a caring way opens the lines of communication and enables the nurse to clinically know the patient.

The next sense is feeling or touch. This is an important sense for nurses because touch can not only be diagnostic; it can be healing. Touching the skin can tell you about fever, decreased circulation, and other clinical aspects of the patient's condition. Touching the hand or laying a hand on the patient's shoulder can convey caring and concern as well as feelings of comfort and calmness. This is especially true with older patients, many of whom do not get touched often because they live alone. A gentle touch can tell the nurse so much about the patient and create an atmosphere of trust and caring.

Healing touch is derived from an ancient technique called *laying on of hands*. It is a biofield therapy that is an energy-based approach to health and healing. Touching someone with the intent to reduce pain and suffering or to promote healing and well-being is a very powerful and useful tool for nurses. Some nurses have training in healing touch therapies, and others simply use touch as a modality for healing. Either way, touch is an excellent tool to promote clinical knowing.

Tasting is a sense that does not seem to apply to nursing; however, if we broaden the definition of taste, it can be used to understand and come to know the tastes of the other. What does the patient like to eat? Has he or she lost the sense of taste? Has the patient got a bad taste in the mouth from an infection or from lack of oral hygiene? All of these are important to assess when making clinical judgments. Health care providers are often concerned about the patient's lack of desire to eat—this is especially true in older adults—when the real problem is that the patient won't eat foods that don't taste good, or the patient can't eat foods that he or she cannot chew well. These assessments are part of clinical knowing, and diets must be adjusted to meet the needs of the patient.

The fifth sense is the sense of smell. Many times new nurses will state that hospital smells are overwhelming and that it is difficult to discern what smell is coming from what patient. Bodily smells in our society are often considered offensive, and we try to cover them up with perfume and room deodorizers. Smells, however, can be very important methods by which to come to know the patient clinically. The odor of wounds and exudates are used to clinically know about the patient's status and whether infection may be a problem. The nurse who clinically knows the patient as a whole and complete person will be able to detect changes in odors quickly and work with other members of the health care team to intervene with appropriate therapies for these problems.

Assessing the patient's sense of smell is also an important clinical knowing tool. The olfactory system is becoming increasingly significant as a clinical tool in the diagnosis of neurodegenerative diseases such as Parkinson's. A number of studies have demonstrated that people with Parkinson's or Alzheimer's disease exhibit olfactory dysfunctions several years before their clinical diagnosis.

Proprioreception is a sense that nurses should have when in the clinical area because everyone has a sense of personal space and when that space is invaded, even by someone trying to assist and help, it becomes uncomfortable. In order to develop a trusting and mutually beneficial relationship with patients, the nurse must explain why he or she is invading that personal space and do so gently and with respect. The sense of being rooted to the earth and yet connected with everyone on the earth should be shared with patients as a part of clinical knowing. Helping the patient know that he or she is not alone and that being human is being linked to all others and to the earth who holds us in her hand is critical to nursing. Both of these other types of senses are important ways to come to know the patient clinically, to build trust between patient and nurse, and to fulfill the responsibility of the nurse-patient relationship.

Example 8.

Nurse Sharon is caring for Mr. T today. She is changing the dressing on a wound on his hip. Before Sharon begins the dressing change, she tells Mr. T that she will be standing over him and asks his permission to do so. He says he is appreciative of her asking because some of the other nurses just treat him like a piece of meat.

As she removes the dressing, she notes an odor that is somewhat sweet and rank. She looks at the wound and notes green-tinged exudate. Nurse Sharon notifies the physician about the smell and look of Mr. T's would. He orders wound cultures to be done and an IV antibiotic started. Nurse Sharon's note of the smell and look of the wound has saved Mr. T from a bad infection, one that may have left him permanently impaired.

Later in the day, Nurse Sharon is speaking to Mr. T, who seems very despondent about his condition and the fact that he may not be able to care for his ill wife any longer. She puts a hand on Mr. T's shoulder and speaks reassuringly to him that she will work with discharge planners to make sure both he and his wife have what they need and that they will include him in all of their planning so that he will be able to have his wishes met. He looks at her and smiles for the first time all day. He tells Nurse Sharon that she is so nice that he actually believes things might be OK.

How have the senses played a part in the interactions between Sharon and Mr. T?

Summary

Clinical knowing can be defined as any process, action, or consideration that affects patients clinically. The concept of clinical knowing can be said to focus on knowing the patient's typical pattern of responses and knowing the patient as a person. This concept is considered central to nursing care and to a nurse's clinical judgment. Since nursing is a practice, professional clinical knowing is at the crux of the nursing discipline. It provides the foundation for what nurses do and how they are seen by society as integral to the health professions.

Knowing the patient encompasses the complex process whereby the nurse acquires understanding of a specific patient as a unique individual, which subsequently enhances clinical decision-making, selection of optimal nursing interventions, and patient outcomes (Whittemore, 2000). Despite these heralded benefits, knowing the patient is severely undervalued in contemporary health care. Benner and Wrubel (1989), in a qualitative study of nursing practice, identified that expert nurses acquired detailed knowledge of habits, preferences, practices, capabilities, and characteristics of patients to facilitate the provision of nursing care. Further examination of this process highlighted the significance of knowing the patient in clinical decision making.

The understanding acquired through knowing the patient is considered central to skilled clinical judgment. Clinical knowing creates an atmosphere where certain aspects of a particular situation stand out as salient and others recede in importance. Clinical knowing allows that nurse to compare the current situation to typical situations, thereby fostering the recognition of relevant changes and early warnings of complications.

The nurse's inability or unwillingness to use clinical knowing has direct consequences for the patient. It places the patient at greater risk for complications associated with a late detection of impending change in physiological status. All medical treatments and procedures carry risks, and knowing the patient has been identified as an important component in early recognition of complications to avert serious sequelae (Minick, 1995). When the nurse does not use clinical knowing, patients can suffer simply because of a standardized rather then personal approach to nursing care.

The nurse who does not use clinical knowing often depersonalizes the patient and creates a feeling of loss of dignity and uniqueness that reduces the patient to object. This can enhance feelings of vulnerability and insecurity rather then the desired feelings of comfort, support, and safety. Therefore, nurses who do not use clinical knowing deny their patients a caring relationship filled with empathy and concern.

Research in clinical judgment in nursing practice strongly supports clinical knowing as an essential core element in the process of decision making (Fitzpatrick, 2002). Because nursing care has become increasingly complex, clinical knowing has become even more important in preventing adverse and/or catastrophic events.

References

Atkins, S., & Murphy, K. (1993). Reflection: A review of the literature. *Journal of Advanced Nursing, 18*, 1188–1192.

Benner, P., Tanner, C., (1996). *Expertise in nursing practice, caring, clinical judgment and ethics.* New York: Springer.

Benner P., & Wrubel, J. (1989). *The primacy of caring.* Menlo Park, CA: Addison-Wesley.

Boyer, D., & Kochinda, C. (2004). Enhancing collaborative communication of nurse and physician leadership in two intensive care units. *Journal of Nursing Administration, 34*(2), 60–70.

Carper, B. (1978). Fundamental patterns of knowing in nursing. *Advances in Nursing Science, 1*(1), 13–23

Ciliska, D., Pinelli, J., DiCenso, A., & Cullum, N. (2001). Resources to enhance evidence-based nursing practice. *American Association of Critical Care Nurses Clinical Issues, 12*(4), 520–528.

Cioffi, J. (1997). Heuristics, servants to intuition in clinical decision making. *Journal of Advanced Nursing, 26*(1), 203–208.

Fitzpatrick, J. (2002). The balance in nursing: Clinical and scientific ways of knowing and being. *Nursing Education Perspectives, 23*(2), 57.

Kilpatrick, K., & Purden, M. (2007). Using reflective nursing practice to improve care of women with congenital heart disease considering pregnancy. *The American Journal of Maternal Child Nursing, 32*(3), 140–147.

Knapp, B. (2004). Competency: An essential component of caring in nursing. *Nursing Administration Quarterly, 28*(4), 285–287.

Lerners, D. (1992). Intuition in nursing practice. *Journal of Holistic Nursing, 10*(2), 137–153.

McCutcheon, H., & Pincombe, J. (2001). Intuition: An important tool in the practice of nursing. *Journal of Advanced Nursing, 35*(3), 342–348.

Meleis, A. I. (2007). *Theoretical nursing: Development and progress.* New York: Lippincott Williams & Wilkins.

Melnyk, B., Fineout-Overholt, E. (2004). *Evidence-based practice in nursing and healthcare: A guide to best practice.* New York: Lippincott.

Minick, P. (1995). The power of human caring: Early recognition of patient problems. *Scholar Inquiry in Nursing Practice, 9*, 303–315.

Nelson, G., King, M., Brodine, S. (2008). Nurse-physician collaboration on medical-surgical units. *MEDSURG Nursing, 17*(1), 35–40.

Nightingale, F. (1860). Notes on nursing: What it is and what it is not. New York: Appleton and Lange.

Oates, S., (1994). A women of valor: Clara Barton and the Civil War. London: Maxell Mcmillian International

Physics: Discovery and Intuition (2007). Albert Einstein Quotes. Found online at http://www.p-i-a.com/Magazine/Issue19/Physics_19.htm first accessed on November 15, 2008.

Retsas, A. (2000). Barriers to using evidence in nursing practice. *Journal of Advanced Nursing, 31*(3), 599–606.

Taylor, C. (1995). Rethinking nursing's basic competencies. *Journal of Nursing Care Quality, 9*(4), 1–13.

Teekman, B. (2000). Exploring reflective thinking in nursing practice. *Journal of Advanced Nursing, 31*(5), 1125–1135.

Whittemore, R. (2000). Consequences of not knowing the patient. *Clinical Nurse Specialist, 14*(2), 79–81.

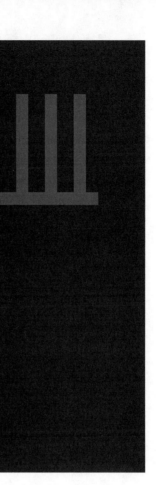

Influences of
Technology
on Knowing
in Nursing

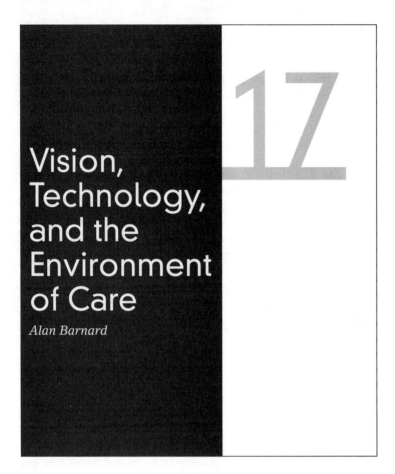

Vision, Technology, and the Environment of Care

Alan Barnard

Chapter Overview

Vision and visual representation are culturally significant phenomena and are central to current Western health care and nursing practice. Clinical practice relies increasingly on vision, and we look often at technology rather than people to assess the people for whom we care. This chapter examines how linear-perspective vision and technology influence the practice of nurses. It seeks to interpret the transformative nature of visual representation within nursing and highlights important implications for caring. In this way, we advance understanding and critical examination of our reliance on vision in technologically intensive environments.

Alternative accounts of current practice(s) are highlighted for further research, practice, and theoretical development.

Introduction

Since the Renaissance, Western culture has experienced an increasing emphasis on vision (Bryson, 1988; Ihde, 1993 a,b; Martin, 1988; Romanyshyn, 1989), and vision has evolved to be a central component of nursing (Barnard & Sinclair, 2006). The Renaissance was a cultural movement beginning around the 14th century in Italy and later spread to the rest of Europe. The period lasted until the 17th century and saw the development of knowledge, learning, and linear perspective in painting. The Renaissance occurred between the Middle Ages and our modern era, and the period witnessed significant cultural and scientific advancements. This era of Western social and cultural development has been characterized as the beginning of an increasing domination and reliance on sight or vision (Ihde, 1993, a,b, 2000; Romanyshyn, 1989). Artists began to understand how to portray linear perspective in their artistic representations and the effect linear perspective vision has on the way that things, people, and events were portrayed in paintings and other visual form. Thus, at this time there emerged an increasing cultural reliance on visual field(s): that is, interpreting the entire scope and nature of what we see when we look at things, people, and events. Examples of artists who were at the forefront of these developments were the Italian artist Masaccio (1401–1428), who was one of the first people to apply the new method of linear perspective in his fresco of the Holy Trinity. Another artist was Andrea Mantegna (1430–1506), who created unusual vantage points in his paintings, often looking at figures from below or at length. In the painting *Lamentation of the Dead Christ,* Mantegna positions the viewer of the painting at the feet of the subject (Christ) in order to stimulate an empathic response. The observer has a sense of witnessing as he or she looks at the person as a result of a heightened sense of space and distance (Urton, 2008).

Romanyshyn (1989) demonstrated that a review of artistic representation throughout history reveals the way that increasing reliance on linear perspective and vision has become a way of knowing that has altered the way we interpret the world and the way we interact with it. In fact, Romanyshyn (1989) argued that since the Renaissance, a new culturally bound conception of the world has emerged that emphasizes our mastery through distance. Increasing space and physical distance has emerged between the observer, who looks; and the things, people, and events that are observed. Linear perspective vision has altered our interpretation of the world from being one in which the depth of matter was one of spatial distance, to one in which horizontal space is emphasized across a visual plane. In order to observe the visual plane and to make judgments about, for example, a person within it, a distance is created between the observer and the observed. That is, as a result of our emphasis on vision, we often step back or step away from people, things, and events in order to comprehend them. (Re)interpretation of health care and nursing praxis is needed in light of the transformations that are continuing to occur.

Nursing has developed a visual culture in which we invest a lot of time looking at people. *Visual culture* in this instance means the predominance of visual forms of media, communication, and information. For example, the development and inclusion of image technology and computer screens is the latest evolution in an increasingly visual health care environment. There has been a social and cultural shift to the visual within what was traditionally an oral/verbal communication culture in nursing. Emerging visual cultures are an appropriate target for analysis. Through technology, we gain perceptual insights into the condition of people for whom we care, and the experience of using technology has an associated sophistication and link with science. Ihde (1993a) describes technology in the modern era as techno-science because of the increasing relations between technology development and scientific advancement.

The cultural orientation of nursing has always been directed toward the care of people, and this has often manifested, or certainly has been romanticized as, care enacted typically through close physical presence to people. Current practice presents many challenges for traditional conceptions of nurse behavior and orientation to care. Today nurses work increasingly in highly technological and often image-based realities that include monitoring systems as part of care delivery. Many clinical environments rely on vision and visual interpretation as a basis for clinical assessment. The modern intensive care and coronary care units rely heavily on monitoring systems. Traditional boundaries characterized by close proximity to the person in a bed are changing. Nurses situate themselves in a range of purposeful positions in order to not only maximize power and control *over* patients (van der Riet, 1997) but also to plan and enact care. The new virtual world of nursing continues to challenge traditional notions of caring as well as our practice habits. In practice, vital signs are increasingly accessed via screens, machinery is increasingly a component of the patient's extended care environment, and body systems are measured and assessed often via technologies that are an extension of the person. It has been noted that image-based practice sometimes appears to represent the progress of the person as a patient with more life than the real thing (Barnard & Sandelowski, 2001; Simon, 1999).

Technology has a major role in transforming the workplace, not only in terms of the machinery and equipment used, but how we do things, how we organize ourselves as nurses, what we value, why we use technology, and what influences our patterns of thinking. For example, nursing practice in hospitals has been transformed into specialties that are organized and defined according to equipment, knowledge, bureaucracy, economics, and behavioral criteria. In observing the transformation, Cooper (1993) went so far as to assert that the process of technological change has advanced to an extent that many nursing environments are defined no longer by human caring but by technology of an area. For example, the machine is a defining technology of renal nursing, and the ventilator is a defining technology for the intensive care nurse.

It is argued here that a measure of the benefit of vision and visual representation in health care is dependent not only on the cleverness and accuracy of technology but also on the place it has within the context of care, our clinical practice, and expressions of caring. *Technology* is defined in this instance as much more than machines, equipment, and tools. Our understanding of technology emerges from the relations between machinery, equipment, tools, utensils, automata, apparatus, structures, and utilities (technical objects) in our practice; and the organizations where we work, the science that informs technological development, the culture(s) that exist as part of our own life experience, social and moral precepts, and the politics that determine which technology is most common and supported in the profession of nursing. Finally, technology must be understood as a non-neutral influence upon what we do, how we act, and what we achieve (Barnard, 1997). It is non-neutral because technology will influence care outcomes that range across the full spectrum of positive to negative experience. Expertise in practice based on person-centered approaches emphasizes the centrality of the individual and by extension the individual's values, choices, and culture. However, the increasing emphasis within health care environments on technological thinking—such as standardization, protocols, and integrated systems to manage health care delivery—can come into conflict with the values and expectations of the person for whom we profess to care.

Technology to a greater or lesser extent can alter our capacity to determine and accomplish individual goals, professional approaches to care, and principles of nursing practice. Technology will influence what Walters (1994) described as the ability of each nurse to "focus" his or her energies on the person and the nurse's ability to "balance" technology with the qualities of caring.

Technology, People, and How Nurses Know

Vision and linear perspective are significant to how we perceive care outcomes in practice and are central to the many strategies nurses use to assess each patient's clinical condition. For example, the experience can be likened to empirical scientific observation because we stand often at a distance observing for relevant and important things of interest. It is not uncommon for nurses to step back and away to observe the progress of care. A significant proportion of health care assessment and intervention is represented now on purpose-designed diagnostic screens for recording such activities as temperature, blood pressure, pulse, oxygen saturation, and the cardiac cycle. Printouts and monitors encourage our need to engage in distancing behaviors such as sitting at a nurses station looking at a monitor or standing away looking over an entire room. Nursing practice involves a lot of clinical time using technology to treat people, to record important aspects of care, and to observe people often at a distance across a ward area or from the foot of a bed. We are surrounded by images, graphic representation, and moving pictures of body functioning; but we have little knowledge of their effect on care provision, human relationships, or our thinking (Barnard & Sandelowski, 2001).

Short (1997) noted that within hospitals, nurses are one of a select group who are able to observe each person's body with impunity. In fact, it has been noted that nurses have a specific and professionally derived angle of vision by virtue of our distinctive epistemological, social, and even moral position at the point of patient care and technology integration (Sandelowski, 1998). Whether looking at a person in a bed, a digital display, an intravenous pump, or a computer screen, it is commonplace to interpret and understand our world(s) via the retina of our eyes. Light, color, and movement are part of our nursing experience and just like society, what we observe has meaning, and an associated language, and it is interpreted in relation to our past and present.

Observation as a methodology is enhanced by technology as it provides the opportunity to repeat or re-visit a phenomenon or scene (i.e., there is opportunity to return to what we have observed previously in order to detect changes and additional features of a patient's condition). We engage in pattern recognition for the identification of clinically relevant phenomena. That is, we use mediated text such as screens, printouts, alarms, and lights as representations of the condition and progress of each person (Barnard & Sinclair, 2006; Green, 1992; Marck, 2000; Sandelowski, 2000; Williams, 1997). Mediation refers to that which is representative or symbolic and stands for meanings and values associated with an aspect of our practice or our patient's current and ongoing health condition. In a semiotic sense, mediating technology are signs that produce images, graphs, and numbers that are signifiers. Signs and signifiers do not present a copy of reality, only a mediated (interpreted) way of knowing a phenomenon (e.g., a person's condition). Interpretation is presented through professionally encoded representations such as significant patterns or numbers displayed by technology. These sign systems are governed by rules and conventions that are shared by a community such as nurses and doctors, and are representative because they have a structure that can be analyzed.

For example, the act of taking a person's temperature demands a repeatable experience because we seek to track changes and look for significant measurement as indicators of a patient's condition over time. In advanced care environments, devices permit temperature to be measured, recorded automatically, and displayed on a screen. Vital signs are presented as accurate representations of the person's condition, and technological devices are an efficient strategy that removes the requirement for a nurse to use a handheld device. In many clinical environments, we look increasingly to image-based realities, which are included to assess the health of a person, state of recovery, changes in condition, and progress of treatment. It is commonplace to observe representation(s) on screens in the form of black and white pictures, colorized images, or digital displays (Barnard & Sandelowski, 2001). We watch attentively to see and note—remark and comment—measure and respond, through an increasing array of special instruments that bring targeted aspects of a person's body and condition perceptively closer to us. In some instances, as a result of monitoring, there is alteration to the actual distance between the observer and the observed, yet distance has a sense of being reduced. The person is sometimes physically at distance yet strangely closer.

Vision, Proximity, and Nursing Care

Technology enhances yet ultimately transforms our experience of people and the environment in which we exist (Ihde, 1995). As a result of the inclusion of technology in care, we perceive and interpret our world in a variety of different ways. For example, we often use automatic instruments to record and display vital signs such as temperature and pulse, and the Internet does not require us to be in close physical proximity to a patient to assess the patient's clinical condition. Although the intensive care and coronary care environments are an obvious example where continuous monitoring occurs, there are many care environments (e.g., general surgical or medical units/wards) where the acuity and complexity of care means that it is increasingly commonplace to witness various instruments and automated technology such as infusion pumps used in care. Physical proximity to a patient can alter because nurses are often *there* but not *here* with the person (Sandelowski, 2002). Many aspects of a patient's ongoing assessment and treatment are displayed and monitored. Body systems are measured and assessed via technologies that are an extension of the person. Visual representation and distancing from people are now commonplace experiences. As a result of an increased emphasis on vision and associated technology, we step back or step away from people, things, and events in order to comprehend them; we are often in physical retreat from the person for whom we care.

Vision, Proximity, and Space

The space between the nurse and the patient as a result of physical retreat is therefore a transformed space, and it must be understood within the context of our abilities as nurses and the experience of each patient. Liaschenko (2003) and Andrews & Kitchin (2005) highlighted that the spatial variation between people is increasing and consequently described clinical environments in terms of "geography of care." Each care environment has geographic characteristics that are related to design, experience, and aesthetics. Just as care relationships are altered potentially by technology, so too the care environment.

An assessment of geographies of care reveals a range of practice modes that involve being with the person in a variety of different ways, and many change our use of space and proximity between persons. For example, in many countries there has been a steady increase in the numbers of patients receiving care at home. A specific group is families caring for in-home, ventilator-dependent children. Medical technology at home creates for this group of children and their families an altered home environment. The inclusion of medical machinery alters usable physical space in the home, introduces foreign technology, and can result in restructuring of the geography of a living space. The experiences of this group are not without significant human cost and involve significant impact upon the meaning of a home, the social meaning of family, and their relationships with a community (Wang & Barnard, 2008; Wang, Barnard & Somerville 2007).

The Dominance of Vision and the Medicalized Body

One interpretation of spatial and geographic changes occurring in our practice is to claim that there is too much dominance and supremacy of vision in health care and clinical practice (i.e., visual hegemony). For example, Romanyshyn (1989) claimed that the body in health care has been transformed from a complete and whole manifestation of our shared cultural life and death, to be a medicalized body that is broken into segmental parts kept at increasing distance from the observer and the observed. The person (patient) observed is broken down into segmental body parts and is redefined as a specimen under observation. The subsequent emergence of a "spectator–spectacle–specimen relationship" is characterized by observational activity described as anatomical gaze (Romanyshyn, 1989).

To illustrate the point, Romanyshyn (1989) made a comparison between medical bodies and pornographic bodies. Both emphasize the range of expression associated with the body as technical function. Each epitomizes the objectification of the body, and each creates a body that is apprehended through a distant, objectifying gaze. The medicalized or pornographic eye of the spectator seeks through humiliation and subjugation of the flesh to reduce the body (person) to that of inanimate thing (object). For example, in its most obscene and objectified sense, the pornographic body is portrayed as a vessel of sexual pleasure, erotic violence, and visual delight through avenues such as the seemingly unlimited visual representation of body parts, sex acts, and anonymous genitalia on the World Wide Web. Nothing escapes the eye of the observer because everything that can be measured and quantified becomes part of the visual experience.

Whether observing machine(ry)—body part(s)—object(s) or a pornographic array of anonymous sexual acts, the exposure is total. Everything measurable can be observed, calculated, recorded, and objectified. The medicalized and pornographic body could be your body, my body—in fact, no-body! The entire experience risks being anonymous and not grounded in the reality that a person is being observed. Limited opportunity emerges for emotional connectedness, and there is limited opportunity for both subjective understanding of experience and achievement of knowing the other in a more complete way. As caregivers there is limited opportunity to awaken in our own understanding discrete personal and specific insights about each individual. Everything anatomical, functional, and quantifiable is exposed for the observer (Henaff, 1995). Subtle differences between people are underrepresented as the interior body of the person is observed via technology within a context of care filled also by furniture, beds, significant others, machines, outputs, and inputs.

Nurses have at times expressed similar conceptions when they have highlighted perceived depersonalization and objectification as a result of the inclusion and use of technology in care. Opinion varies depending upon whether, for example, technology is considered to reduce menial work, increase comfort, emphasize a harmony between technology and caring, and expand knowledge (see Ray, 1987; Simpson, 1990); or undermine patient care, cause fragmentation of health services, and foster uncaring nurses (see Calne, 1994; Henderson, 1980).

From a pessimistic perspective, clinical practice emerges potentially to be a reductionist endeavor that is grounded in a condition of depersonalized care. Care outcomes are measured as a series of urine bags, machinery, techniques, vital signs, cables, and digital display. Body parts are represented for the spectator as graphs, lights, alarms, excrement, and electrical activity. It follows that the spectator (nurse) retreats from the person's body in order to know it not in a holistic and personal sense, but in terms of its composite parts that are displayed for observation at any given moment at a nurse's workstation, on a computer screen, or across a clinical area. According to Romanyshyn (1989), in distancing the self from the person, we gain a spectator's vision of the function of a body. A spectator differs from an observer because there is an implied sense of dispassionate and disconnected watching.

Boykin and Schoenhofer (2001) affirmed that in some circumstances nursing practice environments would seem to support the belief that nursing as primarily a role in which nurses adopt a functional role and are not much more themselves than an instrument, a technology. In such instances nursing practice never seems to progress from being an instrumental endeavor where care risks being depersonalized and characterized primarily as a series of actions and activities that we do to others. For example, a nursing role can be acted out as simply observing and reporting changes that are monitored by technology. Nursing care under these circumstances is described best as a process of doing things.

But does viewing a screen at a distance necessarily signal objectification of person; alter relationships between person, patient, and nurse; reduce caring to an instrumental activity; and discourage nursing practice from being a holistic endeavor? Does viewing a screen, observing a digital display, or looking into a care environment from a distance mean we are not caring; and under these conditions, can knowing a person whole in the moment ever be a realistic outcome?

Vision and Space(s) and Distance

Ihde (1995) differentiated between four kinds of technological knowing or human-machine-technology–world relations. He highlighted that in embodied relationships, the devices we use extend our senses to limits not known previously through "normal" senses, they foster new hermeneutic relations in which interpretation of the real is altered and/or made different, there is development of relationships with technology manifested as the classic love-hate relationship, and they develop whole environments that can be characterized by our relations with technology.

In this final form of technological knowing (background human/technology relations), technology becomes a part of a total environment that we inhabit. As a result of virtual/digital/textual-based technology in health care environments, the person (patient) for whom we care infiltrates into the clinical area or space(s) by virtue of the various monitors and equipment that are associated with the person at any one time. The person is not only here in a bed but extends through technology into the environment of care. The person's body emerges as part of the technology to be included in various ways in the environment of care.

For example, the person may assert ownership of self through the claim that a rhythm observed on a cardiac monitor is *my heart*; a mother might say that an ultrasound picture of a baby is *my baby;* or a postoperative patient may remind the observer that urine collected in a catheter bag attached to their bed is *their urine.* Screens, monitors, bags, and alarms emerge as both representations and extensions of the person's body here in a bed. The experiences highlight ownership of self by the person and reinforce the co-ownership nature of the nurse's responsibility and relationship but also show the way that a person's body is partially extended and represented in other ways. We can interpret a person's cardiac rhythm as it is represented on a monitor, but we do not know if the person is experiencing pain. We can see the temperature of the person at any one time digitally represented on a screen, but we do not know if the person feels hot.

The immediate bed space that once defined the person's body and space no longer confines them as they infiltrate into a much large clinical environment that is part of a complete representation of them. We can see the person's urine as a representation of their bladder and body function. The urine in the bag is a result of the catheter and collection bag that are a quasi-extension of the person's body here in a bed or seated in a chair: in a virtual sense, the urine is still the person's and is part of his or her body as a result of the way that tubes maintain that extension of the body. The material nature of the technology as it extends from the person allows this experience. Therefore it may be the case that when a person (patient) is observed at distance, we see the person and understand him or her better when the person is viewed/interpreted within the context of the whole environment of care and in relation to the manner in which the person's body is represented in discrete but incomplete ways. For example, being up close to a patient who lies in a bed can limit clinical assessment. Lines, cables, and tubes that extend from the person's body move out and away at numerous angles and trajectories into space(s) unseen close up to a bed. The technology moves away from the visual field of the nurse to surrounding areas when the nurse is physically close to the person. Important assessment technology may not be viewed well up close the person because it is located in other parts of the room. An assessment void can be experienced by the nurse as the patient's associated treatment lines, cables, and tubes direct the eye of the nurse away into unseen space that is not always within the nurse's visual field. There can emerge for the nurse and patient a sense of unknowing. Up close physically to a patient, our desire to see all aspects of care delivery during clinical assessment of the person can be limited as our vision is drawn away to other space in the clinical environment that sometimes cannot be seen. A nurse might complain, "I can't see the monitor, the lights, the bag(s), the screen, or the readout."

The numerous vanishing points at the ends of cables and tubes do not at that moment assist to reveal the whole person. It becomes essential for the nurse to move to an alternative position, which sometimes includes retreating back and away in order to know the person in a more complete way at that moment (Barnard & Sinclair, 2006).

Technology and Knowing Person

Phenomenological research (Ihde, 2001) has demonstrated that it takes a deliberate act by a person and a manipulation of nursing practice (Barnard & Sinclair, 2006) to focus on vision by itself. If we do focus only on our visual sense, as is the case sometimes in clinical practice, we do so on purpose in order to focus our attention on a specific aspect of a person at a specific moment. In fact, Ihde (2001) noted that it is not possible to specifically single out your visual sense for extended periods of time because the other aspects of patient care that are interpreted through other senses occur simultaneously within clinical environments. Our patients continue to present clinical information that should tempt all our senses and encourage other ways of knowing.

Focusing only on visual aspects of an environment of care gives the impression of control and emphasizes empirical knowledge; but multisensory dimensions that contain pathways to ethical, scientific, intuitive, and personal ways of knowing remain constant, even if the practitioner is not attuned always to them. For example, observing a cardiac monitor for ventricular tachycardia focuses an observer on viewing a representation of a discrete body part, the heart. If you or I look at the cardiac monitor we might say, "There it is—the arrhythmia!" If this observing and assessing behavior leads the nurse to then return to the person in a physical sense to inquire how the person feels and to assess the person's body further using all senses, then the nurse has made a purposeful choice to focus on the complete person as they present at that moment. In fact, much of our practice is determined by these types of actions and reactions (behavior), but they should not necessarily always be determined as a result of technological mediation. If you do not return to the person at an appropriate moment in their care it is you, rather than the technology, that has made a choice to distance yourself from your patient. It is at that moment that the nurse has made a purposeful choice to focus only on visual information and a partial representation/extension of the person's body, rather than to acknowledge the whole person and use other commonly used senses such as listening and smell. Under these conditions, an illusion of control is created because simultaneously, control is at risk of being lost (Barnard & Sinclair, 2006).

Our understanding of others and their needs has to be informed by an authentic desire to acknowledge and enhance the central tenet of personhood through wise integration and use of technology: that is, we need to develop technological competence. But a central question in that desire is who and/ or what is at the centre of our visual experience? Ihde (1995) noted that vision transformed by increasing technology in the form of monitors, graphs, digital readouts, etc., is destructive to traditional cultures, modes of operating, and ways of knowing. Technologies are not neutral and are transformative by nature. They produce an impetus to change behavior, culture, and relationships.

A response to the question "Who and what are at the centre of visual experience?" is to seek confidently to understand technology and engage in authentic caring. How nurses respond to increasingly visual environments and ongoing alteration to physical proximity and representation of body is important, since it is clear that there will be change in nursing practice. Authentic caring is a reflection of choice, beliefs, and the commitment nurses make to each person they nurse (Boykin & Schoenhofer, 2001). I *am* responsible for who I am as a nurse. To be authentic is to act autonomously and to commit resolutely to a specific course of action and way of being in the world. The inauthentic nurse irresolutely occupies a role. Being a nurse authentically does not necessarily make you a better nurse, but being a nurse becomes explicitly your concern. Thus, ultimately, knowing a person as whole in the moment is an act that is reliant on a personal commitment and intentionality despite changes inherent in an environment of care. It is informed by a desire to do better for others and a commitment to understand the implications of technology for care.

Final Words

Visual cultures of nursing have a role to play in relationships between people. Further research and scholarship is required to investigate caring relationships within the context of emerging technology. It is clearly the case that nursing has an increasing emphasis on visual representation and that technology alters bodily experience and representation. Mediated text and visual representation are part of what postmodernists might describe as polymorphic seeing (Ihde, 2001).

What is emerging at this time is a proliferation of numerous ways of seeing, witnessing, representing, and viewing phenomena as a result of an increasing emphasis on vision and textual image.

This chapter highlights a significant and shared experience of practice(s). It emphasizes the importance and scope of our visual sense. It also exposes different and important interpretations of nursing practice(s) within approaches to care that stress vision and sometimes distancing between the nurse and the person receiving care. The idea of nurses stepping back and away from someone sick may not fit with accepted proxemics (the use of space). Intimacy, personal distance, polite distance, etc., are enacted across conventional boundaries, and it is clearly the case that new conventions and boundaries are emerging at this time. It is noted that technology is transformative in its intention and produces change. Amidst all the change, it is unclear at this point if many nurses practice in ways characterised best by anatomical gaze or how often nurses return to the whole person at opportune and appropriate moments.

Explanation of the ways nurses practice and patient experiences of caring will assist to improve clinical practice and health care. Walters (1995) highlighted correctly that the importance of understanding technology in nursing cannot be underestimated because "as nursing is practiced in the midst of technology, acknowledging the material world of health care involves developing an understanding of technology used by nurses in their daily practice" (p. 339). How each nurse responds to our evolving visual culture and distancing from persons is an important question, especially given changes in nursing and health care to traditional caring boundaries and space. We live and practice increasingly in environments of care that are representative of reality, and a major issue remaining for us is to understand the relationships between persons and the influence of changing contexts on care.

References

Andrews, G. J., & Kitchin, R. (2005). Geography and nursing: Convergence in cyberspace? *Nursing Inquiry, 12*(4), 316–324.

Barnard, A. (1997). A critical review of the belief the technology is a neutral object and nurses are its master. *Journal of Advanced Nursing, 26*, 126–131.

Barnard, A., & Sandelowski, M. (2001). Technology and humane nursing care: (Ir)reconcilable or invented difference? *Journal of Advanced Nursing, 34*, 367–375.

Barnard, A., & Sinclair, M. (2006). Spectators & spectacles: Nurses, midwives and visuality. *Journal of Advanced Nursing, 55*(5), 578–586.

Boykin, A., & Schoenhofer, S. O. (2001). *Nursing as caring*. MA: National League for Nursing.

Bryson, N. (1988). The gaze in the expanded field. In H. Foster (Ed.), *Vision and visuality* (pp. 87–114). WA: Bay Press.

Calne, S. (1994). Dehumanisation in intensive care. *Nursing Times, 90*(17), 31–33.

Cooper, M. C. (1993). The intersection of technology and care in the ICU. *Advances in Nursing Science, 15*(3), 23–32.

Fairman, J., & D'Antonio, P. (1999). Virtual power: Gendering the nurse-technology relationship. *Nursing Inquiry, 6*, 178–186.

Green, A. (1992). How nurses can ensure the sounds patients hear have a positive rather than negative effect upon recovery and quality of life. *Intensive and Critical Care, 8*, 245–248.

Henaff, M. (1995). Sade, the mechanization of the libertine body and the crisis of reason. In A. Feenberg & A. Hannay (Eds.), *Technology and the politics of knowledge* (pp. 213–235). Bloomington: Indiana University Press.

Henderson, V. (1980). Preserving the essence of nursing in a technological age. *Journal of Advanced Nursing, 5*(3), 245–260.

Ihde, D. (1993a). *Philosophy of technology*. New York: Paragon House.

Ihde, D. (1993b). *Postphenomenology*. Chicago, Illinois: Northwestern University Press.

Ihde, D. (1995). Image technologies and traditional culture. In A. Feenberg & A. Hannay (Eds.), *Technology and the politics of knowledge* (pp. 147–158). Indianapolis, Indiana University Press.

Ihde, D. (2001). *Bodies in technology*. Minneapolis St. Paul: MN, University of Minnesota Press.

Liaschenko, J. (2003). At home with illness: Moral understandings and moral geographies. *Ethica, 15*, 71–82.

Locsin, R. (1995). Machine technologies and caring in nursing. *Image: Journal of Nursing Scholarship, 27*(3), 201–203.

Locsin, R. (1995). Technological competence as caring in critical care. *Holistic Nursing Practice, 12*(4), 50–56.

Locsin, R. (Ed.). (2005). *Technological competency as caring in nursing: A model for practice*. Indianapolis: Sigma Theta Tau International Press.

Marck, P. (2000). Recovering ethics after "technics": Developing critical text on technology. *Nursing Ethics, 7*, 5–14.

Martin, J. (1988). Scopic regimes of modernity. In H. Foster (Ed.), *Vision and visuality* (pp. 3–28). Seattle, WA: Bay Press.

Ray, M. A. (1987). Technological caring: A new model in critical care. *Dimensions of Critical Care Nursing, 6*(3), 166–173.

Romanyshyn, R. (1989). *Technology as symptom and dream: Technology as vanishing point*. London: Routledge.

Sandelowski, M. (1998). Looking to care or caring to look? Technology and the rise of spectacular nursing. *Holistic Nursing Practice, 12*, 1–11.

Sandelowski, M. (2000). Devices and desires: Gender, technology and American nursing. Chapel Hill: The University of North Carolina.

Sandelowski, M. (2002). Visible humans, vanishing bodies, and virtual nursing: Complications of life, presence, place, and identity. *Advances in Nursing Science, 24*, 58–70.

Short, P. (1997). Picturing the body in nursing. In J. Lawler (Ed.), *The body in nursing* (pp. 7–9). South Melbourne: Churchill Livingstone.

Simon, C. (1999). Images and image: Technology and the social politics of revealing disorder in a North American hospital. *Medical Anthropology Quarterly, 13*, 141–162.

Simpson, R. L. (1990). How to survive the next decade. *Nursing Management, 21*(12), 24–25.

Urton, R. (2008). Key innovations and artists of the Italian renaissance. Art History Pages. Retrieved July 2, 2008, from http://www.eyecon-art.net/history/Renaissance/early_ren.htm.

van der Riet, P. (1997). The body, the person, technologies and nursing. In J. Lawler (Ed.), *The body in nursing* (pp. 95–108). South Melbourne: Churchill Livingstone.

Walters, A. J. (1994). An interpretive study of the clinical practice of critical care nurses. *Contemporary nurse, 3*, 21–25.

Walters, A. J. (1995). Technology and the lifeworld of critical care nursing. *Journal of Advanced Nursing, 22*, 338–346.

Wang, K, & Barnard, A. (2008) The experience of caring for a ventilator dependent child at home: a phenomenographic examination. *Qualitative Health Research, 18*(4), 501–508.

Wang, K,, Barnard, A.. & Somerville, M. (2007) Paediatric Community Nursing: The experience of caring for technology-dependent children at home. In Barnard, A. & Locsin, R. *Technology and Nursing Practice* (p. 60–72). London: Palgrave-Macmillan.

Williams, S. (1997). Modern medicine and the "uncertain body": From corporeality to hyperreality? *Social Science & Medicine, 45*, 1041–1049.

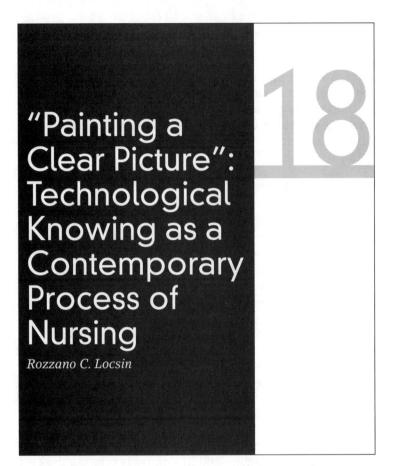

"Painting a Clear Picture": Technological Knowing as a Contemporary Process of Nursing

Rozzano C. Locsin

Chapter Overview

This chapter describes and explains technological knowing as a contemporary process of nursing. As an intentional and mutual process, the goal is to advance the understanding of health and well-being. Knowing in nursing is critical such that while it may be important to know that a comatose patient on a ventilator may not care very much about a gowned, masked, anonymous nurse, this masked nurse in the ICU essentially becomes unmasked in the sense of revealing a compassionate person to the vulnerable patient. In this nursing, the focus is mutual affirmation of what matters most to the nurse and nursed. With technological knowing as a deliberative activity, evidences derived from technologies are representations that illuminate the person paradoxically both as object and as subject. With technological knowing, advancing health care technologies fosters "painting a clear picture" of the nurse and nursed—the hoped-for premise—enabling mutual knowing of persons as participants in their care rather than as objects of our care.

Introduction

> *It is in moments of illness that we are compelled to recognize that we live not alone but chained to a creature of a different kingdom, whole worlds apart, who has no knowledge of us and by whom it is impossible to make ourselves understood: Our body. (Proust. http://www.brainyquote. com/quotes/authors/m/marcel_proust.html)*

Technological advances have increasingly influenced the distinct valuing of contemporary health care. Hospitals and health care institutions are known for their sophisticated technologies, which promise to enhance the knowing of persons with great efficiency and immediacy. Possession of these machine technologies contributes to the reputation and intrinsic value of the institution—with hallmarks of technology that cultivate an image of quality and reliability in sustaining human health, and in ostensibly offering the best in human care. Supporting this image are health care professionals who also demand the latest technology as the ultimate way toward the efficient practice of knowing persons. This is clearly evident in prolific advertising of the wonders and marvels of lifesaving machines available in institutions that is broadcast in television, print, and Web-based media. What process provides credibility to the professional practice of nursing in the use of these leading-edge technologies that are now taken for granted as integral and vital to quality human health care? Importantly, should nurses frame their practice in technological milieus from within an explicit epistemological process grounded in nursing? Are nursing and high-tech, mechanistic apparatus mutually exclusive?

Person and technology. A person is defined as a whole, dynamic, and unpredictable human being who is complete in the moment (Boykin & Schoenhofer, 2001). This qualified definition of *person* brings to light the realization of knowing persons as a practice of nursing. Of great importance to knowing a person is the condition that the person concomitantly wishes to be known by the nurse or other. This is a critical component to the practice of nursing in whatever milieu the care is enacted in.

Technology qua technology allows the nurse to know the represented aspect of the nursed. This is the nature of the knowing process, for although technology allows the knower to know the other with efficiency, the reality that is presented as the known is only a representation of the real. This legitimizes the consistent and continuing innovation in nursing and health care to spur creation of technologies that can enable the nurse to know more about the person in the moment. The consistency, value, and morality of appreciating the person in a nursing relationship are critical to the well-being of both the nurse and patient. To continually know more about the person allows the nurse to practice nursing more fully. The achievement of nursing expertise that is an expression of the merging of nursing and health care technologies is through and within the process of technological knowing in nursing.

Representations and nursing. History has preserved for millennia the representations of ancient personalities such as King Tutankhamun, Inca Atahualpa, and the mythical Greek gods Perseus and Medusa. We know that King Tut, the 14-year-old king enshrined in a gold sarcophagus, was one of the most celebrated pharaohs of the ancient Egyptian realm. Perseus we know as the fabled son of Zeus who slew Medusa. Their lives, both fact and fable, have been made known to us through stories recorded on parchment, tablets of clay, and dwelling walls and transmitted orally for generations. We come to know these characters as people through the details imprinted on the graphic artifacts that artisans have handed down through the ages.

In today's era of virtual iconography, access is rapidly gained to imagery that is startling in its ability to bring to vision and cognizance what was hitherto unimaginable. In contemporary nursing, nurses in high-tech situations routinely create and preserve virtual pictures, stories, and graphic representations of the patient that pertain to health. The artisan with chisel or quill of ancient times is effectively paralleled in the nurse and technology of these latter times: both lend unparalleled expertise to the technology of the times in artfully preserving a record. In nursing, can it be said then, given the sheer amount of technological equipment and information available in practice, that nurses truly know their patients? Must technology be the primary focus in order for the potential of the machinery and for the expectation of the patient to be fulfilled? How then do nurses really know the one nursed? Is the patient an extension of the technology, or is the nurse? What matters, and what is the primary focus? These questions provide provocative considerations about the close association of technology and person.

Constrained within the technology and human association is the notion of persons in their biological completeness, that is, human beings whose composition is maintained by innovative technologies in health care providing for altered and alternative views of persons as whole. Without doubt, human beings are preoccupied with appearances. With the proliferation and reliability of medical advances, the popularity of alterations in human parts, especially surgical cosmetic alterations, has likewise burgeoned. Technological human parts answer to a call from an increasingly affluent market. The comparative ease with which technological human parts can be acquired represents, for many, a reality that can be altered and manipulated efficiently by a surgeon's knife. Artificiality continues to receive societal affirmation: artificiality is acceptable and has become a norm that is seldom questioned. What, then, is real? Is our understanding of the person superficial if we dwell only in the person's former reality?

Health care options almost always border on questioning continuity of being healthy or simply being alive. Organ donation has launched a new description of human beings, creating an even greater issue of what constitutes artificiality: *neomorts* are posited to be persons who are organ donors but considered to be brain-dead. Their bodies are kept alive with machine technologies until needed or harvested—with the ultimate gift of this ambiguous state being that their organs enable other persons to live longer lives. Essentially, such composite of a nonliving human being with a nonhuman living device is a cyborg—for all intents and purposes living, but techno-mechanically sustained.

A techno sapiens is humanlike, mimicking human forms. Techno sapiens appears human although composed of artificial and technical parts, simulated but normalized. Technological parts such as robotic limbs are often functionally engineered with self-perpetuating computer programs, like those in artificial hearts or computers that function as intelligent machines. Do these "human" beings fit the description of persons? Consequently, will it be appropriate then to ask the question, is the future of nursing the continuous practice of knowing and valuing of human beings as persons? Advancing nursing to care for future human beings is critical to understanding a legitimate practice of nursing in a subsequent technological world.

Technology, Image, Representation

How can we know the reality of the substance or the existence of a concept? How do we know that human beings are composites of parts?

Forming a preconceived image of the person can be done using sensory information such as aural and tactile sensation. Nonetheless, the popular way of verifying the image and the knowing of the person is precisely done and confirmed by visualization. One can often ask these questions: If this is the only acceptable way that one can know another person, then how can those who have differently abled sensations know the other? What happens when one is without visual sight or is perhaps color-blind? Does the image of the visualized other change? Are perception and knowing dependent upon accuracy of sensory stimulation and input? Should all sensory inputs point to the right or correct image? Who decides what is right or correct? Should technology be a major instrument assigned to deliver this verdict?

The ascription of being real is generally applied to any thing that can be appreciated as true, provided there is evidence that it is real and existing. Often used as evidence in support of these conditions is the form of the substance or concept. One source to turn to is Plato, who provided grounding arguments in his philosophical descriptions of forms. Through sensory evidence of the existence of the form, the reality of the substance or concept is appreciated. A visual expression of a wished-for form from the story *The Little Prince* illustrates this formalization. The Prince asks the narrator to draw a sheep.

> *Not knowing how to draw a sheep, the narrator draws what he knows, a boa with an elephant in its stomach, a drawing which previous viewers mistook for a hat. "No! No!" exclaims the Prince. "I don't want a boa with an elephant inside! I want a sheep." He tries a few sheep drawings, which the*

Prince rejects. Finally he draws a box, which he explains has the sheep inside. The Prince, who can see the sheep inside the box just as well as he can see the elephant in the boa, says, "That's perfect." (The Story. http://en.wikipedia.org/wiki/The_Little_Prince#Viewpoint.)

Furthering this discourse, another example of using sensory input as basis for claiming the existence of something *real* is the story of the three blind men: Three men who have not seen an elephant were asked to describe an elephant based on their sensory input. The formation of an image and the ultimate description of an elephant are founded on the sensory input. These blind men (or men in the dark) touch an elephant to learn what it is like. Each one touches a different part, but only one part, such as the side or the tusk. They then compare notes on what they felt and learn they are in complete disagreement.

This story is used to indicate that reality may be viewed differently depending upon one's viewpoint. What seems an absolute truth may be, in the moment, a relative truth due to the deceptive nature of half-truths.

18.1

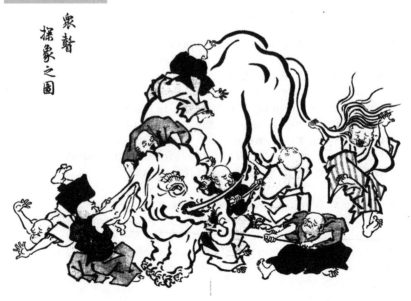

Knowing Person

One of the critical issues on the practicality of the concept of knowing person as a process of nursing is its use as a concept that can be interpreted in two ways. As an adjective, *knowing* is used to describe one who is an inquisitive, motivated, and stimulated person whose objective is to increasingly know the other. Nevertheless, *knowing* is also a concept that pertains to an activity—a process beyond the bounds of temporality that allows the nurse and nursed to fully understand each other in the moment. In nursing, it is the latter description of knowing the person that serves well the profession and discipline—as the nurse-patient activity of mutually understanding each other as persons.

How this knowing occurs has been the subject of study by scholars of nursing. In 1995, Radwin reviewed the nursing literature with the aim of describing the emerging concept of knowing the patient. In the literature, Radwin found two components of this concept: the nurse's understandings of the patient and the therapeutic choices the nurse selected for the patient. Furthermore, three specific factors were observed: the nurse's experience with caring for patients, chronological time, and a sense of closeness between patient and nurse.

In delineating the process of understanding the patient, Alexander (1990) declared that knowing the patient is for the purpose of appreciating the particulars of the patient that makes him or her different from all other patients who may have the same health care condition. Important in the consideration of knowing the patient are therapeutic choices that the nurse makes relative to the patient's condition. In knowing the patient, interventions are chosen so that the patient is treated as a unique individual. Essentially, knowing the patient is "important to nursing practice. It actualizes a cherished value in nursing, treating the person as an individual… and may be an important characteristic of expert nursing practice" (Radwin, 1995, p. 1146).

One of the concerns voiced by nurses and other health care professionals regarding the practicality of the concept of knowing person as a focus of nursing is the concept itself. Two of the most common usages include its use an adjective and the other as a verb. When used as an adjective, a knowing person is an individual who is inquisitive and erudite, and whose objective is to increasingly to know more about others. Another meaning ascribed to knowing person is as a concept pertaining to an—knowing persons is a practice process aimed at understanding a person or persons in the moment.

In nursing, the concept of knowing person better serves the profession and discipline when it is recognized as an activity in the practice process of nursing. Knowing person as a contemporary process of nursing provides diverse ways of appreciating persons as active participants in their care. This process is best explicated and evidenced in technological knowing.

Knowing the person well. One of the essential demands of professional nursing is for its practitioners to know their patients well. The expectation is entrenched in practice situations to the extent that repeatedly, nurses profess that they are able to know their patients well only when they are given more time to be present with them. Often contributing to this problem is the institutionalized documentation procedure wherein the nurse expends important nursing care time recording information that is required in maintaining the medical records system. Why is this textual documentation required?

The ideal reason is ostensibly to preserve the recorded authenticity of the changes that occur in patient health and wellness situations. Documenting patient activities and nursing actions helps guarantee continuity of care. Rationalizing the time required to know the person, a technological device is supposedly available in order to make more time available for actually being with the patient. However, the rigid demands for documenting nursing activities have taken a different turn, from enhancing certainty and continuity of care to providing accuracy for legal reimbursement to prevent legal ramifications. Inasmuch as the nurse's authentic presence with patients is to come to know who they are as persons and what matters to them, this is frequently concealed and not accomplished in a timely manner.

With these unceasing documentation formalities, the practice of documenting nursing care has accordingly assumed different forms. An even wider opportunity is provided for the development and integration of multiple technologies of care that are now merged with these same computer-based machines on which nurses enter patient documentation.

From computer-dominated equipment in nurses stations (such as handheld computers at the patient's bedside) to portable computers on wheels that nurses wheel to the patients' bedsides, or from voice-activated electronic recordings to multiple transcription techniques in textual forms, these machine technologies (Locsin, 1995) influence the realization that nurses use technologies in order to know patients more fully as persons.

Nurses' persistent demands for ways to reduce the time they spend on documenting evidence of their care in textual forms are all too real and understandable. From the perspective of knowing persons, receiving affirmation for these demands requires use of a technology-based design and form of documentation. However, perpetuating the task of documenting nursing actions through the narrative process as in handwritten nurses' notes or narrative notes on computer may only guarantee that nurses spend more time away from patient care.

Advancing Technologies in Practice

Technology extends us into the world and, in the process recreates it. Technology is thus both revealing and transforming of nature. (Sandelowski, 1997)

In advancing technologies in nursing practice, the ultimate questions one can ask about the process of knowing persons should include the idea of chronicity: How much time is needed to know the person? Is time a matter of measurement in hours and minutes? In the process of knowing persons, what information is necessary in order for the nurse and nursed to know each other more fully and participate more effectively in their knowing?

Within the intention of knowing the other, the information one can often ascertain is about the object and subject of the person. The initial phase of the traditional nursing process consisting of assessment, planning, intervention, and evaluation (APIE) subscribes to the activities that serve to know the composite aspects of human beings; that is, their bio-psycho-socio-cultural-physiological and chemical status.

Clinical laboratory testing and head-to-toe assessments are examples of nurses' activities guided from a popularized, linear nursing process that is appreciated as the best way to address the use of technologies to capture the representations and the essences of the invisible parts of the human body. In order to measure the arterial blood pressure using the sphygmomanometer or the electrical activity of the heart using the EKG, instruments and tools are used. All these gadgets, instruments, and tools allow nurses to know the valuable but invisible composition of the human being, even if their measurements are only the representations of the real, functioning human beings.

Although technological parts also may complete human beings and become integral to living quality lives, advancing health care technologies that determine this quality of life is also essential. Technological advancements measuring the physiological, anatomical, and biochemical systems of human beings are critical to knowing persons as functioning human beings. Knowing how these technologies function and ascertaining the nurses' competency with these technologies often dictates the quality of knowledge the nurses can possess about those who are nursed. The idea of knowing the person has the one nursed as focus, for knowing persons is a deliberate and intentional process of nursing in which persons are consciously acknowledged as whole, dynamic, and unpredictable in the moment (Barnard & Locsin, 2007).

Technological Knowing in Nursing: A Contemporary Process of Nursing

New needs need new techniques (Pollack, (http://thinkexist.com/quotes/jackson_pollock/2.html)

The following assumptions frame the concept of knowing person. These are also the overarching assumptions of technological knowing as a contemporary process of nursing:

Assumptions.
■ Persons are unpredictable and irreducible, thereby demanding the development of creative, innovative, and imaginative nursing practice activities so that nurses may come to know the persons fully as human beings with hopes, dreams, and aspirations.
■ All nursing takes place in nursing situations—shared experiences between the nurse and the one nursed, allowing each other to grow and know one another.

> The one nursed allows the nurse to enter his or her world so that the nurse may support, affirm, and celebrate the patient's personhood.

- Technological competency is an expression of caring in nursing, the ideal of nursing practice using technologies to know persons fully as complete in the moment.
- Nursing is a discipline and a profession. As such, the practice of nursing is based on knowledge developed by a community of nurse scholars and derived evidences from theory and research.

To make known the person is to present him or her in the best possible way, using the best mechanisms that clearly depict distinguished self. This presentation or representation can be illustrations as in descriptions and explanations about the person using narratives, graphic or visual depictions, or audio expressions, all authentically depicting the person as real. With nursing technologies, depicting the real person is to paint a clear picture of him or her, especially those aspects that cannot be appreciated as real when using human sensory mechanisms. Technological knowing is demanded for the ultimate purpose of knowing the real person.

Derived from the theoretical perspective of "technological competency as caring in nursing," (Locsin, 2005), the concept of technological knowing is construed as the practice process of using technologies of care to acknowledge the value of knowing the one nursed through contemporary technological advancements.

Technology allows the nurse to know human beings as persons (Locsin, 2005). Important with technology use in nursing is the condition that the one nursed allows himself or herself to be known as a person.

Technological knowing is a process of nursing that provides opportunities for persons to know each other through technological competency as an expression of caring in nursing (Locsin, 2005). Technological competency in nursing fosters the recognition and realization of persons as participants in their care rather than objects of care. The idea of participation in their care stems from the recognition of active engagement, in which the nurse enters the world of the one nursed and through available and appropriate technologies attempts to know the nursed more fully in the moment.

In this practice, the assumption is understood that the one nursed allows the nurse to enter his or her world so that together they may mutually support, affirm, and celebrate each other's being. In this relationship of the knower and the "knowee," technology provides the efficiency and the valuing that marks their mutual and momentary reality. Because of technological advancements, this efficiency is enhanced, and immediate and simultaneous knowing is experienced.

Illustrated in Figure 18.2, technological knowing as a practice of nursing is advanced within the context of three integrated concepts: technological caring (Ray, 1987), a focus on caring nursing with the ethico-moral conditions of nursing practice in critical care settings; technological dependency (Sandelowski, 1993), the focus on the potency of the force that extends between valuing technology and caring; and technological competency (Locsin, 2005) as the expression of caring in nursing.

Two concepts advance the valuable and significant use of technologies in nursing: (a) *technological nursing*, described as the nursing of persons with lives that are dependent on

18.2

The relationship between technological caring, technological dependency, and technological competency

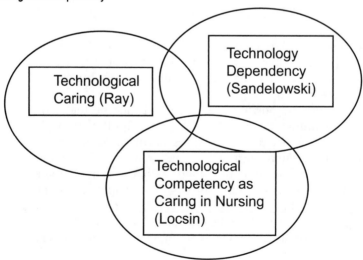

technology, and (b) *knowing persons*, the process through which nurses come to know persons more fully through technologies within the practice of technological competency as caring in nursing (Locsin, 2005). Each of these concepts provides the essentials of technology in nursing and health care. These essentials direct the understanding of persons as experiencing life as human beings, regardless of living as dependents of technologies. Many unanswered questions demand substantive answers regarding one's experiences with dependency on technologies and the experiences of persons who care for them.

These concepts composing technological knowing are based on Locsin's (2005) middle-range theory of "technological competency as caring in nursing." This is the "practice of using health care technologies for the purpose of knowing persons in an efficient and appropriate manner" (Barnard & Locsin, 2007, p. xv). The understanding of persons as participants in their care rather than as objects of our care permeate the voicing of nursing as an expression of caring nursing, one in which the purpose of nursing is nurturing the one nursed uniquely as a person.

Technological knowing prompts the nurse to participate in knowing persons in the moment. The ultimate purpose of technological knowing is to continuously acknowledge persons as whole and complete regardless of various human parts. Such an acknowledgment compels redesigning the processes of nursing—those ways of expressing, celebrating, and appreciating the practice of nursing as continuously knowing persons as whole moment to moment. In this practice of nursing, technology is used not to know, what is the person? but rather to know, who is the person? While the former question alludes to the notion of persons as objects, the latter addresses the uniqueness and individuality of persons as human beings (Locsin & Purnell, 2007).

How does the nurse know the person nursed? In knowing the person, the nurse reflects on the nursing situation, focusing on the uniqueness of the person being nursed. Although traditional patterns of knowing (Carper, 1978) contribute toward providing answers to nursing questions, there also exist other patterns of knowing in nursing. For example, in simulations technology, questions may succinctly be asked and answered through *technological knowing* as a distinct pattern of knowing, fluidly relating to a world immersed in

18.3

Technological knowing as contemporary process of nursing

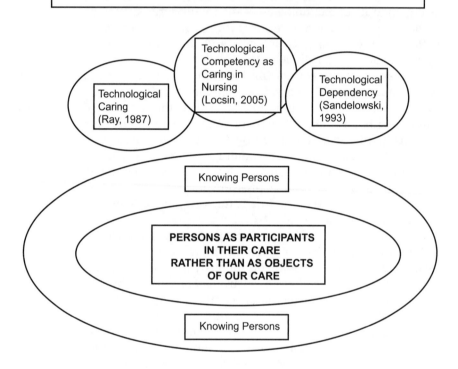

technology and more particularly, to a practice of nursing grounded in caring (Locsin, 2008).

In nursing, technological knowing can be an essential, re-envisioned aspect of knowing the one nursed; or technological knowing can simply be knowing via the gadgets or tools that the nurse uses to know the nursed as a person. Regardless, technological knowing invokes the use of technology to know persons fully as participants in their care rather than as objects that require knowing.

There are various technologies that are essential components of the nursed, especially if the person's quality of life is dependent upon these technologies, such as implantable pacemakers, AICDs, and other mechanical or electronic parts. The reality is upon us that the number of persons who are now dependent upon technologies is growing exponentially and that more will be in this group as casualties of devastating wars such as those in Afghanistan and Iraq. Soldiers coming home with missing human parts that are replaced with mechanical or electronic prostheses are vivid reminders that technology has a human value beyond its function. Limbs are often the most evident because of the bipedal mobility expected of human beings. Although mobility can be achieved with wheelchairs, now with cutting-edge machines with mechanical and electronic components, the expectation continues to hold fast that human beings are ambulatory as a norm. Inability to walk provides questionable appreciation of the quality of human living as experienced by the person who is not able to do so.

Concluding Statements

> *Technology is designed to be invincible, invulnerable, objective, and predictable, in contrast to the human characteristics of vulnerability, subjectivity, and unpredictability. It is in this context that the nurse is challenged to care. (Cooper, 1993, p. 26)*

In the 21st century, the concept of patient and its corresponding role as a care recipient no longer serves as the perfect example of a patient individual (one who waits to receive care and is told what to do); rather, the patient is a person who is very well informed and knowledgeable about his or her health, and who rightfully demands the best possible health care as a human right. Such demands evolving from easily accessible data and other resources regarding health and illness care are now fluidly retrieved in seconds. In situations such as these, the one nursed demands participation from the nurse in designing, implementing, and evaluating his or her care. Truly cognizant of the changing health care environment, the nurse creates opportunities of care together with the nursed, by using contemporary technologies to know him or her in the moment. This is the ultimate situation of anticipated care, in which the nurses can truly and meaningfully know the nursed as a participant in the nursed person's care.

Contemporary health care is about the informed and knowledgeable person who uses all available resources to know more about his or her health, and to identify and demand the most appropriate care necessary to living life more rightfully and meaningfully as a participative person.

How can technology facilitate or assist the nurse so that he or she can come to know the person? The process of technological knowing promotes the understanding of human health and well-being. The focus of the nurse and nursed is their continued affirmation of what matters most to them. Technological knowing is therefore necessary and critical to knowing persons as participants in their care, instead of being simply the objects of our care.

References

Alexander, L. (1990). Explication of the meaning of clinical judgment in nursing practice using Ricouerian hermeneutics. *Dissertation Abstracts International*, UMI No. ACC9119796.

Barnard, A., & Locsin, R. (2007). *Technology and Nursing: Practice, process, and issues*. Hampshire, United Kingdom: Palgrave-Macmillan.

Boykin, A., & Schoenhofer, S. (2001). *Nursing as caring: A model for transforming practice*. Sudbury, CT: Jones and Bartlett Press.

Carper, B. A. (1978). Fundamental patterns of knowing in nursing. *Advances in Nursing Science, 1*(1), 13–23.

Cooper, M. (1993). The intersection of technology and care in the ICU. *Advances in Nursing Science, 15*(3), 23–32.

Locsin, R. (2005). *Technological competency as caring in nursing: A model for practice*. Indianapolis, IN: Sigma Theta Tau International Press.

Locsin, R. (2008). Caring scholar response—Grounding nursing simulations in caring: An innovative approach. *International Journal for Human Caring, 12*(2), 47–49.

Locsin, R., & Barnard, A. (2007). Technological competency as caring: A model for nursing. In A. Barnard & R. Locsin (Eds.), *Technology and nursing: Practice process and issues* (pp. 16–28). London: Palgrave-Macmillan.

Locsin, R., & Purnell, M. J. (2007). Rapture and suffering with technology in nursing. *International Journal for Human Caring, 11*(1), 38–43.

"New needs need new techniques." http://thinkexist.com/quotes/jackson_pollock/2.html. Accessed January 10, 2009.

Proust, M (n.d.). http://www.brainyquote.com/quotes/authors/m/marcel_proust.html. Accessed January 10, 2009.

Radwin, L. (1995). Knowing the patient: An empirically generated process model for individualized interventions. *Nursing Research, 44*, 364–370.

Ray, M. (1987). Technological caring: A new model in critical care. *Dimensions in Critical Care Nursing, 6*(30), 166–173.

Sandelowski, M. (1993). Toward a theory of technology dependency. *Nursing Outlook, 41*(1), 36–42.

Sandelowski, M. (1997). Knowing and forgetting: The challenge of technology for a reflexive practice science of nursing. In S. Thorne & V. Hayes (Eds.), *Nursing praxis: Knowledge and action.* Thousand Oaks, CA: Sage.

Swanson-Kauffman, K. (1986). Caring in the instance of unexpected early pregnancy loss. *Topics in Clinical Nursing, 8*(2), 37–46.

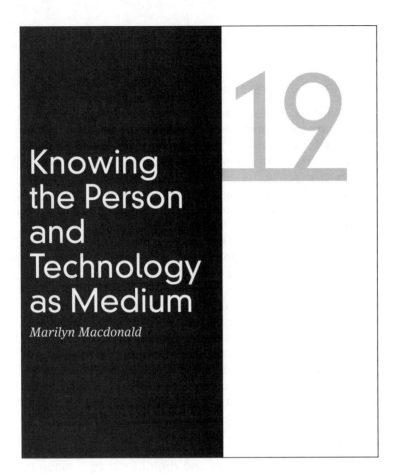

19

Knowing the Person and Technology as Medium

Marilyn Macdonald

Chapter Overview

This chapter illuminates three conceptual statements: knowing the person, technology as a medium in this process, and human science views. Issues from the integration of these concepts arise when the human science perspective intersects with the technological/biomedical perspective in the practice of care. Emphasizing the development and use of health care technologies, this chapter focuses on technology as a conduit of care grounded in a human science perspective, so that nurses may come to know persons in their care.

Knowing the Person or Knowing the Patient?

This chapter focuses on technology in nursing as a conduit of care grounded in the human science perspective. Issues arise when the human science perspective intersects with the technological/biomedical perspective on the practice of human care.

Much of the nursing literature reviewed focused on the importance of knowing the patient and supported the assumption that the terms *patient* and *person* were inter-changeable. Liaschenko (1997) has argued that knowing the person in nursing is composed of three layers of knowing: case, patient, and person. *Case* is the general biomedical knowl-edge regarding diagnoses, prognoses, and treatment, and is unrelated to any particular person. Knowing the *patient* was understanding the various physical and emotional responses of patients to treatments, and knowing the *person* was to have both of the above as well as a much deeper understanding of what life means to the person, to have a sense of the person's values, beliefs, and sense of agency. While the term predomi-nantly used in the literature was *knowing the patient*, it was clear in the work presented that the nurses were speaking about the importance of knowing the person.

More than a decade ago, nurse researchers studied what knowing the patient meant and the difference it made in nursing care (Tanner, Benner, Chesla, & Gordon, 1993). This remains the most salient work on the topic. These researchers found that knowing the patient meant knowing how patients responded to all aspects of care and treatment, and it meant knowing the patient as a person. The effect of this knowing on nursing care was central to clinical judgment. It enabled advocacy, allowed for the acquisition of knowledge applicable to specific populations, and necessitated personal engage-ment with the person. In this work, the researchers explained in detail that during change-of-shift reports, nurses gathered the biomedical information on the patient but did not really know the patient yet. This work was with ICU nurses who wanted to have the first hour of the shift alone with the patient to get to know them, know their responses to touch, to move-ment, to medications, and to interventions in general. Nurses preferred not to have to report on how the patient was until they established some degree of knowing the patient. Getting to know patient responses at the beginning of the shift often enabled nurses to detect subtle changes in responses before hemodynamic parameters changed (Ibid).

Researchers in the remainder of the literature reviewed did not set out to study knowing the patient. Each set out to study the answers to a different question, but it is significant to note that in each of the studies (discussed below), the researchers discovered the concept of knowing the person embedded in the results.

One of the earlier quests to uncover the concept of knowing the person was that of Fisher (1989), who studied the notion of "patient dangerousness" as described by psychiatric nurses and found that nurses described patients as dangerous based on the degree to which they knew the patient. Nurses with little knowledge or understanding of the patient as a person were more likely to describe the patient as dangerous than nurses who had a comprehensive understanding of the patient as a person.

Equally intriguing was the work of Jenny and Logan (1992), who studied ventilator weaning and discovered that successful weaning depended on how well the nurse knew the patient. They readily admitted that the various technologies employed in the care of patients revealed a set of parameters that described biomedically how the patient responded but that patient responses were mediated by the degree to which the nurse knew the patient. Knowing the patient meant that the nurse knew what the patient could tolerate, when the patient hurt, and/or how much the patient could endure. When nurses knew the patient, a trust was established between them that enabled the patient to participate in the weaning process: the patient knew that the nurse would know when things were not going well and would help. Nurses also advised physicians when certain patients were not ready to begin weaning.

Further evidence of the importance of knowing the person in nursing surfaced in a study of nurses' decision-making strategies (Radwin, 1995). In this grounded theory study, the core category that explained the process of decision making was knowing the patient. Knowing meant familiarity and intimacy. The strategies used by nurses in the process were empathizing, matching a pattern, getting the big picture, and balancing preferences with difficulties. When the nurses had less time for patients or had less nursing experience, they would employ empathizing and matching a pattern. Matching a pattern meant that based on what worked in the past with other patients, nurses would employ these interventions in the situation at hand. In situations where they truly knew the patient, they described knowing the person's responses as well as knowing about who the person was in daily life; and based on as much information as possible, they would plan interventions that were tailored to the person. Subsequent to this study, Radwin (1996) conducted a review of literature on the concept of knowing the patient and concluded that there were "three specific factors related to knowing the patient, the nurse's experience with caring for patients, time, and a sense of closeness between patient and nurse" (p. 1143).

Additional evidence of the importance of knowing the person emerged from a study (Henderson, 1997) exploring the factors that influenced patient participation in their own care. Knowing the patient emerged as a central factor illustrating that when nurses knew patients both professionally and personally, patients more readily participated in their care. Also discovered in this study were the factors necessary to get to know patients: "mutual trust and rapport, positive nurse-patient attitude, sustained nurse-patient contact, and meaningful interaction" (Henderson, 1997, p. 112). Patients wanted to have meaningful conversations with nurses, wanted to get to know nurses, and wanted to feel as if the nurses knew them as the people they were, not as people in certain beds with certain diagnoses. When patients felt that the nurses knew them, they trusted them and would participate in their own care, accepting guidance from nurses. Nurses felt that as they got to know patients as persons, they were more successful in selecting interventions appropriate to the patient, and that the patients experienced greater comfort. Equally important in the study findings were factors that prevented nurses from getting to know patients. These included lack of time, negative nurse-patient attitudes, and a focus on tasks. A lack of time prevented nurses from engaging in small talk with patients to get to know them. In fact, when they were pressed for time, nurses used closed-ended questions to limit the conversation with patients and focused on the tasks to be done.

The importance of knowing the person was not limited to studies of hospital patients; it emerged in a study of the quality of care, in particular the quality of the palliative care in a community setting. Study findings revealed that knowing the patient was central to high quality palliative care, and that in order to establish this, nurses needed to make early contact with patients and families, sustain the contact, and ensure that the contact was more than physical care. Care needed to involve the whole person, including spending time with him or her and getting to know the person beyond his or her disease. This type of nursing care is not quantifiable and as such may be considered unnecessary, yet it is precisely this type of care that characterizes the human-becoming perspective.

Nurses in this study felt conflicted to be working in health care at a time when nursing is supportive of a holistic approach to care. The health care system is exploring how to incorporate less skilled/knowledgeable workers in the provision of direct physical care (Luker, Austin, Caress, & Hallett, 2000). A follow-up to this work (Speed & Luker, 2004) studied the effects of health care restructuring on the work of district nurses in the United Kingdom. They used Carper's (1978) framework of knowing in nursing and concluded that restructuring had the effect of privileging knowing about and empirical knowing over aesthetic and personal knowing. Simply stated, nurses were being limited to case and patient knowing, and this prevented them from actually knowing the person.

More recently this author (Macdonald, 2005) conducted a grounded theory study to explore the origins of difficulty in nurse-patient encounters and discovered that central to the construction of difficulty was knowing the patient. In situations where the nurse had taken the time to get to know the patient, the family, how the patient and family interacted, and what was of importance to the family, nurses rarely encountered difficulty. In contrast, when nurses were pressed for time, did not listen to the patient, and made decisions unilaterally about what was best for the patient, difficulty almost always happened. Patients in this study eloquently described how they needed to know that the nurses knew their story and knew about their situation. Only then did they believe they could tell the nurses how they felt, what was bothering them, and the reassurance that everything would work out somehow. When patients did not feel as though the nurses knew them, they worried about whether they were getting the care they needed and hesitated to ask for things.

Similar to what happened with the preceding studies, time was a factor in getting to know patients. Additional factors that emerged in this study and that varied from previous work included who is working, the availability of supplies and equipment, the patients' families, and changes in the care environment/setting. Patients noticed that certain groups of nurses worked better together than others, and they explained that when nurses worked well together, you could feel it in the air. The atmosphere was relaxed and patients felt comfortable making requests and sharing thoughts with the nurses. Nurses also described how much better it was to work when everyone helped each other and how they also felt they were able to give the patients the best possible care under these circumstances. No one left until all the care was done, and everyone left with a sense of satisfaction in their work.

Limited availability of supplies and equipment consumed precious time that nurses may have spent with their patients. During the course of this study, the pharmacy made a change in their information system software anticipating that the change would reduce by half the time pharmacy would spend dispensing medications. The opposite happened and nurses described situations where they spent extended periods of time trying to procure medications, waiting for medications, explaining to patients why the medications were not available, and going to the pharmacy themselves to collect medications for their patients. There were other examples related to this factor; however, the point was that all systems supporting patient care needed to be functioning efficiently, otherwise nursing time with patients was affected.

Nurses also spoke about the importance of families and spending time with families; and when this did not happen, relationships were strained between the nurse, the patient, and the family. In terms of care space changes, one of the major changes was the reduced lengths of patient stays. This made getting to know patients more challenging because often when patients were admitted, they were too ill to interact extensively with nurses; and as soon as they were stable, they were discharged from the care space. Nurses expressed that they felt they had not adequately prepared patients for discharge and noted that often, these patients were readmitted, as evidenced by the revolving-door syndrome.

The evidence presented was gathered using qualitative research approaches in which both nurses and patients had the opportunity to explain what knowing the patient meant to them. This capturing of meaning is central to a human science perspective and will be explained later in the chapter. Also evident in the literature was the importance of time in getting to know the patients. Saving time is central to the capitalist enterprise of the Western world; encouraging nurses to mount arguments for more nurses to spend more time with patients, although laudable, may not be deemed as the best use of their time. The single greatest driving force for change in the past three decades has been technology. The promise of technology has been to save time. It seems, therefore, worth exploring the opportunities that technology offers that can contribute to gaining time in nursing work in order to regain time to get to know patients.

Technology as a Medium

Before describing some of the many ways that technology saves time and contributes to improved patient care, it is important to briefly discuss the often heard- and written-about aspects of technology, such as those concerning the caring debate, and the idea that technology dehumanizes care (Almerud, Alapack, Fridlund, & Ekebergh, 2008). Nurses often report spending more time on the computer than with patients. This preoccupation with the belief that computers contributed to dehumanizing patient care was soundly put to rest 25 years ago. Gadow (1984) explained that any intervention, whether by machine or human, had the potential to objectify human beings. When a strict interpretation of hemodynamic measures is accepted as portraying the clinical status of the person, it may well represent the clinical status of the objectified person. Measures such as these are stripped of the meanings and values that the illness has for the person. Once this occurs, the person is also stripped of autonomy over the body, and the professional and the technology reign. Gadow maintained that any act or intervention that objectifies the person is problematic and not unique to technology. It is how we are and how we perceive and use technology in our care of patients that determines whether the person is objectified and dehumanized.

Evidence of the humanizing influence of technology was provided by Mullen (2002) in a study of how technology and nursing influenced one another with a focus on the cardiac monitor as technology. Mullen found that nursing care was not at odds with technology, but rather, technology provided the nurse with additional patient information and enabled the individualizing of care. Technology has contributed to improving and enhancing patient care, person care, and nursing care in many significant and innovative ways. For example, telehealth has been used extensively in the care of persons with congestive heart failure (CHF), diabetes, and asthma. Using telehealth in the management of CHF has reduced the overall use of health care resources by 41%, physician visits by 43%, emergency department (ED) visits by 33%, and hospitalizations by 29% (Lehmann, Mintz, & Giacini, 2006). Telehealth technology includes the use of video monitors, video cameras, speakerphones, blood pressure and pulse meters, pulse oximeters, scales, and glucometers. Health professionals provide patients with this equipment and instructions on how to use it so they can perform their assessments remotely, thus reducing the number of in-person visits. According to Waldo (2003), not only were health outcomes better in individuals in which the technology was used, but better quality of life was also reported.

Asthma is common in children and necessitates frequent ED visits. Appropriate use of medications is often the source of difficulty. Researchers have found that educating children and families on the proper use of inhalers and rescue medications using digital videos via the Web was as effective as face-to-face visits. They also found that those who learned via the Web reported improved quality-of-life scores over those receiving face-to-face visits, and ED visits were reduced (Chan, Callahan, Sheets, Moreno, & Malone, 2003).

The benefits of preoperative education for patients were well known for many years. Historically, patients awaiting surgery received this education in hospitals. Many years ago, individuals began attending preoperative education prior to surgery on an outpatient basis. Individuals who were very debilitated or lived in rural or remote areas were frequently not able to access clinic settings. Now, however, they can receive preoperative education via interactive telehealth networks (Thomas, Barton, Withrow, & Adkisson, 2004). In addition to telehealth technology, mobile phone technology has demonstrated effectiveness in health promotion and monitoring in interventions such as dietary modification, smoking cessation, and physical activity, as well as in monitoring patients with cancer, and the frail elderly (Blake, 2008).

There is a great deal to be excited about on the technology front for nursing home residents. They too can benefit from telehealth technology. When the nursing home resident's health status changes, EKGs can be performed, lung auscultation and heart sounds can be evaluated using an electronic stethoscope, ears can be assessed using an e-otoscope, and blood can be drawn and transported for testing. Nursing homes have struggled to attract nurses as the overall registered nurse (RN) shortage has grown (Masterson, 2004). Live video is available, providing nursing homes with the possibility of having greater nursing input in the assessment of residents without the resident needing to be moved unless the necessary care cannot be provided in the nursing home. This same technology will allow the nursing home to schedule a wound assessment by an enterostomal therapist, have a physiotherapist assess a resident's gait, and arrange for a family visit via video for those who are unable to visit in person (Daly, Jogerst, Park, Kang, & Bae, 2005).

Technology also has a great deal to offer the elderly who choose to remain at home or to live longer in independent or assisted-living apartments. Living spaces can be equipped with motor-sensing devices to control lighting, electrical locks for doors, door and window openers, blind and curtain openers, smoke and gas detectors, and temperature controls. Computerized medication dispensers can dispense the medications as needed and have voice capability to remind residents to take medications. This technology also can provide artificial pets and robots. Robots are equipped with information to respond to frequently asked questions to help residents who are forgetful and do not like to keep asking the same questions over and over (Rantz et al., 2005).

Technology is also shaping nursing and being shaped by nurses in significant ways. Technology that can record the vital signs of a person and interface with the electronic medical record to download this information offers a vital saving of time for nurses (Simpson, 2004). In many situations, nurses still take all vital signs, manually record them on notepaper, and then record them a second time on the patient record. This represents a clear waste of nursing time that could be spent with patients.

This author observed the outdated nurse call systems in hospitals during a field study (Macdonald, 2005). Present systems allow the nurse to interact with patients via the intercom, but the nurse cannot see the patient and cannot easily determine if there is a need to reprioritize and leave the person they are attending to attend to the person calling. This can lead to lost time or failure to attend to patients who are most in need. Technology available in home care allows nurses to perform both visual and physical assessments remotely and decide what to do. On hospital wards, nurses can be down the hall from a patient and not have access to technology that allows remote assessment.

Technology provides nurses with more information about their patients than ever before, allowing for more comprehensive assessments (Peck, 2005). Medication administration is an area in which nurses frequently are frustrated with the potential for medication errors. Technology has now made possible bar coding that is linked with the patient identification bracelet and the electronic medication record. This supports the "five rights of medication administration" and creates the possibility of further reducing the likelihood of medication administration errors (Hurley et al., 2007).

While nurses readily recommend and support the use of technology that works and saves time, they also do not hesitate to report technology that causes them to lose time or that takes more time than a manual application. This illustrates how important it is for nurses to be part of technology and software development so that the product really does save time and improve processes of care (Courtney, Demiris, & Alexander, 2005). The existence of telenursing has allowed nurses to work longer in nursing or to work in the presence of previously debilitating physical injury (Peck, 2005).

The use of personal digital assistants (PDAs) offers tremendous opportunity for nurses to have more up-to-date information in their hands at all times. This technology represents having a reference library that includes drug formularies, lab and diagnostic manuals, textbooks, and journals (George & Davidson, 2005). Every day, nurses encounter patients and families who have electronically gathered information and have a series of questions. Health care providers need to be able to respond, and devices such as PDAs permit this. In addition to what PDAs already offer, researchers have noted these devices can contribute to helping nurses further improve patient care. Software programs have been created containing patient outcomes assessments and feedback as well as best-practice guidelines. The hope is to encourage nurses to use evidence and to be able to verify patient outcomes in real time, thus reinforcing the value of the evidence or demonstrating the need for further evidence gathering (Di Pietro et al., 2008; Doran et al., 2007; Doran & Sidani, 2007). The preceding examples represent a small number of the many ways in which technology has contributed to enhancing the lives of patients and of nurses. How then can technology be at odds with the human-becoming perspective?

Human Becoming Meets Technology

According to Parse (1998), the human-becoming theory originated from the human science perspective; compared to the view of the person in the natural science perspective, it represents a very different way of viewing the person and how the person is in the world. In the human-becoming perspective, health care professionals are "concerned with the quality of life from the perspective of the people they serve" (Parse, 1998, p. x). Human becoming posits that humans create meaning in all situations, freely choose how to be in the world, and co-construct health and illness in constant interaction with all that surrounds them.

Parse recognized that nurses and most health care professionals are products of education programs rooted in the totality paradigm. This is the paradigm of the natural sciences that believes that persons can be studied, treated, and cured part by part (reductionism), and that the mind and body can be considered separately. In this paradigm, laboratory tests, scans, and all information emanating from technology take precedence over information provided by the person. Health care professionals believe that access to health care determines the health of the person and the randomized clinical trial information is privileged over all others (Pincus, 2000).

Clearly the evidence emanating from clinical trials is important and serves all persons at varying times in their lives; however, clinical trials do not capture the meaning that phenomena have for the person. The human science perspective places the person at the center in the health care system and seeks to uncover the meaning that illness has for the person, accepting that meaning will vary from situation to situation. Meaning is in the foreground as well as learning about the person's values and relationships. Concepts central to human science are meanings, patterns and relationships, and the hopes and dreams of the person (Parse, 1998).

Health care professionals (HCPs) practicing from a human science perspective do not unilaterally decide what is best for the person (unless the situation is an emergency) and then proceed to carry out an intervention. The health care professional would suspend judgments, labels, and opinions and journey with the person, inviting the person to share situational meanings and joining the person where they are. Human scientists believe the person carries the answers to their questions inside and that HCPs need to practice being present with the person in order to assist the person to reveal or imagine how they will plan to do things (Parse, 1998).

In a story relating the influence of nursing, Bolte Taylor (2006) described her rehabilitation from a stroke. This description clearly confirmed that within the human science principle, the agency rests with the person. She explained that the greatest lesson for her was that rehabilitation was up to her; she had to decide to do it or not. Central in helping her with the process were health professionals, specifically those who connected with her. She described connecting as "touching me gently and appropriately, making direct eye contact with me, and speaking with me calmly" (p. 82). Bolte Taylor further explained that when the connections were not made with HCPs, it drained her energy, and she would not participate in her care.

Practicing being present with the person is definitely congruent to knowing the person and to a human science perspective. Nurses who described the importance of knowing the patient also described how they could individualize care by knowing the person. Getting to know the patient meant considering the individual first and enabling the individual to decide—a central principle of human-becoming theory. Health care providers will, however, struggle to practice in this paradigm in many health care settings and will encounter a variety of issues.

Evidence-based practice is a mantra in the delivery of health care. Emerging from the evidence are best-practice guidelines (BPGs) based on the evidence. BPGs typically do not include a section that recommends consulting with the patient in the process of implementing the BPG. This action sets up the possibility of health care providers having a set of expectations of what the person will do or how the person will be when what is being proposed may have no meaning or a different meaning for the person. In crisis situations, standard practices are implemented, and this is as it should be; however, as soon as we begin to announce to the person that he or she needs to alter how he or she lives, and we proceed to give an education session on how this is done, we may find the person's needs and reality of life falling outside our plan. Getting to know the person by being present with him or her will allow us to find out what the illness means to the person, including hopes and fears, and how the person envisages proceeding with his/her care.

Interprofessional learning is currently a priority in many universities, encouraging student health care professionals to learn together in order to be better able to work together in the workplace (Craddock, O'Halloran, Borthwick, & McPherson, 2006). The totality or natural science perspective is woven throughout the learning of all health professionals, including nurses (Parse, 1998). Very few nurses are prepared at the entry to practice level in the human science perspective, and with the advent of interprofessional learning, they will be influenced by the natural science perspective not only in their clinical education, but also in the classroom. The challenge will be great to orient nursing education and practice to the human science perspective, and to work to introduce this perspective in other health disciplines.

Technology itself emerged from the totality or natural science paradigm and has revolutionized the way almost everything is done. Some of the issues that HCPs practicing in the human science perspective may encounter involve computer software, as well as unquestioned reliance on the numbers registered by a piece of technology. Nurses often encounter frustration with the software provided in the work setting. Practicing from a human science perspective, the nurse journeying with the person will find out what the person identifies as challenges and how the person envisions proceeding. When the nurse attempts to document care and encounters a computer program that only allows the entry of one patient problem and then requires entry of the proposed intervention, the practice can be frustrating because the software technology is driving the nature of the practice. This is where it becomes evident and important that nurses be the developers and the decision-makers regarding the software that health care organizations invest in for patient-care delivery.

Technology has a seduction for many, and HCPs will readily admit that they can become totally focused on the machine and forget the person who is attached to the machine. Providing care from a human science perspective means keeping the person as the central focus, yet will be frequently challenged in settings where the natural science perspective is dominant.

Designers of technology and the accompanying software often view the products as neutral, yet the philosophical perspective of the developer is ever present. A meaningful example of this was reported by Forsythe (1996), in which a research team designed an education program for sufferers of migraine. As individuals presented to the physician's office, they electronically entered their personal history; in response, the computer program provided educational information based on the data entered. The software education program was developed on the basis of what medicine knew about migraines. Fortunately, during the study researchers also collected observational and verbal data from participants and discovered that the educational programs covered very little of what was important to the person. The aim of the program was to help migraine sufferers, yet the person was never involved in the development. The program, therefore, was of little use and may well have served to undermine human beliefs regarding the usefulness of technology.

Partnering with patients and families is also a current trend in health care, and technology such as the World Wide Web has allowed the persons in our care to be even better equipped to participate in their care and to decide what they see as best for themselves. A Canadian survey (Martin, 2002) of patient views on the patient-provider relationship found that more than 50% of patients believe they have the primary responsibility for decisions regarding their health; an additional 35.6% expect decision making to be shared between themselves and their health care provider. Canadian patients seek and expect to receive information regarding their health condition (Anthony & Hudson-Barr, 2004; O'Connor et al., 2003). This was confirmed in the Canadian Health Services Research Foundation and Canadian Institutes of Health Research (2007) consultations that identified values-based decision making and public engagement as the most important issues.

Further evidence of a shift in thinking from provider-only solutions to thinking about patient involvement has come from the literature on patient-centered care. Three robust documents that confirm the importance of patient-centered care are the Registered Nurses of Ontario (2002), Best Practice Guideline on Patient Centered Care; the American College of Critical Care Medicine (Davidson et al., 2005) Clinical Practice Guideline for Patient Centered Intensive Care Units; and the Picker Institute and Commonwealth Fund–sponsored report on patient-centered care (Shaller, 2007).

Many health care delivery centers describe the care they provide as patient centered. Patient-centered care encompasses respect for human dignity, the belief that patients are experts of their own lives, and respect for patient goals. Patient care based on values of continuity, consistency, timeliness, responsiveness, and universal access will also be safe care (RNAO, 2002). Asking patients about what they want and how they see their health care is part of patient-centered care. This approach can also lead to improved partnering with patients in care delivery and in sharing accountability with patients. True partnerships are congruent with the human science perspective and foster the notion of journeying with the person through the illness experience.

The Future

This author has argued that technology and the human science perspective are complementary, and that technology and its products can be developed to support a practice of nursing from a human science perspective. Although no debate was entertained regarding the replacement of health care professionals with varying forms of technology, technology has been considered as a medium. We do know, however, that many tasks formerly carried out by humans are now completed by varying forms of technology.

The spectre of robots in living spaces for the elderly was advanced in illustrating the benefits of technology. These robots also had voice capacity and could provide answers to a number of frequently asked questions that the elderly avoided bothering others with. Futurist and natural scientist Kurzweil (2005) noted that the most important thing to remember about technology is the exponential rate at which it develops. We presently predict future events based on what has happened in the past 50 years, yet "most advanced mammals have added one cubic inch of brain matter every thousand years, and we are doubling computational capacity yearly" (p. 16).

Kurzweil also predicted, "Machine intelligence will become indistinguishable from that of its human progenitors within the first half of this century" (2005, p. 3). Bolte Taylor (2006), neuroanatomist and natural scientist, eloquently described how HCPs needed to be with her in order to facilitate her with doing the work of rehabilitating herself. Despite being a natural scientist, she captured perfectly how the human science perspective lived and practiced by HCPs facilitated her rehabilitation.

At this moment in time, it seems unlikely that a robot could be created that would develop relationships with humans and journey with them through their health and illness processes. Earlier the claim was made that the development of technology and its products needed to be guided by a human science perspective in order to support the practice of HCPs working from a human science perspective. Is it logical to entertain the idea that developing a robot from a human science perspective could result in creating a machine with humanlike intellectual and caring capacity? The question is ours to entertain.

Summary

Knowing the person in our care has been taken for granted—his or her care needs to be elevated in the consciousness of HCPs. This chapter began by presenting the work of researchers who studied myriad health-related concerns experienced by persons who received health care. Interestingly, these studies revealed the importance of knowing the person in the process of researching patient problems or concerns. An important factor in knowing the person was time. The human-becoming perspective considers the person to be the central focus of care. It is reasonable to assume that if health care practice is oriented to include a human science perspective, the person will then become the center of what we do and nurses will strive to protect this.

Technology offers the promise of realizing time efficiencies, and when conceived and designed with the aid of the intended user, it has delivered on this promise. Technology was portrayed as a medium to aid HCPs in the delivery of person-centered care. Tensions at the intersection of technology and the human science perspective were discussed, and possibilities were outlined. Given the exponential growth of technology, readers were challenged to entertain the futuristic question, is it logical to entertain the idea that technologically developing a robot from a human science perspective could result in creating a machine with human-like intellectual and caring capacity?

References

Almerud, S., Alapack, R. J., Fridlund, B., & Ekebergh, M. (2008). Beleagured by Technology: Care in technologically intense environments. *Nursing Philosophy, 9*, 55–61.

Anthony, M. K., & Hudson-Barr, D. (2004). A patient centered model of care for hospital discharge. *Clinical Nursing Research, 13*(2), 117–136.

Blake, H. (2008). Innovation in practice: Mobile phone technology in patient care. *British Journal of Community Nursing, 13*(4), 160–165.

Bolte Taylor, J. (2006). *My stroke of insight*. New York: Penguin.

Canadian Health Services Research Foundation and Canadian Institutes of Health Research. (2007). Priority Research Themes. Retrieved February 28, 2008, from http://www.chsrf.ca/other_documents/listening/direction-3-themes_e.php

Carper, B. (1978). Fundamental patterns of knowing in nursing. *Advances in Nursing Science, 1*(1), 13–23.

Chan, D. S., Callahan, C. W., Sheets, S. J., Moreno, C. N., & Malone, F. J. (2003). An Internet-based-store-and-forward video home Telehealth system for improving asthma outcomes in children. *American Journal of Health System Pharmacists, 60*, 1976–1981.

Craddock, D., O'Halloran, C., Borthwick, A., & McPherson, K. (2006). Interprofessional education in health and social care: Fashion or informed practice? *Learning in Health and Social Care, 5*(4), 220–242.

Courtney, K. L., Demiris, G., & Alexander, G. L. (2005). Information technology: Changing nursing processes at the point-of-care. *Nursing Administration Quarterly, 29*(4), 315–322.

Daly, J. M., Jogerst, G., Park, J. Y., Kang, Y. D., & Bae, T. (2005). A nursing home telehealth system. *Journal of Gerontological Nursing, 31*(8), 46–51.

Davidson, J. E., Powers, K., Hedayat, K., Tieszen, M., Kon, A. A., Shepard, E., et al. (2007). Clinical practice guidelines for support of the family in the patient centered intensive care unit: American College of Critical Care Medicine Task Force 2004–2005. *Critical Care Medicine, 35*(2), 605–622.

Di Pietro, T., Coburn, G., Narissa, D., Doran, D., Mylopolus, J., Kushniruk, A., et al. (2008). What nurses want: Diffusion of innovation. *Journal of Nursing Care Quality, 23*(2), 140–146.

Doran, D., Mylopolus, J., Kushniruk, A., Nagle, L., Laurie-Shaw, B., Sidani, S., et al. (2007). Evidence in the palm of your hand: Development of an outcome-focused knowledge translation intervention. *Worldviews on Evidence-Based Nursing, 4*(2), 69–77.

Doran, D., & Sidani, S. (2007). Outcome focused knowledge translation: A framework for knowledge translation and patient outcomes
improvement. *Worldviews on Evidence-Based Nursing, 4*(1), 3–13.

Fisher, A. The process of definition and action: The case of dangerousness. *Dissertation Abstracts International,* UMI No. 8917915.

Forsythe, D. E. (1996). New bottles, old wine: Hidden cultural assumptions in a computerized explanation system for migraine sufferers.
Medical Anthropology Quarterly, 10(4), 551–574.

Gadow, S. (1984). Touch and technology: Two paradigms of patient care.
Journal of Religion and Health, 23(1), 63–69.

George, L., & Davidson, L. J. (2005). PDA use in nursing education: Prepared for today, poised for tomorrow. *Online Journal of Nursing
Informatics, 9*(2).

Henderson, S. (1997). Knowing the patient and the impact on patient
participation: a grounded theory study. *International Journal of
Nursing Practice, 3,* 111–118.

Hurley, A. C., Bane, A., Fotakis, S., Duffy, M. E., Sevingy, A., Poon, E. G.,
et al. (2007). Nurses' satisfaction with medication administration
point-of-care technology. *Journal of Nursing Administration, 37*(7/8),
343–349.

Jenny, J., & Logan, J. (1992). Knowing the patient one aspect of clinical
knowledge. *Image Journal of Nursing Scholarship, 24,* 254–258.

Kurzweil, R. (2005). *The singularity is near.* New York: Penguin.

Lehmann, C. A., Mintz, N., & Giacini, J. M. (2006). Impact of Tele health on
healthcare utilization by congestive heart failure patients. *Disease
Management & Health Outcomes, 14*(3), 163–169.

Liaschenko, J. (1997). Knowing the patient? In S. Thorne & V. E. Hayes
(Eds.), *Nursing praxis knowledge and action* (pp. 23–38). Thousand
Oaks, CA: Sage.

Luker, K. A., Austin, L., Caress, A., & Hallett, C. E. (2000). The importance
of "knowing the patient": Community nurses' constructions of quality in providing palliative care. *Journal of Advanced Nursing, 31*(4),
775–782

Macdonald, M. T. (2005). Reconciling temporalities: A substantive explanation of the origins of difficulty in the nurse-patient encounter.
Dissertation Abstracts International, 1397B, UMI No. 3169430.

Martin, S. (2002). Shared responsibility becoming the new medical buzz
phrase. *Canadian Medical Association Journal, 167*(3), 295.

Masterson, A. (2004). Towards an ideal skill mix in nursing homes.
Nursing Older People, 16(4), 14–16.

Mullen, K. C. (2002). Nursing, technology, and knowing the patient.
University of North Carolina, Chapel Hill. *Dissertation Abstracts
International,* AAT 3047044.

Parse, R. R. (1998). *The human becoming school of thought: A perspective
for nurses and other health professionals.* Thousand Oaks, CA: Sage
Publications.

Peck, A. (2005). Changing the face of standard nursing practice through
Tele health and telenursing. *Nursing Administration Quarterly,
29*(4), 339–343.

Pincus, T. (2000). Challenges to the biomedical model: Are actions of
patients almost always as important as? *Advances in Mind Body
Medicine, 16*(4), 287–294.

Radwin, L. E. (1995). Knowing the patient: A process model for individualized interventions. *Nursing Research, 44*(6), 364–370.

Radwin, L. E. (1996). Knowing the patient: A review of research on an emerging concept. *Journal of Advanced Nursing, 23*, 1142–1146.

Rantz, M. J., Marek, K. D., Aud, M., Tyrer, H. W., Skubic, M., Demiris, G., et al. (2005). A technology and nursing collaboration to help older adults age in place. *Nursing Outlook, 53*, 40–45.

Parse, R. (1998). *The human becoming school of thought: A perspective for nurses and other health professionals.* Thousand Oaks, CA: Sage.

RNAO Best Practice Guideline. (2002). Client centered care. Retrieved June 25, 2006, from www.rnao.ca

Shaller, D. (2007). *Patient centered care: What does it take?* Retrieved February 27, 2008, from http://www.commonwealthfund.org/publications/publications_show.htm?doc_id=559715

Simpson, R. L. (2004). The softer side of technology: How IT helps nurses care. *Nursing Administration Quarterly, 28*(4), 302–305.

Speed, S., & Luker, K. A. (2004). Changes in patterns of knowing the patient: The case of British district nurses. *International Journal of Nursing Studies, 41*, 921–931.

Tanner, C., Benner, P., Chesla, C., & Gordon, D. (1993). The phenomenology of knowing the patient. *Image Journal of Nursing Scholarship, 25*, 273–280.

Thomas, K., Barton, D., Withrow, L., & Adkisson, B. (2004). Impact of a preoperative education program via interactive Tele health network for rural patients having total joint surgery. *Orthopedic Nursing, 23*(3), 39–44.

Waldo, B. (2003). Tele-health and the electronic medical record. *Nursing Economics, 21*(5), 245–246, 210.

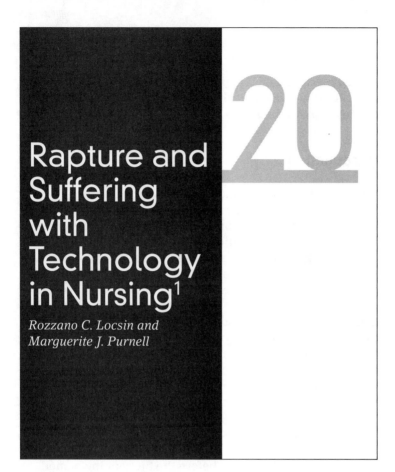

Rapture and Suffering with Technology in Nursing[1]

Rozzano C. Locsin and Marguerite J. Purnell

Chapter Overview

Technological advancements have shaped human life. As technology has become increasingly sophisticated, philosophers such as Heidegger have carefully pondered the worth of its influence on the quality and duration of life. Concerns about technology encompass the experiences of persons whose lives depend upon technologies, and the experiences of those persons who care for them. Accompanying the rapture of technologies in nursing is the consequent suffering or the price of advancing dependency with technologies that critically influence human lives. With increased use of technologies and ensuing technological dependency experienced by recipients of care, the imperative is to provide

technological competency as caring in nursing, guided by a
formalized practice model such as *Technological Competency
as Caring in Nursing*.

Introduction

Technological advancements have shaped human life. As
technology has become increasingly sophisticated, philosophers have carefully pondered the worth of its influence
on the quality and duration of life. In healthcare, issues of
the good, utility, and cost are foiled by the often fatal attraction of a glamorous drug or "technoluxe" cosmetic procedure
(Frank, 2003) that promises rapture, but instead delivers horror and suffering. From a Heideggerian philosophical view
concerning technology and its "revealing," and complemented
by Locsin's (1995) theory of Technological Competency as
Caring in Nursing as framework, this paper will accentuate
and discuss the effects of modern technology on healthcare,
and focus its influences primarily on nursing. The beneficial
effects of technology are traced as integral to health care, not
only for nurses in professional practice, but also for other
professional caregivers who are faced with the burden of
caring for persons in high-tech settings, including the home.
      Over 50 years ago, well before the burgeoning of modern
healthcare and specialized healthcare technology, the philosopher Martin Heidegger (1993) prophetically spoke of the
danger of uncritical acceptance of technology and of disregard for its "ambiguous" (p. 338) essence. In dry, meaningful
language, he described how technology may not appear to be
what it really is—coercive and consuming, and how human
beings are simultaneously needed both to bring order to or
be ordered or used by technology. In describing the ways
that modern technology is revealed, Heidegger observed
that, "The energy concealed in nature is unlocked, what is
unlocked is transformed, what is transformed is stored up,
what is stored up is in turn distributed, and what is distributed is switched about ever anew" (p. 322). Heidegger's central
concern is that future generations will not realize that this
technological metamorphosis will create a *standing-reserve*
(p. 322) which waits solely upon and for the technology. In
this standing reserve are not only nature, but *human beings*
both as sources and re-sources, for example, as Heidegger

witnessed so many years ago, the "supply of patients for a clinic" (p. 323) was a standing reserve. It is precisely the idea of human beings in this duality, influencing, and being influenced by healthcare technology, its iterations and various metamorphoses, and the challenges experienced in nursing caring in a technological environment, that form the justification for this paper.

The tension between the technological assessing of persons as objects, despite anthropomorphic "user friendly" external appearances, and the caring intention of nurses to know the person as whole and complete in the moment, obliquely pay homage to Heidegger's conception of the *ambiguity* (p. 338) of the essence of technology. Can this tension be ameliorated or reconciled?

Person or Object of Care?

The focus of nursing ought to be the understanding of patients as participants in their care, rather than as objects of care. Often, the perspective of wholeness of person denotes the appreciation of the whole person as composite or derived from the understanding of an object-self. The object body is understood as that which can be known by an observer, a material entity while the subject self is the phenomenological body: "the body known from the inside, the body that is experienced, the lived body, the body as 'me'" (Sakalys, 2006, p. 17). The conception of person as whole is predicated on the various understandings of this distinctive term. The fundamental differences among knowing the composition of the person stem from the philosophical perspectives through which these terms are viewed. Commensurate with technology, from a positivist philosophical perspective, persons are appreciated through their component parts, recognizing the completeness of the person from a 'lens' that is dependent upon human sensory perception. The person is a whole being because the sensory (visual, hearing, touch, smell) data obtained by the observer, and which are able to be machine replicated, reflect a "complete" person with physical composites and human physiological functioning. Consider the subject of Shelley's (1919/1969) novel, *Frankenstein*. Frankenstein was a composite being, and known for committing gruesome crimes. Created from several human body parts that were in turn obtained from as many different human beings, Frankenstein was put together, completed, and made whole, then brought to life. This human replica *that* was put together using various human parts was created biologically and humanly complete, and eventually, when brought to life appeared "more" human. Frankenstein came to be regarded as a human, albeit grossly distorted as a monster, with characteristics "inherited" from the multiple donors of organ and limb to his life.

When viewing persons as participants in their care, instead of objects of care, biological wholeness and completeness as sensory evidence are not primary sources of knowledge. Rather, it is the relationship with others, and the understanding of the value placed on life that allows nurses to know persons fully as "being cared for."

Influence of Technology on Practice

Such a conception may seem rhetorical, that a person is a person. However, in nursing, views of persons range from the view of persons as whole in the moment, to notions of persons as made up of parts. This latter understanding illustrates nursing practice as "fixing" persons to make them wholes again, and does not serve nursing well as a discipline of knowledge and practice profession. Rather, it perpetuates the understanding of nursing as a practice technique with a recipe to follow as guide to produce an outcome of care. Yet, the Heideggerian (1965) notion of "enframing" (p. 324) – the coercive perpetuation of technology - forces nurses to objectify persons in order to care, and challenges understandings of persons who are participating within the shared experience of a nursing situation. A glimpse of the influence of contemporary technology, with its extraordinary hold over human care and ethics, and the potential for nursing practice may be well perceived from the following exemplar:

> *Nearing the end of a legal struggle concerning the rights of a woman in a persistent vegetative state, the U.S. Congress decided that the case could be heard in Federal court. One legislator, who was convinced and unwavering in his declaration that the person in a "vegetative" state was a living human being, described her condition and "responses" to parental stimulation as "like a human being."*

Given this statement, dare it be asked, *When did this person cease being a "real" human being?* —To the extent that her current responses were "like a human being?" How often do similar objectifications and characterizations of persons not recognized as "a real human being" occur? In contrast, distinct and apart from this view of person as object, dwells the particular idea of persons who are fully human, despite suffering endured and ensured by dependency on technological advances.

Punctuating this discussion of wholeness is a poignant story of an infant born in 1995 to migrant farmers working in the fields of South Florida. The infant was beautiful and healthy, but was born without any arms or legs. It was totally dependent then and now, on being cared for to supply every want and need. Yet, the infant is a whole person regardless of the missing parts. The customary technological resources used in assessing the health of persons created a distinct and limiting realization that with appendages missing, those vital "parts" around which the technologies were designed, for example, blood pressure cuffs, rendered the technologies deficient and immaterial. Physicians and nurses were concerned about how they could perform the usual but necessary technological care such as performing laboratory tests and the use of contraptions that traditionally require access through the limbs. This situation emphasized Sandelowski's (1993) concern about the practice of nursing and the advent of technological dependency. While the existence of modern, sophisticated, and advanced technologies were critical to modern nursing and health care, none of these technologies were up to the challenge of a person requiring unusual health care technological demands. "Knowing" the infant who is a living and functioning human being, a person who is whole and complete in the moment regardless of the missing parts, was a reality, and coping with this reality was another challenge.

The focus of nursing is to know persons (Locsin, 2005). Ways of knowing persons are manifold, and include empirical, ethical, aesthetic, and personal (Carper, 1978), as well as the symbolic and integrative ways of knowing (Phenix, 1965). In knowing persons, the imperative is for nurses to focus on the "objective" composite of persons, and more important, on the "subjective" nature of being human. In a nursing encounter, this particular view includes the moral imperative to know "who" is the person, rather than the objectifying "what" is a person.

Coming to know the person is critical to nursing. Competently using technologies to achieve this goal is essential in order to appreciate nursing practice more fully as an integral aspect of human health care.

Human-Technology Interface in Nursing: Source or Re-source?

The paradoxical enchantment/disenchantment of society with technology continues to spur the tension between subject and object, person and technology, source or resource, and the need for unified and integral care of the whole person. This disenchantment ripples from consumer to manufacturer, and to investor, and is ultimately reflected in decreasing financial gains, far removed from the plight of the person experiencing the technology. In a report to over 700 investors, reporters, and entrepreneurs, the following statements were made:

> *Making realistic robots is going to polarize the market, if you will....You will have some people who love it and some people who will really be disturbed....Individuals are becoming overwhelmed and worse, I believe that this state of being overwhelmed has moved the personal computing market to the point of diminishing returns.*
>
> *(C. Shipley, 2006).*

The question arises: Does the disenchantment emanate from the view of technology as mere technology, or is it something far deeper and primal? Is the acceptance of technology in various forms assisted by creating "user friendly" anthropomorphic attributes and human look-a-likes, or as this excerpt below recounts, a human *feel*-alike?

> *After more than 2 1/2 years of physical therapy and electronic stimulation, stroke victim Mike Marin still couldn't open a door with his left hand. Now, thanks to a robot, Marin can open a door. His atrophied left arm isn't completely useless anymore. Marin is at the forefront of what may seem an unlikely use for robots: providing the caring human touch.*
>
> *(C. Hogan, 2006)*

This suggestion that robots and robotics-based technologies are designed to "provide the caring human touch" is intriguing. While the goal is to provide the best quality of life for a person lacking the essential composites of a fully functioning human being, emulating a human through a provision of a robotic "caring human touch," although a technological advancement, seems to be a paradoxical answer to the challenges of human-computer interaction. Nevertheless, Hogan (2006) claims being able to show consistently improved therapy outcomes after using robots versus humans providing conventional, standard care. This is a far cry toward achieving even minimal "care" for persons who are technology-challenged.

"Nursebot", a robot which alternately can assume the male and female personalities of Earl and Pearl by changing the voice gender, was tested among elderly patients (Online News, Yahoo, 2006). Despite the stereotype of older people being "technology phobic", the seniors accepted the robots. Their major concern was that the robots would not be able to do enough to provide adequate help for them. However, while robotic assistants are better suited for repetitive tasks, such as escorting persons to restrooms, or reminding them to take medications, these same functions are now accomplished more cheaply by watches, and radios, and the ubiquitous walker frame with tennis ball "gliders" on the legs.

The answer of society to the traditional ontological question, "What is nursing?" does not adequately reflect either the growth and development of nursing as a discipline of knowledge or as an expert, complex, practice profession. The need to continuously raise this question can be ascribed to the perennial use of the word "nurse" as narrowly referring to the routine performer of tasks, and as a consequence, to the image of nursing practice in all its complexity persisting as merely the performing of tasks. The creation of the robo-nurse—a complex piece of machinery that, in human fashion, is made to perform technical nurse activities such as taking a person's temperature (Gutierrez, 2000)—perpetuates this image. The robo-nurse simply facilitates completion of tasks for people, as does the nursebot described above. The persistent image of nursing as accomplishing tasks undeniably makes the nurse appear to be an automaton (Locsin, 2001). The essence of technology whether enframed (Heidegger, 1993, p. 324) in complex anthropomorphic machinery, or in graphic "live" viewing of functioning internal body parts, coerces and challenges caring as the essence of nursing in the expression of nursing practice.

Much can be said about technology in nursing, from its fascinating essence allowing greater dimensions of efficient and competent practice, to the creation of phenomenal opportunities for persons in order to live more fully. From the appreciation of care practices as the skillful performance of activities for making persons well or healthy, to the use of instruments and tools for promoting health and preventing illness, technology in nursing is critical to fostering health and wellness in contemporary times. The results of these technologies, however, also increase opportunities for care and cure activities, to the extent that contemporary health care appears to exist only because of the advantages of technological advances. While technology captures our fascination with visions of an idyllic life, living out a life that is dependent on technology can, likewise, lead to deep suffering. In doing so, understanding the ambiguity of the essence of technology and the consequences it evokes are befitting the revealing or poiesis (p. 317) of which Heidegger (1993) wrote. With increasing persistence for technological advancements, and the dependency that these technologies create for recipients and the users of the technologies, the imperative is to recognize and provide prospects for nursing guided by a framework of practice such as technological competency as caring (Locsin, 2005).

Two foci dictate the significance of technologies in nursing: *technological nursing* described as the nursing of persons with lives that are dependent on technology, and *knowing persons* - the process through which nurses come to practice nursing using technological competency as caring in nursing to know persons more fully (Locsin, 2005). In each of these foci, nursing provides the essential recognition of the influences of technology in nursing and health care. These essentials are directed toward the understanding of persons who experience life fully as human beings, regardless of being dependent with technologies.

Theory-based Practice

Unraveling and acknowledging the allure of technology and the suffering occurring as a consequent of technology and its use are essential to nursing and its critical practice nature. *Technological Competency as Caring in Nursing* (Locsin, 2005) is a practice framework that allows for knowing the other as person, and for providing self and the other opportunities to come to know through appreciating, affirming, and celebrating each other as person.

The Practice of Nursing as Knowing Persons

How will the practice of nursing as knowing persons engage future human beings through caring, while simultaneously recognizing the often limited physical and psychological form and function of being human? How is competency with technology expressed in knowing persons as whole in the moment? The ultimate purpose of technological competency is to acknowledge persons as whole. Such acknowledgment compels the redesigning of processes of nursing — ways of expressing, celebrating, and appreciating the practice of nursing as continuously knowing persons as whole from moment to moment. In this practice of nursing, technology is used not to answer the question, "What is a person?" but rather, to come to know "Who is a person?" While the former question alludes to the notion of persons as objects, the latter addresses the uniqueness and individuality of persons as human beings.

The advent of medical technology and its domination as a major influence in healthcare places nursing in an awkward position; being dependent upon competencies for these technologies in order to engage in practice. The practice of nursing as technological competency—an expression of caring in nursing—is the achievement of knowing persons as whole moment to moment. It is the authentic, intentional, knowledgeable, and efficient use of technologies of nursing. These technologies influence the recognition of nursing as integral to healthcare. As such, this practice recognizes the role technology has on the practice of nursing. Technological competency allows the nurse to participate in the process of knowing persons as whole in the moment; the ultimate purpose of which is to *continuously* acknowledge persons as whole.

Nonetheless, in such a contemporary environment, there is the possibility and likelihood that the nurse will be able to predict, and prescribe for the one nursed. When this occurs, these situations forcibly lead nurses to appreciate persons more as objects than as person. Such a situation can only occur when the nurse has assumed to "have known" the one nursed. While it can be assumed that with the process of "knowing persons as whole in the moment," opportunities to continuously know the other become limitless, there is also a much greater likelihood that having "already known" the one nursed, the nurse will predict and prescribe activities or ways for the one nursed, and objectification of person ultimately occurs. This is the coercive yet elastic tension between the essence of technology and caring as the essence of nursing: Both are mediated by the thoughtful, technologically competent and caring nurse. While it is necessary to understand the operation of machine devices in order to understand the functioning human being, the use of these technologies should not consign persons to be regarded as objects. The objectification of persons becomes an ordinary occurrence in situations wherein the practice of nursing is merely understood as achievement of tasks.

Technological competency as caring involves intentionality (Purnell, 2003) with compassion, confidence, commitment, and conscience as requisites to caring in nursing. Intentionality, in which are embedded patterns of values, ideals, and unique professional knowledge which distinguish nursing, is active in shaping, guiding, and directing practice (Purnell, 2006). This is where the process of nursing takes on a focus different from the traditional series of problem-solving actions. By donning the lens of Nursing as Caring (Boykin & Schoenhofer, 2001), technological competency as caring in nursing is acknowledged. Through this lens, nursing is expressed as the simultaneous, momentary interconnectedness between the nurse and the nursed (Locsin, 1995). The nurse relies on the patient for calls for nursing. These calls are specific mechanisms that patients use, and they provide the opportunity for the nurse to respond with the authentic intention to know the other fully as whole person. Calls for nursing may be expressed as hopes, dreams, and aspirations. As uniquely as these nursing situations are expressed, the nurse is challenged to hear these calls for nursing and to respond authentically and intentionally in nurturance. These appropriate responses may be communicated as patterns of relating information, such as those derived from machineries like the EKG monitor, in order to know the physiological status of the person in the moment, or to administer life-saving medications, institute transfers, or to refer patients to other healthcare professionals as advocate for the patient in the moment.

The challenge of nursing is expressing technological competency as caring, ably focusing on the other as caring person, whole and complete in the moment, and growing in caring from moment to moment. Every human being uniquely responds to personal conditions in the moment. The nurse understands that the process of nursing occurs without preconceived views that categorize persons as needing to fixed, like fitting the individuals into boxes of predicted conditions. By allowing the patient to unfold as a person and to live fully as a human being, the nurse facilitates the goal of nursing in the "caring between" and enhances personhood (Boykin & Schoenhofer, 2001) of both the nursed and the nurse.

Nursing practitioners long for a practice of nursing that is based on the authentic desire to know persons fully as human beings rather than as objects. Through this authentic intention and desire, nurses are challenged to use every creative, imaginative, and innovative way possible to appreciate and celebrate the person's intentions to live more fully and grow as a human being. Only with expertise with technologies of nursing can technological competence as an expression of caring in nursing be realized. The nurse as artist overcomes the essence of the technology with its continuing influence on the object or part, and reveals what Heidegger calls *physis* (p. 317) - a higher essence of poeisis, the unfolding of something into what it is, such as a blossom opening, or a call to a more primal truth (p. 333). In nursing, this primal truth is coming to know the one nursed through intention to care for wholeness of person, and for the whole person (Purnell, 2003), where in authentic presence, the nurse brings all that he or she is to the nursing situation, and attends to what matters.

It is evident from this description that describing nursing practice as the completion of tasks does not answer to the unfolding fullness of nursing. Nurses are urged to value technological competency as an expression of caring in nursing and as integral to healthcare. Otherwise, the image of the robo-nurse, simply facilitating completion of tasks for people, will render the nurse an automaton. The nurse will have fulfilled Heidegger's (1993) depictions of persons as standing-reserves, standing ready in endless cycles to serve the technology through a task-oriented practice.

Artificial Emotions and Evocative Objects

How will nursing be practiced in the future when human beings are partly machines? Turkle (2004) tapped into a side of technological dependence that is seldom addressed; that of emotional attachment. She stated, "What has become increasingly clear is that, counter-intuitively, [human beings] become attached to sophisticated machines not for their smarts but their emotional reach. They seduce [human beings] by asking for human nurturance, not intelligence. [Humans] are suckers not for realism but for relationships" (n.p.)

The advent of technological marvels in sustaining human lives, viewed from the ideals of persons as whole and the many ways nursing practice is grounded in caring perspectives, underscores nursing as a caring discipline. Nursing theories vicariously view human beings as whole and complete in the moment, as nursing transpiring between the nurse and the one nursed, and the appreciation of health as quality of life. The appreciation of these concepts dictates the understanding of how nursing is recognized, how it is practiced, and how nursing is integral to healthcare.

Reconciliation or Rift—Technology and Caring in Nursing

The focus of nursing is the person. However, technological advances, especially in modern medical and nursing practice, continue to challenge definitions of person. Through the lens of nursing as caring, all persons are understood as caring by the virtue of their humanness (Boykin & Schoenhofer, 2001). Persons are held to be whole in the moment, with health as quality of life understood by the person being cared for. As human beings move closer toward the *posthuman* (Hayles, 2000), caring nursing theories must be flexible enough to accommodate new understandings of person. Traditionally, the central focus of nursing care has dealt with the human being as person. However, as modern and future advances in technology push toward our technological evolution, depending upon our perspective, we will see partly human beings or partly human machines – cybernetic organisms (cyborgs) and other techno-sapiens as recipients of nursing. What will be this nursing? How will nursing be experienced by the nurse and the one nursed? Will caring as the essence of nursing hold sway over technology? Heidegger (1993) said it best:

> *The closer we come to the danger, the more brightly do the ways unto the saving power begin to shine and the more questioning we become. For questioning is the piety of thought. (p. 3)*

References

Brazeal, C. (2001). A sociable machine, *USA Today*.

Boykin, A., & Schoenhofer, S. O. (2001). *Nursing as caring: A model for practice*. Sudbury, CT: Jones and Bartlett.

Carper, B. A. (1978). Fundamental patterns of knowing in nursing. *Advances in Nursing Science, 1*(1), 13–23.

Frank, A. W. (2003). Connecting body parts: Technoluxe, surgical shapings, and bioethics. Paper presented at the *"Vital Politics"* conference, London School of Economics, September, 2003.

Gutierrez, L. (2000, March 1). Robo nurse? *The Palm Beach Post*, 3D.

Hayles, K. (2000). Visualizing the posthuman. *Art Journal, 59*(3), 50–54.

Heidegger, M. (1993). In D. F. Krell (Ed.), *Martin Heidegger: Basic writings*. San Francisco: Harper Collins.

Hogan, C. (2004). *The Boston Globe,* February 29, 2004.

Locsin, R. C. (2001). *Advancing technology, caring, and nursing*. Westport, CT: Auburn House.

Locsin, R. C. (2005). *Technological competency as caring in nursing, a model for practice*. Indianapolis, Indianapolis, IN: Sigma Theta Tau International Honor Society of Nursing.

Locsin, R. C. (1995). Machine technologies and caring in nursing. *Image: Journal of Nursing Scholarship, 3*(27), 201–203.

Phenix, P. H. (1964). *Realms of meaning*. New York: McGraw Hill.

Purnell, M. J. (2003). *Intentionality in nursing: A foundational inquiry*. Dissertation Abstracts International, 64, 639.

Purnell, M. J. (2006). Development of a model of nursing education grounded in caring and application to online nursing education. *International Journal for Human Caring, 10*(3), 8–16.

Sakalys, J. S. (2006). Bringing bodies back in: Embodiment and caring science. *International Journal for Human Caring, 10*(3), 17–21.

Sandelowski, M. (1993). Toward a theory of technological dependency. *Nursing Outlook, 41*(1), 36–42.

Shelley, M. (1969). *Frankenstein: Or the modern Prometheus*. New York: Oxford University Press.

Shipley, C. (2006). *Washington Post*. Accessed February 8, 2006. http://www.washingtonpost.com/wp/dyn/content/article/2006/02/08/AR2006020802239.html

Turkle, S. (2004). A published interview by S. Allis. In *The Boston Globe* (February 29, 2004)

Yahoo Online News. "Nursebot". Accessed November 22, 2006. http:// news.yahoo.com/s/ap/20061122/ap_on_hi_te/robots_health_care.

---

[1] Reprinted:

Locsin, R., & Purnell, M (2007). Rapture and suffering with technology in nursing. *International Journal for Human Caring, 11*(1), 38–43. With permission from the International Association for Human Caring (publisher).

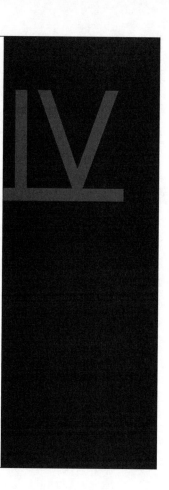

Knowing the Person Through Lenses of Culture and Community

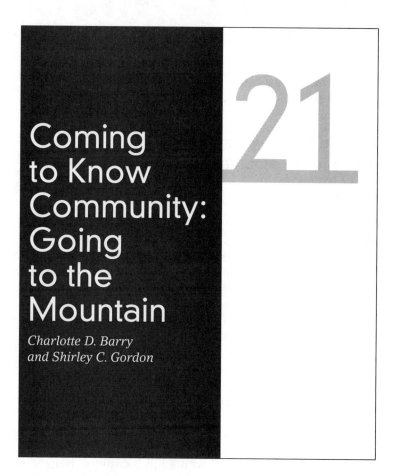

Coming to Know Community: Going to the Mountain

*Charlotte D. Barry
and Shirley C. Gordon*

21

Chapter Overview

This chapter offers a thoughtful approach to knowing community guided by a particular model of Community Nursing Practice. The model is grounded in the transcendent values of respect, caring, and wholeness and the actualizing values of access, essentiality, empowerment, intersectoral collaboration, and community participation. The Model is depicted in a hand-drawn watercolor to illustrate creativity in nursing practice and to inspire using creativity in coming to know and in designing ways to be in community that reflect the community's hopes and dreams for well-being. The Celebrity Chef Cooking Club and the Head Lice Prevention and Treatment Program illuminate elements of the Model and demonstrate its usefulness in a community nursing practice that is both ordinary and profound.

Coming To Know Community: Going To The Mountain

Introduction

The experience of building a school in an extremely poor mountain village in Pakistan serves as an introduction to community health nursing. Greg Mortenson, a nurse and mountain climber, described his coming to know community in the book *Three Cups of Tea* (Mortenson & Relin, 2007). In a breathtaking account, Mortenson described his nearly fatal attempt to climb the second highest mountain in the world the notorious K2 in the Karakoram Mountains of Pakistan and his daring rescue. The focus of this chapter is Mortenson's subsequent return to the remote village of Korphe, deep in the heart of the mountains.

One year after Mortenson's ill-fated climb, he returned to the village. His intention was to fulfill a promise made out of gratitude for the care and concern he received during his long recuperation process: to build a school for the village children. Mortenson described his fund-raising activities in the United States for the school, the purchase of building supplies, the precarious journey up the mountains, and the discovery that the only bridge to the village would not be strong enough to carry the supplies. Mortenson was shocked but allowed the reality to sink in: They needed to build a bridge before the school could be built. After raising funds again—this time for the bridge—Mortenson obtained the needed supplies and made the long trek back up to the village to begin the process of collaborating with deal makers and village elders. The bridge finally was built.

Then his real drive to build the school was ignited. Mortenson served as the overseer of the building, measuring brick sizes and block heights and keeping accurate notes on the progress and delays. His dream was to get the school built before the winter set in. But the delays frustrated Mortenson: the men working on the school had to work their fields before winter. Many also worked in mountaineering, guiding and carrying for various mountain-climbing groups.

Although Mortenson kept responding to the various calls for caring from the village, his hopes and dreams to get the building completed collided with the villagers' desperate need to ensure they had fundamental provisions to survive a fierce winter. Mortenson's frustration showed. Finally, the village chief asked him to come for a walk with him. Together they climbed up the mountain in near silence. After an hour, as Mortenson caught his breath, the chief finally uttered these words: "I thank all merciful Allah for all you have done, but the people of Korphe have been without a school for 600 years, what is one more winter?" (p. 139) A little later came the invitation of acceptance: "Dr. Greg, you must take time to share three cups of tea, we may be uneducated but we are not stupid. We have lived and survived here for a long time (p. 150).

Being offered three cups of tea, in Pakistan, is an honor. An invitation to share a cup of tea is offered as a norm of social behavior. A second cup is offered to extend a visit and share the experience of companionship. And a third cup, a special offer, is reserved for family and close friends who have been drawn into an inner circle. The third cup is drunk in thoughtful communion allowing for silence, dialogue, collaboration, or negotiation.

The professional practice of community health nursing is much like Mortenson's experience: Inspired by caring for others, feeling compassion for their well-being, energized by commitment, and grounded in a large dose of patience. And as Mortenson did, in our efforts to care for others, we have many times let our own hopes and dreams obscure the hopes and dreams of those we serve.

Coming to know a community is a process of intentional presence and respectful exploration inspired by caring, compassion, commitment, patience, and humility. Humility guides the nurse in understanding that although the nurse is an expert on community health matters, the community members are expert in their hopes and dreams for well-being.

Purpose

The purpose of this chapter is to describe a specific theoretical approach to knowing community. The Community Nursing Practice Model (CNPM) (Parker & Barry, 2006), grounded in the values of caring, respect, and wholeness, provides a framework for nursing practice that inspires knowing the promise of communities by understanding the community's hopes and dreams as well as its strengths and capacities.

Theoretical Approach

The Community Nursing Practice Model (CNPM) (Parker & Barry, 2006), is grounded in nursing values of respect for person, caring, and appreciation of wholeness. The basis of the CNPM was formed from transcendent values explicated in the mission and philosophy statements of the Florida Atlantic University Christine E. Lynn College of Nursing (2002, para 1), which guide the teaching, learning, and practice of nursing. Transcendent values, present in each nursing situation, include respect, caring, and wholeness of persons. The actualizing values of the CNPM, which are thought to guide practice (Barry, 1993), were adopted from the World Health Organization (1978) and include access, essentiality, community participation, empowerment, and intersectoral collaboration.

The CNPM illuminates the transcendent and actualizing values in four interrelated themes—nursing, person, community, and environment—that form the traditional paradigmatic view of nursing (Parker & Barry, 1999).

Nursing. The focus of nursing reflects the philosophy of Florida Atlantic University's (FAU) Christine E. Lynn College of Nursing: Nurturing the wholeness of persons and environments through caring (FAU, 2002/para 1). From this perspective, nursing is practiced within a context of nursing situations and understood as the lived experience of caring between the nurse and the one nursed. Nursing knowledge is created, lived, and embedded in the nursing situation, illuminating a synthesis of values, shared meaning, and the integration of multiple patterns of knowing and understanding.

Person. The respectful question, how can I be helpful to you? guides the nurse's approach to knowing persons, based on respect and humility, and inspires openness to learn and grow (Parker & Barry, 2006). The person defines what is necessary for his or her well-being and determines priorities that are meaningful. Conceptualizing persons "at promise"

21.1 Illuminating the Elements of the Community Nursing Practice Model

CNPM Element	Description
Nursing Situation	Lived experience in which the caring between the client and nurse nurtures wholeness of both.
Calls for Nursing	Communications, either articulated or silent, from the client that make known hopes and dreams for well-being.
Nursing Responses	Nursing actions that are created in response to the calls for nursing.
Transcendent Values	Values present in each and every nursing situation.
Caring	Understanding that to be human is to be caring. Nursing actions that nurture the wholeness of the other.
Respect	Valuing the inherent dignity and uniqueness of the other.
Wholeness	State of being described by the other in the moment, living connected to family and environment.
Actualizing Values	Values present in nursing situations as needed.
Access	The availability of consistent health care that is competent, respectful, culturally sensitive, and cost effective.
Essentiality	The client/patient describes what is necessary for his/her well-being.
Community Participation	The active engagement with members of a community fostered by openness to listening to calls for nursing and to creating nursing responses.
Empowerment	The client's awareness of making individual choices that influence health and well-being.
Intersectoral Collaboration	Refers to the openness to seek and honor the expertise of providers and agencies to potentiate the outcomes of services essential to well-being.

Adapted from Barry and Gordon (2006).

rather than persons "at risk" further inspires moving from a problem-oriented, "fix-it" approach to a holistic nursing practice approach (Swadener & Lubeck, 1995).

Community. Community is defined by its members and is characterized by shared values, respect for members, and a sense of personal security in membership (Smith & Mauer, 1995; Peck, 1987). Knowing the other in relationship to his/her community offers the opportunity to understand and participate more fully with individual and collectives hopes and dreams (Parker & Barry, 2006).

Environment. The traditional notion of environment is expanded within the CNPM beyond the immediate context of patients' lives to consider the relationship between health, social issues, and the natural environment, which influence and create conditions for heath, well-being, and/or illness (Chooporian, 1986). The Community Nursing Practice Model is presented in Figure 21.1.

The model is envisioned as "3 concentric circles around a core." (Barry & Gordon, 2006, p. 31; Parker & Barry, 2006). The model, a vector diagram of a hand-drawn watercolor, illuminates the unique creation of nursing situations in the core and the seamless interconnections of relationships, collaborations, structures, and institutions within and across the concentric circles of empathetic concern. The core and concentric circles are not bound by impenetrable perimeters, but rather are fluid, allowing movement of persons and services from the core outward and the concentric circles inward. The core represents a nursing situation defined as "the lived experience of caring between the nurse and the one receiving care" (FAU, 2002/para 1). Each concentric circle represents a widening group of individuals, groups, and agencies that share a concern for and support of the well-being of persons and communities. The first concentric circle includes concerned persons such as family members and community members.

Categories of services in the core consist of the design and coordination of care, including primary care, health promotion, health screening, and early intervention, as well as tertiary prevention. The concentric circles represent the ever-widening involvement of persons and groups drawn together by similar interests to provide and evaluate care.

21.1

The Community Nursing Practice Model: Concentric Circles of Empathetic Concern

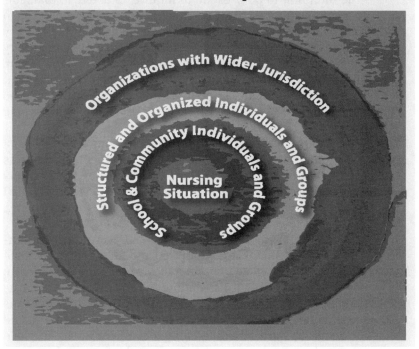

Copyright–FAU 2006

The second concentric circle widens the concern to include community organizations such as a school district, local health department, or other community or social service agencies. The third concentric circle includes state, regional, and national organizations that support or direct the provision of care by nurses. These organizations may include state boards of nursing, state and national nursing professional organizations, and other governmental agencies overseeing the implementation of professional care and supportive services. Unique expressions of caring in the nursing situation are created in response to calls for nursing. Essential care activities provided within and across the concentric circles include primary health care; primary, secondary and tertiary prevention; consultation;

collaboration; coordination; consortium building; consensus building; political activism; and leadership.

Inquiry Group Method

Within the CNPM, coming to know a community begins with the intention to be present, to inquire, to listen, to dialogue, and to partner with as an equal. How can I be helpful to you? This respectful question forms the basis of the inquiry group method developed to assess and evaluate community strengths, hopes, and dreams (Parker, Barry, & King, 2000). Defined as a "route of knowing," this community-assessment approach illuminates individual and community strengths and needs, while giving inspiration for the creation of nursing responses (Parker & Barry, 2006).

As a type of focus group, the inquiry group method uses a group interview format centered on a specific focus that was facilitated by moderators. The purposes of the group interview are to generate qualitative data reflective of individual group members' caring activities and hopes for well-being, as well as to evaluate program effectiveness.

Here is how an inquiry group works. Upon entering a community, stakeholders are identified and invited to participate in a focus group. The invitation may be extended personally, by word of mouth, by distributing flyers, or by hanging posters in prominent places. Many times various focus groups need to be conducted to assure that all voices are heard. The focus groups are scheduled at a convenient time and place determined by the co-participants, moderators, and community members; and a time limit is determined with respect for individuals' busy schedules. The moderators determine who will be the recorder or if the group allows tape recording of the group session.

When the group is assembled, a circular seating pattern is created to invite a sense of communion. Introductions follow with the moderators stating that although they are experts in health matters, the co-participants are expert in their caring and their hopes and dreams for well-being for self as well as the community. The members are informed about the group process. The session will be recorded either by hand or by audio tape, and the four questions below guide the process. When the session begins, each participant is asked to write his or her response to the questions that may serve as a prompt when the session begins. Each is invited to speak and each may contact us later with more ideas.

The first question is, how do you care for yourself day to day? Each is asked to write down his or her response (to be kept by the individual) so thoughts are not lost as others answer. Then silence follows as co-participants reflect. After a few moments, a volunteer is requested to begin. When each person has responded, the second question is asked: how do you care for your family day to day? And the same process ensues. The third question is, how do you care for your community? And the last is, how can we be helpful to you? Summarize the results at the end and ask, "This is what we heard. Is this how we can be helpful to you?"

This same format can guide a program evaluation. The inquiry group introduction may begin with, this is what we heard at the initial focus group: that we could be helpful by (fill in the blank with specific program information). This is how we responded to your request. Has this been helpful? How could it be improved or changed?

The values guiding the CNPM are essential in creating the environment for the inquiry groups in which individuals feel respected, feel listened to, and feel they have a voice in creating community well-being. The inquiry group method has been very useful in hearing calls for nursing from the community and in creating unique responses to the calls. The following provide descriptions of programs created in response to the voice of specific communities.

Usefulness of this Approach

The Celebrity Chef Cooking Club was created in response to voices heard over and over again in inquiry groups: "Help us feed our children" (Barry, 1998).

Beginnings

The Celebrity Chef Cooking Club. At the invitation of the public health nursing director, we as directors of Community Nursing Project of FAU were asked to consider establishing a school-based health room at an alternative middle/high school. The school had been recently renovated and was scheduled to open as a full-service school, with many social-support agencies available on the campus. The school was located in an under-served, multicultural, low-income neighborhood in southeast Florida. We accepted and began identifying stakeholders in the development of the health room program. Parents/guardians, community members, children enrolled in after-school programs, school and public health nurses, nursing faculty, directors of social service agencies, directors of the aftercare programs, and school faculty/staff were identified and invited to participate in inquiry groups.

The Community Nursing Project directors were the group moderators. As nurses and experts in health care, we had expected to hear in response to the question, how can we be helpful to you?, ideas such as blood pressure screenings, diabetes screenings, health education, health fairs, physical examinations, or immunizations. But instead we heard from each group, help us feed our children. The community members were mostly the working poor, working long hours and often two jobs to provide for their families. The children were in school all day and in aftercare programs often until 9 p.m. When the children got home at night, they often found exhausted parents/guardians, if they were home yet, and usually no hot supper.

We were shocked with the call from the community but knew in our hearts that we would have to respond to begin to establish trust with this community. We reflected and dia-logued among ourselves about how we would do this. The decision was made to do it, to create a Celebrity Chef Cooking Club, and to invite local celebrities to come and cook or to pro-vide the money to cook a hot meal for the children. The focus would be health promotion: serving healthy, nutritious food; role modeling as nurses and other community professionals; and building community. The school principal gave permis-sion to use the cafeteria kitchen facilities, the FAU student nurse association provided the first meal, and two after-school programs—the Boys and Girls Club and MAD DADs—brought the children. We were up and running in 1 week's time.

Over the course of 10 years, the Celebrity Chef Cook-ing Club served a hot meal once a week to as many as 120 children. Celebrity chefs who volunteered included a uni-versity president, local ministers, the police, school nurses, health department nurses, firefighters, directors of local social service groups, faculty, church groups, and physicians. Local shops and farms donated food, and various churches gave money each year to support the program. The program evolved over time and became a service project for the teenagers in the neighborhood. They helped in every aspect of the program, from meal preparation to serving the food and the cleanup. The hours served could be applied to their high school service requirement.

The Celebrity Chef Cooking Club was created in response to the community's hopes and dreams to feed their children, and it sparked the creation of a school-based wellness center. The Wellness Center provides school- and community-based primary health care, health promotion, health screenings, and immunizations. It remains a center for nursing education, research, development, and evaluation.

The Head Lice Treatment and Prevention Project. In the previous exemplar, coming to know community began with a direct invitation to open a school health room in a middle school. This exemplar describes the importance of coming to know community and empowering a community to come to know itself when there is a call for nursing in response to a stigmatized condition.

The Head Lice Treatment and Prevention Project was developed in 1996 in response to a community call for safe and effective head lice treatment options. Through the project an invitation was extended to attend an elementary school parent meeting in which the agenda was focused on a recent head lice outbreak at the school. This outbreak was the third one of the school year. Guided by an openness to listen and willingness to come to know the community, the meeting began with the respectful question, how can we be helpful to you? Parents, guardians, and the school nurse described their frustration and anger in response to having another head lice outbreak at their school. The group believed that there were a handful of students, referred to as "licers," who were frequently infested with head lice and therefore responsible for the repeat outbreaks. They described this group of students and their families as a threat to the well-being of the rest of the school community. The group collectively voiced a desire to have the entire school screened for head lice and wanted all children, faculty, and staff found to have lice or nits removed from school until they were "clean."

In many countries, head lice are a highly stigmatized condition. This is particularly true in the United States. In the setting described above, students experiencing head lice and those students' families faced significant social stigma. In his classic work on stigma, Goffman (1963) described stigmatized persons as being socially discredited on the basis of an undesirable attribute that sets them apart from normal society. Persons who are stigmatized are not accepted by "normal people" and are often considered not quite human—inferior and dangerous (Goffman, 1963). At this elementary school, the stigma dramatically increased if head lice treatment strategies were unsuccessful, if reinfestation occurred, or if the infestation became persistent. Interestingly, some of the students with head lice were seen as victims, whereas other students were considered the source of the problem.

After respectfully listening to the group, we shared the following assumptions to verify if they reflected the beliefs of the group:

- Head lice were a school-based problem.
- Head lice are highly transmissible.
- A small number of students were responsible for the outbreaks.
- Parents of children with persistent head lice were neglectful in allowing the condition to continue.
- Removing children, staff, and faculty who had head lice from school would control all future outbreaks and make the school environment safe for their children.

The limitation of each assumption was addressed during a brief educational presentation of what was currently known about head lice and the efficacy of available treatments. Building on their concern for the well-being of the school community, we led a dialogue on what it meant to be a member of their school community. This dialogue led to a refocusing on how to care for each other during a head lice outbreak. The group decided to form a committee to develop a plan of approach that was respectful of all members of the school community.

Over the course of the next few months, we worked with the committee, school nurse, and school administrative staff to send educational information to all families, with the objective of increasing head lice awareness and decreasing stigma. Guided by the value of intersectoral collaboration, in that it provides a conduit for working together, we identified community resources available to help families with head lice education and treatment such as the local nonprofit treatment facility, college of nursing Head Lice Treatment and Prevention Project, local county health department, and community churches. In addition, a fund-raiser was held to help provide families with treatment products, lice combs, and, when needed, access to lice and nit removal services for persistent cases. Recognizing head lice is endemic in the community; families are now encouraged to screen their children once a week to identify and treat head lice early. Transmission of head lice is controlled through early recognition and treatment rather than forced absences.

Discussion

What started out as an event that threatened the wholeness of the school community became an opportunity to learn and grow (Parker & Barry, 2006). Grounded in the nursing values of respect for person, caring, and appreciation of wholeness, the Community Nursing Practice Model (Parker & Barry, 2006, 1999) was useful in coming to know the community's hopes and dreams. A shared understanding of community, based on respect for all persons, empowered the group to work toward creating a safe school environment.

The creations of the two nursing situations—the Celebrity Chef Cooking Club and the Head Lice Treatment and Prevention Program—were like climbing a mountain. They required thoughtful preparation, passion about being present in the community; a willingness to risk; courage; humility; and most importantly, patience. The CNPM values guided the development of these nursing situations and inspired our commitment to stay with them despite obstacles such as funding issues and location issues.

Other Leadings

The CNPM, offers the grounding to seek new heights and insights in community nursing practice. The route to knowing, in inquiry group method, moves nurses to the persons and communities served to engage in a respectful approach: We are experts in nursing and you are an expert of caring for yourself and your community. How can we be helpful to you?

The values of the CNPM inspire and invigorate partnerships of caring that focus on the strengths and hopes and dreams for well-being of the other. Just as if we were climbing a mountain, let us be patient with ourselves and those nursed as we work together to plan and implement nursing responses. And let us strive to be invited to share three cups of tea: each as honored guest, nurse, and client, each in communion.

References

Barry, C. (1993). Nursing values expressed in caring rituals. In D. Gaut & A. Boykin (Eds.), *Care as healing: Renewal through hope.* New York: National League for Nursing Press.

Barry, C. (1998). The Celebrity Chef Cooking Club: A peer involvement feeding program promoting cooperation and community building. *Florida Journal of School Health, 9*(1), 17.

Barry, C., & Gordon, S. (2006). Theories and models of school nursing. In J. Selekman (Ed.), *Comprehensive textbook of school nursing.* Scarborough, ME: National Association of School Nursing.

Chooporian, T. (1986). Reconceptionalizing the environment. In P. Mocia (Ed.), *New approaches to theory development* (pp. 39–54). New York: National League for Nursing Press.

Florida Atlantic University Christine E. Lynn College of Nursing. (2002). Philosophy. Retrieved January 10, 2009, from Florida Atlantic University, Christine E. Lynn College of Nursing Web site: http://nursing.fau.edu/index.php?main=1&nav=76

Goffman, E. (1963). *Stigma: Notes on the management of a spoiled identity.* Englewood Cliffs, NJ: Prentice-Hall.

Mortenson, G. & Relin, D. O. (2007). *Three cups of tea.* New York: Penguin.

Parker, M., & Barry, C. (1999). Community practice guided by a nursing framework. *Nursing Science Quarterly, 12*(2), 125–131.

Parker, M. E., & Barry, C. D. (2006). Developing a community nursing practice model. In M. Parker, (Ed.), *Nursing theories for nursing practice* (pp. 389–396). Philadelphia: F. A. Davis.

Parker, M., Barry, C., & King, B. (2000). Use of inquiry method for assessment and evaluation in a school-based community nursing project. *Family and Community Health, 23,* 54–61.

Peck, S. (1987). *The different drum: Community making and peace.* New York: Simon & Schuster.

Smith, C., & Mauer, F. (1995). *Community health nursing: Theory and practice.* Philadelphia: W.B. Saunders.

Swadener, B., & Lubeck, S. (1995). *Children and families "at promise": Deconstructing the discourse of risk.* Albany, NY: State University of New York Press.

World Health Organization, Alma-Ata. (1978). *Primary health care.* Geneva, Switzerland: Author.

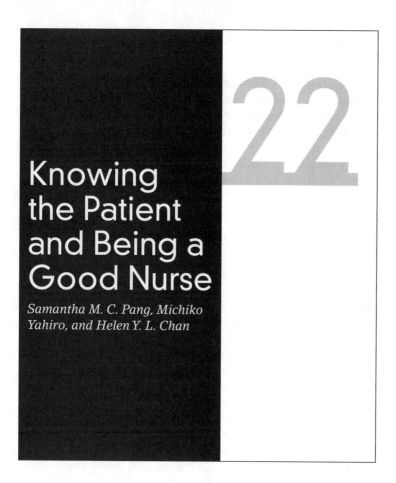

Knowing the Patient and Being a Good Nurse

Samantha M. C. Pang, Michiko Yahiro, and Helen Y. L. Chan

Chapter Overview

Drawing on the patients' personal responses in the study "How Patients Characterize the Good Nurse," this chapter presents what the patient knows about "good" nurses and how listening to the patient's voice is related to being a good nurse. In sharing their encounters with nurses who had most impressed them during their cancer treatments and hospitalizations, patients expressed their vulnerabilities in terms of existential, experiential, and relational changes. Good nurses were those who could acknowledge these changes occurring in patients, whereas nurses who failed to meet the threshold of goodness were those who could not see their patients in the midst of these vulnerabilities.

The relationships between good nurse effects and positive patient outcomes are well articulated within the emergent themes of empowering the patient to deal with life positively, optimizing the patient's relational well-being, and relieving the patient of negative emotions and discomfort. The chapter also examines the role of listening to patients' voices in knowing how to be a good nurse.

Introduction

Research studies on knowing the patient have revealed the importance of understanding the phenomena fostering expert nursing judgment and individualized patient care (Henderson, 1997; Luker, Austin, Caress, & Hallett, 2000; MacDonald, 2008; Robin, 2000; Takemura & Kanda, 2003; Tanner, Benner, Chesla, & Gordon, 1993). Examination of factors affecting knowing the patient in the clinical context, and the relationships between knowing the patient and positive patient outcomes, has been primarily focused on what knowing the patient means and how understanding the patient is related to individualized intervention (MacDonald, 2008; Radwin, 1996). In this chapter, a new dimension is extended to the knowledge base of knowing the patient: knowing what the patient knows about good nurses and how being a good nurse is related to knowing the patient.

Listening to Patient Voices

A group of nurse researchers from Asia gathered in Nagano, Japan, in November 2003. They held a common interest in developing several new understandings of nursing ethics based on Asian values and cultures. In contrast with Anglo-American-European cultures, which have their roots in the Judeo-Christian tradition, many Asian cultures find their roots anchored in Confucian philosophies. Confucian moral theories are fundamentally virtue based (Pang, 2003), and incorporating an Asian perspective can enrich the international dialogue on normative virtue ethics for nurses. Further, the approaches to ethics found in the textbooks for Asian nurses are predominately based on Western medical bioethics. In searching the literature, it was found that most studies focusing on what constitutes good nursing rarely included the patient's perspective. A question was raised as to whether we could develop an understanding of the good in nursing practice, as articulated by patients in our own cultures.

In his discourse on the possibility of developing a normative virtue ethics for the health professions, Edmond Pellegrino (1995) argued that we have to start with expounding the phenomena of patient and health professional interactions by focusing on "fact of illness," "act of profession," and "act of healing" grounded in the realities and actualities of the clinical encounters. Because the primary responsibility of nurses is to people who require nursing care (International Council of Nurses, 2006), explicating patients' perceptions of good nurses in their clinical encounters would be the most relevant starting point for developing an understanding of the good. This good is intrinsic to nursing practice. The possession and exercise of the qualities (virtues) of character enable nurses to move forward toward achieving that good, but the lack of thereof (vices) prevents it (Hursthouse, 2006). Inspired by Pellegrino's discourse, the research team affirmed the importance of listening to the patient's voice in arriving at an understanding of what constitutes good nurses. In this paper, a good nurse is a nurse who is both excellent (being competent) and ethical (having a moral quality) in practice. In engaging the patients to articulate the goods in nurses whom they had encountered in their illness and health care experiences, we hope to arrive at some understandings of the admirable traits of character in nurses that would positively influence the patients' health and well-being.

In 2004, the research team embarked on a phenomenological inquiry to explore the ways in which patients characterized the good nurse (Pang, 2008). This journey was started by interviewing cancer survivors and listening to their first-person experiences of good and bad nurse encounters during the course of their cancer treatments and hospitalizations. Van Kaam's (1966) controlled explication method was used to analyse the merged dataset of interview transcriptions gathered from 97 cancer survivors in Japan; Korea; Taiwan; and Suzhou, China. We also verified the analysed findings of 2,630 questionnaire responses from both cancer patients and patients with multiple hospitalizations in Japan; Korea; Taiwan; and Suzhou and Hong Kong, China. Regardless of cultural variations, the findings revealed that the patients highly valued a person-to-person relationship with nurses, and because they felt vulnerable due to their illness and hospitalization, they felt safe in these relationships that helped them cope with their situation. The nurses who had most impressed the patients as being good demonstrated the behaviour of "knowing the patient," and the reverse were those nurses who failed to meet the threshold of what constituted good in the patients' eyes. The study has elicited rich descriptions of what knowing the patient means in relation to being a good nurse.

This chapter illuminates this phenomenon of knowing the patient by drawing on the experiences of Japanese and Chinese cancer patients (Izumi, Konishi, Yahiro, & Kodama, 2006; Wang, Yahiro, Pang, & Xue, 2007). Given the nature of the illness they experienced, the first section focused on knowing patients' vulnerability. The second section described how the good nurse influenced patient vulnerability. In delineating the relationships between positive patient outcomes and the influence of a good nurse, the implications of knowing the patient and being a good nurse will be expounded.

On Knowing the Patients' Vulnerability

Vulnerability in the broad sense implies the capability of being wounded or susceptibility to injury. In this sense, all patients are in a state of vulnerability aggravated by the illnesses from which they suffer, with some being more vulnerable than others. In the analysed transcriptions of patients' positive and negative encounters with nurses during the course of their cancer treatments and hospitalizations, the patients expressed their sense of vulnerability in three aspects: existential, experiential, and relational change.

Existential change. Existential change is relating to the change of the fact or state of living after becoming a patient. The Chinese ideogram "病" for "being sick" means having the heart hanged on a weighing scale. Wandering between fear and hope is a common emergent theme in phenomenological studies of people living with cancer or degenerative diseases (Charmz, 2002; Mizusaki, 2004; Wong, 2008). They experience fear of deterioration, weighing this against the hope for functional improvement; fear of social isolation, weighing this against hope for acceptance by others; fear of the unknown, weighing this against hope for informed management; fear of threats to their health, weighing this against hope for stable health status. In describing their good and bad nurse encounters, patients in this study also revealed their state of being as analogous to hanging on a weighing scale. In contrast to good nurses, nurses considered by the patients as bad were those who not only failed to acknowledge the patients' changing state of being, but also behaved in deplorable ways that made the patients feel more burdened or harmed.

The illness changed not only the relationship of the patient with the people around him or her, but also the way the patient looked at himself or herself. They had come to realize how much they depended on nurses. Feelings of being care dependent were shared by many patients. Following are some examples that illustrate this feeling of care dependency.

A 73-year-old man with prostate cancer shared,

> *I was like a bedridden, elderly person ... If I could do it by myself and go to the bathroom freely, naturally I would have liked to do so. It might be very nice, but unfortunately I could not do that in the hospital. All my personal needs were attended to by the nurses.*

Reluctantly the patients found themselves being "treated like an old or sick person." They expressed the view that no one wants to be dependent on others, yet they had been held captive by the situation. Forced dependence on others negatively impacted patients' evaluation of self-worth, as a 44-year-old patient with breast cancer expressed:

> *No one wants to be looked after by others; no one wants to stay in hospital, but when the diagnosis was made, and after I am named "patient," I realized that "patient" did not rank equally with other normal peoples. In fact at the time, I unequivocally thought I had to forfeit everything such as my status, identity, and freedom. We have to keep staying in the hospital and we are displaced by the hospital at the status. We are mortified at our situation as we have to be under the nurse's care. Patients, especially patients with cancer, are not only losers in health, but also*

losers in society. Therefore, patients are vulnerable, not just in front of medical staff, but also in front of people in general.

In order to give life a chance, patients found that they did not have much choice but to receive aggressive treatments that rendered them dependent on nurses' care during the course of treatment. When the patients were asked to share their experiences of good and bad nurse encounters, it was noteworthy that they met with nurses in these life moments of wandering between fear and hope, and with feelings of powerlessness and helplessness.

Experiential change. Substantial work has been done to unfold the lived experiences of cancer patients in relation to their illness and treatment trajectories (Mizusaki, 2004; Tschudin, 1996; Wong, 2008). Cancer itself makes a serious assault on patients' physical well-being, leading to changing anatomy and deteriorating functions that result in patients having to modify their lifestyles, such as coping with swallowing difficulties after receiving radiotherapy to treat nasopharyngeal cancer (NPC). For these patients, eating becomes progressively hard work. Rather than experiencing eating as a pleasure, patients with NPC find eating an exhausting process. They have to learn how to work out the difficulties, including being forced to implement diet modification. When patients are confronted with more and more swallowing problems, their typical reactions include withdrawing from social interaction, reducing leisure activities, and avoiding eating in public places.

Similarly, in our study, in eliciting patients' views of their experiences with good and bad nurses, it is interesting to note that their narratives also revealed this phenomenon of experiential change. Patients recounted their experiences, such as pain, nausea, poor appetite, and malaise; but in addition to these physical discomforts from their diseases, uncertainty regarding the disease progress and treatment regimen placed further psychological burdens on them. The patients were perplexed and helpless because of the unknown, and they counted on the health professionals to help them find a way out. A patient with malignant lymphoma explained, "Feeling bad due to illness is just a common feeling among patients in the hospital. It is to be expected for patients ... Patients always worry that their doctor will give up on them."

Another patient who was newly diagnosed with colon cancer stated vividly he was feeling down after his operation. He said that he thought many cancer patients found themselves "in a hole with no end" as he did.

Uncertainty was shared by many patients with cancer because of the nature of their disease. With diseases related to internal organs, they felt their fate was uncertain from one day to the next.

In recalling their positive and negative encounters with good and bad nurses, it is in this context of experiential changes that the patients told their stories about what the nurses had done that most impressed them.

Relational change. The diagnosis of cancer brings obvious change to the patient's physical health and even more subtle changes in how he or she relates to others. Patients expressed concerns about whether their attending nurses could understand these subtle changes. Being admitted into hospital and becoming a patient is a drastic change, as explained by this 44-year-old woman with breast cancer, who wished to speak for her fellow patients:

> *As patients, we were downcast after hospitalization. Hospital was definitely an alien environment for us, so we always had to say to everyone, "excuse me," "thank you," "thank you" ... Originally, almost all of us had had some social status, but after becoming patients, we forfeited almost everything.*

Patients felt they had become anonymous people whose social identity and status became meaningless assets for them in adapting to this strange hospital environment. As classless strangers pleading for help, their survival skills were to relate to others by acting humbly and submissively.

Besides being deprived of their social status, they found themselves turned into statistical probabilities in the eyes of the physicians. One patient vehemently protested, "Often, the medical staff eyed me in [terms of] statistical percentages. I am not an experimental mouse. I am a patient and have no relationship with statistical percentages."

The overwhelming sense of unfamiliarity and strangeness made patients feel stunted. One patient recalled the moment when she was newly diagnosed with breast cancer:

Just after my admission as a patient, it was really difficult for me to know how I should deal with my problems and how to spend my time. I could find out nothing about the treatment in the hospital. All of the people in the hospital were strangers to me. It is hard for a cancer patient to be sure which road is better to take with regard to therapy. Also, a cancer patient always feels uncertain as to what to say to doctors or nurses.

Rather than a lack of opportunity to seek more information from the health professions, the crux of the problem for patients was in not knowing what to ask or how to ask. Similar difficulties were encountered by patients in sharing their concerns with even their close family members, as illustrated by a 46-year-old woman with gastric cancer: "Although my father visited me, I could say nothing. I didn't know what was going on anymore ... When I was discharged from the hospital, a nurse asked me, 'Do you have any queries or worries?' I had so many worries, but I could say nothing."

In a medical culture in which physicians are seen as elite and as having high authority, patients incur a heavy sense of inferiority that inhibits them from seeking information. This is especially true of the older generation, who grew up in an age when paternalism was the norm in medical practice. Patients are hesitant about questioning the nurse or doctor. For example, one patient shared, "When I ask my doctor a question, I say something like: 'Forgive my ignorance, but ...' Therefore, elderly people may have difficulty asking the doctor questions because the physician has a very high status in his/her generation."

Although nurses were more likely to be viewed as equals and therefore approachable in the eyes of patients, patients found that nurses were often so occupied with their tasks that they dared not disturb them. Some patients confided their need for help among themselves: "All patients are in a vulnerable state and in need of help. We know nurses are busy, so we have an unvoiced wish in our mind, and always have this unspoken fear."

In order to cope with their sense of alienation and fear, patients were concerned about whether they could maintain a good relationship with nurses, who were the only health professionals with whom they came in contact most of the time in the hospital.

After admission, patients enter a room that contains nothing noteworthy. Everyone wants to have some kind of comfort or some kind of relationship with others, and for patients in the hospital, there is the nurse only. Therefore, every patient looks to the nurse.

Since patients identified nurses as their coping resource, they seized every opportunity to get access to them, such as picking up on the nurses' words that might provide clues about their condition, and turning them over in their minds.

Patients were care recipients and also observers of how care was being delivered in the clinical setting. What they observed happening in the ward had a direct bearing on their sense of vulnerability and well-being. Patients counted on the health professionals; consequently, every word uttered by either doctor or nurse was noted by patients. In one patient's words,

Patients are very susceptible to a nurse's or doctor's gentle words, which seize hold of the patient's heart (⬛⬛). A heartfelt word can heal patients. When I hear the nurse's kind words and look at her smile, I feel that I can get better. On the other hand, strong words make patients feel more miserable.

In observing what was going on in the ward, patients found that some nurses were not aware of these feelings of vulnerability that are so prevalent in patients. Patients were always waiting for nurses or doctors to approach them. If a nurse or doctor passed in front of a patient's bed without saying a word, the patient felt lonely. One patient further elaborated:

The effects of physicians' and nurses' expressions on patients were tremendous. We tended to think too much. For example, I thought, 'I might be fine because my doctor

*seemed to be smiling,' but it was probably because the
doctor had just finished an enjoyable phone call with his
girlfriend. When the doctor was hard-faced, he might just
have been hungry. But we patients were so sensitive that we
assumed that all of the physicians' and nurses' expressions
were directly related to our own illness.*

*In becoming a patient who required hospitalization and
cancer treatments, the sense of vulnerability in the aspect
of relational change primarily emerged from patients'
understanding of their dependence on the health professions in order to have positive health outcomes. Their former relational network underwent such a dramatic change
that they became classless strangers in the medical world,
where patients have to rely on the health professions to
restore their health and well-being. In this transition, nurses came into their lives as an important coping resource
because nurses were seen as more approachable, as well as
the most accessible for help. This may explain why patients
were mindful of being on good terms with nurses, and why
they were observant of and sensitive to what nurses said
and did.*

On Knowing the Effects of the Good Nurse on Patient Vulnerability

In this phenomenological inquiry of cancer patients' experiences of good nurses, rich descriptions were elicited about the
ways in which good nurses help to alleviate patients' feelings
of vulnerability in the midst of existential, experiential, and
relational changes. Three themes of the influences of a good
nurse emerged: empowering the patient to deal with life positively, relieving the patient from negative emotions and discomfort, and optimizing the patient's relational well-being.

Empowering the patient to deal with life positively. Patients
are required to make decisions about treatment options as
well as life and family arrangements about which they do
not have prior knowledge and experience. The patient narratives revealed that meeting with a good nurse, with whom
the patient feels his or her existential change is understood,
produced positive patient outcomes. These included making
the patient willing to share his/her personal matters with

the nurse, helping the patient to banish pessimistic thoughts, making the patient feel that life is valuable, and helping the patient to restore hope and confidence so that he/she can make decisions on treatment and life matters. The following narrative illustrates how a 64-year-old woman with breast cancer felt about being understood by the nurse at her cross-roads between returning home or continuing treatment:

> *One day, after completing her morning rounds, the nurse came back to my bedside and said, "How are you, Ms. A? I can see you are experiencing something unusual." I was so surprised. Although I had said nothing to her, Nurse B had observed my expression. In fact, my nerves were on edge because I was worried about the progress of my chemo-therapy. I was also facing a dilemma as to whether I should continue to receive my treatment in the hospital or go home to take care of my mother-in-law, who was over 80 and now in an elderly home because of my hospitalization. I really wanted to care for her and she was already being prepared for going back home. Nurse B listened and responded to the suffering I expressed, then checked and gave me some useful information about my discharge period—this meant when I could get the final results of my chemotherapy. At this time, I had not talked about my worries with any family members or friends because I thought they did not under-stand much about my health problems. In this case, Nurse B could help me because she was a professional, so she could understand my actual situation, including the condi-tion of my cancer and also my mental state. I knew that the good nurse could offer suggestions that would enable the patient to improve his or her life. Nurse B helped me to reduce my worries and doubts. She then helped me to make my decision and also eased my mind. Yes, I could make a decision by myself.*

In this narrative, the patient felt understood by the nurse, who was able to appreciate what kind of illness and treat-ment experience that patient was going through, and who had the wisdom to address the patient's wishes and concerns as a unique person. Other than feeling understood by the nurse, the patient was impressed by the nurse's willingness to spend time with her and listen to her suffering.

By contrast, nurses who only seem to be concerned about getting their tasks done would never be able to produce this positive patient outcome, since the patient would not be willing to share his/her personal matters with such a nurse. A patient said,

> *I met another nurse who I think was competent, but she just performed her own duties speedily and efficiently, without more. When she came into my room in the morning, she always walked quickly and only said, "Good morning." Later, she silently did the minimum work required and left quickly. She did what was necessary, but nothing that was nice, unnecessary, or extra. I did not feel good when I perceived that she was clearly intending to go to perform her next task soon; I could not ask her for anything then. Often my timing was inappropriate when I wanted to say something or ask some questions. Even if she had talked more, it would not have taken too much time. I guess it would have taken around a minute.*

Indeed, patients always solicited information actively from nurses. However, if nurses did not spend time with their patients or communicate with them, the patients felt more vulnerable. They could not rely on their attending nurses when they needed to know more about their problems or seek out solutions.

Relieving the patient from negative emotions and discomfort. As demonstrated in the section on experiential change, patients became care dependent and relied on nurses to help them find a way out. The following personal interviews show both the negative patient outcome in relation to meeting with a bad nurse and the positive patient outcome in relation to meeting with a good nurse.

> *I vomited several times after the operation but could not get out of bed. I called a nurse immediately because my kidney basin was already full. When I asked the nurse to help, she looked very displeased. Of course I would have liked to wash the basin by myself. I would have done it if I could. I thought I would never ask for help again … The next time, I tried to do it myself. Another nurse came and was surprised, saying, "No, no, stop! This is my job! You don't need to do such a thing." I felt very grateful and I cried.*

Whereas meeting a bad nurse increased the patient's sense of vulnerability, the patient felt relieved to meet a good nurse. Positive patient outcomes from meeting good nurses included relief from pain or discomfort; alleviation of worries; and a calm, peaceful, and cheerful feeling. These positive outcomes also included the nurse making the patient feel that his or her condition was not so bad and hence giving the patient courage to go on.

Optimizing the patient's relational well-being. A sense of vulnerability emerged from patients' understanding of their dependence on nurses for yielding positive health outcomes. Meeting with a good nurse on whom the patient could rely provided the best assurance of optimal recovery, as indicated by this 54-year-old man with gastric cancer and liver metastasis:

It was the most impressive event in my hospitalization. On the first day after my operation, Nurse K said that I should take walks. I know it now, but I think I had no time to understand how important it was in the true sense. So I said to her, "No way, how can I walk in this condition? I will start tomorrow." She then said, "Well, but let's walk now, instead of tomorrow. Just around this ward, let's walk, Mr. A." I was pleased that she was encouraging me, but I really didn't want to walk. I had already made my decision, using many excuses, such as I cannot walk because I am in pain; I am quite helpless, suffering; or today is just the first day post-operation. She said again and again that I needed to walk and why I should walk, and then I walked. After I finished making one circuit of the ward, Nurse K said, "Mr. A, that isn't enough. You can walk round at least three times today." That was really hard exercise. While walking around the ward, I thought, "What a large hospital!" Finally, I walked round the ward three times! As the days went by, I came to appreciate her. She always accompanied me when I walked. She said hello to me cheerfully, even from afar, whenever she saw me.

Nurse K earned Mr. A's confidence, so that he finally listened to her advice regarding early ambulation because she had demonstrated compassion, consideration, knowledge, cheerfulness, and optimism in relating to the patient. In establishing a trusting relationship with good nurses, patients' feelings of unfamiliarity, strangeness, and fear were relieved; and positive feelings of warmth, security, safety, and love were ensured instead, making a positive impact on patients' health and relational well-being.

Conclusion and Nursing Implications

Drawing on patients' narratives about their experiences of good and bad nurse encounters during hospitalization and the course of cancer treatment, this chapter aimed to arrive at some understanding of what patients know about good nurses and how knowing the patient is related to being a good nurse. Elicited from the patients' voices are rich descriptions of their feelings of vulnerability in the midst of existential, experiential, and relational changes. Good nurses are those who can acknowledge these changes that are occurring in their patients, whereas nurses who fail to meet the threshold of goodness are those who cannot see their patients in the context of these vulnerabilities. The relationship between good nursing and positive patient outcomes is well articulated in the patients' recorded narratives. When they meet good nurses, patients' relational well-being is optimized, negative emotions and discomfort are relieved, and patients are empowered to deal with life positively.

Patients' voices as feathers and cartloads of firewood. The further question is how we make sense of these patient voices to arrive at a better understanding of how to be a good nurse. We would see these patient voices as feathers and cartloads of firewood, which appeared in the dialogue between Mencius and a feudal king. This story appeared in a Confucian classic titled Mencius written around 400BC, in which the teachings of Mencius are deliberated through interrogations between the master and his followers who would like to seek his wisdom in dealing with their problems. This king came to seek Mencius' advice about the way to become a good king who could benefit his people. Mencius responded to his question by making an analogy which implied that the king could only find the answer through critical self-introspection.

> *"Should someone say to you, 'I am strong enough to lift a hundred chun [about 70 kg] but not a feather; I have eyes that can see the tip of a new down feather but not a cartload*

of firewood,' would you accept the truth of such a state-
ment?" (Mencius, 400BC/2003, p. 17)

Drawing on this analogy made by Mencius we would like
to construct a dialogue between the patient and the nurse
who wants to become a good nurse.

Nurse: What makes you think that the ways nurses perform
their work accord with whether or not they are good
nurses?

Patient: Should someone say to you, "I am strong enough to
lift a 70 kg object but not a feather; I have eyes that
can see the tip of a new down feather but not a cartload of firewood," would you accept the truth of such
a statement?

Nurse: No.

Patient: Why should it be different in your own case? Your
professional education is sufficient to enable you
to reach the core competencies required of a nurse,
yet patients fail to benefit from the work you do for
them. That a feather is not lifted is because one fails
to make the effort; that a cartload of firewood is not
seen is because one fails to use one's eyes. Similarly,
patients cannot recognize the good in your work
because you fail to listen to their voices. Hence, your
failure to become a good nurse is due to a refusal to
act, not an inability to act.

Nurse: What is the difference in form between refusal to
act and inability to act?

Patient: If you say to someone, "I am unable to do it," when
the task is striding over the North Sea with Mount
Tai under your arm, then this is a genuine case of
inability to act. But if you say, "I am unable to do it,"
when it is what we have shared with you about how
good nurses help to alleviate our vulnerabilities,
then this is a case of refusal to act, not of inability.
Hence your failure to become a good nurse is not
the same in kind as striding over the North Sea with
Mount Tai under your arm, but the same as the nurse
understands my concern.

The good nurse is the one who is able to see the patient in
a vulnerable state of being (cartload of firewood) and is able to

make an effort to address the patient's need in that particular context with the embodiment of the good nurse's works (lift a feather). By contrast, a nurse who fails to meet the threshold of goodness is one who fails to see the "cartload" and fails to make an effort to "lift a feather." It is interesting to see that these patient voices did not touch on the kinds of clinical situations characterized by conflicting values and competing role requirements that often catch nurses in ethical dilemmas or workplace distress and render them unable to act. The inclusion of patient voices reflecting on our good and bad practices will help to discern what belongs to refusal to act and what belongs to inability to act on the part of nurses in fostering the good that is integral to nursing practice. This discernment will help us to focus on what is important in nursing and therefore worthy of our efforts.

References

Charmz, K. (2002). Stories and silences: Disclosures and self in chronic illness. *Qualitative Inquiry, 8*(3), 302–328.

Henderson, S. (1997). Knowing the patient and the impact on patient participation: A grounded theory study. *International Journal of Nursing Practice, 3*(2), 111–118.

Hursthouse, R. (2006). Are virtues the proper starting point for morality? In J. Dreier (Ed.), *Contemporary debates in moral theory* (pp. 99–112). Malden, MA: Blackwell.

International Council of Nurses. (2006). *Code of Ethics for Nurses.* Geneva: Author.

Izumi, S., Konishi, E., Yahiro, M., & Kodama, M. (2006). Japanese patients' descriptions of "The Good Nurse": Personal involvement and professionalism. *Advances in Nursing Science. Philosophy and Ethics, 29*(2), 14–26.

Luker, K. A., Austin, L., Caress, A., & Hallett, C. E. (2000). The importance of "knowing the patient": Community nurses' constructions of quality in providing palliative care. *Journal of Advanced Nursing, 31*(4), 775–782.

MacDonald, M. (2008). Technology and its effect on knowing the patient: A clinical issue analysis. *Clinical Nurse Specialist, 22*(3), 149–155.

Mencius. (2003). *Mencius Book I.* (Lau, D. C., Trans.). Hong Kong: The Chinese University Press. (400BC).

Mizusaki, T. (2004). *Meaning of patients diagnosed with cancer to know about their illness in Japan: To understand their narratives from phenomenological hermeneutics.* Doctoral dissertation, Nagano College of Nursing, Nagano, Japan (in Japanese), 2004.

Pang, S. M. C. (2003). *Nursing ethics in modern China: Conflicting values and competing role requirements.* New York: Rodopi.

Pang S.M.C. (2008). Inclusion of patients' voices in a virtue ethics for nurses. Editorial comment, *Nursing ethics*, 15 (5), 571-572.

Pellegrino, E. D. (1995). Toward a virtue-based normative ethics for the health professions. *Kennedy Institute of Ethics Journal, 5*(3), 253–277.

Radwin, L. E. (1996). "Knowing the patient": A review of research on an emerging concept. *Journal of Advanced Nursing, 23*(6), 1142–1146.

Robin, M. (2000). Consequences of not "knowing the patient." *Clinical Nurse Specialist, 14*(2), 75–81.

Takemura, Y., & Kanda, K. (2003). How Japanese nurses provide care: A practice based on continuously knowing the patient. *Journal of Advanced Nursing, 42*(3), 252–259.

Tanner, C. A., Benner, P., Chesla, C., & Gordon, D. R. (1993). The phenomenology of knowing the patient. *Image: Journal of Nursing Scholarship, 25*(4), 273–280.

Tschudin, V. (Ed.). (1996). *Nursing the patient with cancer* (2nd ed.). London: Prentice Hall.

Van Kaam, A. (1966). *Existential foundations of psychology*. Pittsburgh, PA: Duquesne University Press.

Wang, H., Yahiro, M., Pang, M. C., & Xue, X. L. (2007). A qualitative study on cancer patients' perception of the good nurse. *Journal of Continuing Education for Nurses, 22*(1), 21–23 (in Chinese).

Wong, K. R. (2008). *Living with dysphagia: Striving hard to preserve oral feeding*. Unpublished master's thesis, The Hong Kong Polytechnic University, Hong Kong SAR, China, 2008.

Acknowledgments

Good Nurse Research Team: H. F. Wang and X. L. Xue (Suzhou, China), S. Izumi, M. Kodama and E. Konishi (Co-PI, Japan), S. C. Chou, S. Y. Chen (Co-PI, Taiwan), Y. S. Hong and Y. R. Um (Co-PI, Korea).

Continuous Knowing of Patients: The Japanese Nursing Perspective

Yukie Takemura and Katsuya Kanda

23

Chapter Overview

Japanese nurses who have gained the reputation of good nursing practice from patients and colleagues tend to have problem-solving skills and also aim to help patients find meaning in their lives with illness. How well the nurse knows the patient influences the quality of patient care, and thus it is extremely important for the nurse to know the patient continuously from both the patient's perspective and the his or her own perspective. Nurses who are able to do both have the ability to switch between modes of getting to know the patients and are able to use different conversation styles.

Introduction

There was once a patient who suffered from cerebral hemorrhage and was half-crippled. She always had a grim expression on her face and was quiet. She refused to take any anti-hypertensive drugs or receive nursing care. I asked how she was feeling and tried to plan out a nursing care plan. She simply kept saying, "You would not know what it is like or how I feel. Just leave me alone." One day when I was not on duty, I decided to talk to her, just to have a conversation. Gradually she began to talk about herself, what she was like before, what she was thinking now, and her visions for the future. She looked very calm. I stared at her and felt a very warm connection between the two of us. She stared back at me with a smile on her face. From that day onwards, she began to change. She started talking to nurses, laughing, and becoming receptive of nurses' suggestions. The nursing care, which was out of synch before was finally in place. I realized that I used to understand patients according to a nursing framework. Then I began to understand how to use the framework as an excellent tool. This is when I decided to research the nursing process.

The Process of Nursing Practice by Japanese Nurses

The nursing process for problem-solving has contributed to the development of nursing as a whole, such as the realization of scientific, systematic and continuous nursing intervention, standardization of nursing practice, facilitation of documentation, encouragement of nurses' autonomy and so on. This traditional nursing process is now widely adapted in nursing practice and education (Leddy, 1998 p. 215), which has been used since the 1980s in Japan. However, the limitations of this nursing process have recently been identified. (Henderson, 1987; Colleen, 1996; Pesut & Herman, 1998; Leddy, 1998, p. 215). Yura and Walsh (1983, p. 132) point out that nurses must have intellectual, interpersonal, and technical skills in order to carry out the nursing process, and that problem-solving is entailed in the intellectual skills. However, it is not yet clear if the problem-solving process is appropriately utilized as a tool in the art of nursing in Japan because some

Japanese nurses have the idea that the problem-solving process itself is the most important part of nursing.

The Elements and the Process of Good Nursing Practice

We aimed to describe the process of good nursing practice carried out by the Japanese nurses, which probably includes problem-solving procedures (Takemura & Kanda, 2001). For the research, we interviewed 24 nurses, 12 patients, and one of the patient's spouse in Japan, and came up with the below observations.

Our analysis shows that nurses feel they have carried out good nursing practice as a result of the following factors: On one hand, the patients realize the meanings and values of their experiences with illness and are content; they change for the better; they participate in decision-making; they place their trusts on nurses. On the other hand, the nurses know the patient, attend to the patient, and use available resources. Each of these factors can individually enable the nurse to carry out the good nursing practice, though they are all related to one another. More effective results can be produced when they are used in combination.

The first factor, helping patients explore and realize meanings and values of their experiences with illness, means that the patients admit that their experience of their illness or its treatment has meanings and values in their lives, therefore they are satisfied and relieved. Knowing the patient is to understand the patient's subjective world, which the patient actually experiences and interprets, and the holistic patient, the nurse's assessment of the patients using their professional knowledge and experience in relation to all patient information so that the nurse can help better understand the patient. Attending to the patient means that nurse takes good care of the patient, treats him/her as a valuable individual, shows interests in, interacts with, and is concerned about the patient. In addition, there are two subcategories attached to this category: the nurses interact with the patient and care for the patient. To interact with the patient means to ensure sufficient attention is paid to the patient and sometimes includes the patient's family, his/her colleagues, or those people around him/her. Caring for the patient means that the nurse puts his/her self in the patient's position and is concerned about the patient, and that the nurse shows consideration for the patient.

A patient changing for the better refers to positive physical, mental, or environmental changes in the patient. The nursing intervention therefore is carried out with the aim of making positive changes for the patient now and in the future. Patient participation points out that the patient accepts his/her own condition, so that he/she can participate willingly in the decision-making, treatment, and care process. To use available resources means that every resources is fully utilized to reach the goal of improving the patient's condition so he/she changes for the better. Resources include collaboration and cooperation with colleagues and people in other types of occupation and the preparation of human and material resources during the implementation of nursing intervention. A patient's trust of a nurse refers to the situation whereby a patient trusts and likes a nurse, and wants to rely on the nurse. In this category, there are two subcategories: one is that the patient distinguishes one nurse from other nurses and recognizes him/her as a special person that the patient trusts and likes; the other one is that the patient recognizes and acknowledges the role and capability of the nurse and relies on the nurse.

The study reveals that the factors for good nursing practice have a lot in common with the features and outcome of high quality care (See Figure 23.1) and the factors reflect the type of nursing quality demanded by patients (Radwin, 2000). In many ways, good nursing practice corresponds to the concepts of caring (Morse et al., 1990), however, good nursing practice also includes factors such as a patient's realization of the meaning and value of his/her experience with illness or a patient's changing for the better, which corresponds to the outcome of caring. Good nursing practice particularly emphasizes a patient's realization of the meaning and value of his/her experience with illness, therefore it is different from the concept of caring.

Sato (1986) notes that, "the nursing process for problem-solving has changed nursing into a practice where there is an absence of any feeling of existence or of reality, such as the reality of understanding or of being together." On the contrary, good nursing practice emphasizes that a patient realizes the meaning and value of his/her experience with

23.1

A cycle of factors for "good nursing practice"

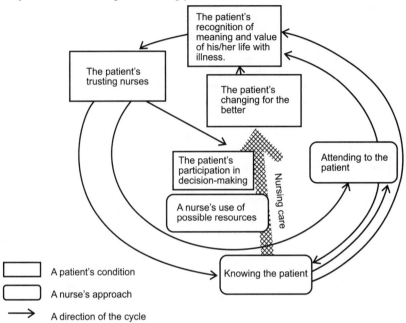

illness. Furthermore, in order to actualize it, it is essential not only to improve the condition of the patient, but also to get to know the patient and to attend to the patient. These features are supplementing the boundary of problem-solving procedures. Therefore it is useful when the factor for good nursing practice and the procedures are used correctly to improve the process of nursing practice.

The Process of Nursing Practice

We did the research for the purpose of identifying the details of the implementation of nursing care process, which began with knowing the patient, and moved towards the goal of changing the patient for the better (Takemura & Kanda, 2003). Figure 23.2 is an image of the process for better understanding, though it was not attached in the published thesis to

23.2

A process of Japanese nursing practice

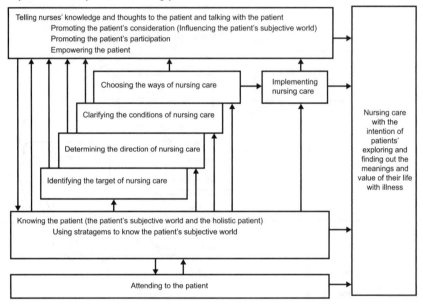

avoid confusion as it seemed the process was on the straight line though it was actually a very complicated process.

Our analysis shows that before a nurse implements the nursing care, there are five procedures: (1) know the patient, (2) identify the targets of nursing care, (3) determine the direction of nursing care, (4) clarify the conditions of nursing care, and (5) choose the ways of nursing care. Our analysis points out that in order to provide high quality nursing care, it is important to have the ability as a professional to clarify the conditions of nursing care, to choose the ways of nursing care, and to understand the ethical point of view such as knowing the patient, identifying the targets of nursing care, and determining the direction of nursing care. The nurses equipped with these abilities are able to know the patient quickly, accurately, and automatically, and are able to implement adequate and sufficient nursing care to the patient without any problems.

To know the patient refers to the process whereby a nurse builds up the patient image by getting information about the patient. This is the crucial part in the process of nursing practice. When a nurse gets the information of the patient for the first time, he/she quickly forms the first image of the patient and then alters the first image gradually when he/she obtains new information. The patient image can be divided between the patient subjective world and the holistic patient. We described the patient subjective world as the patient's subjectivity as perceived by nurses and that it is an infinite world experienced only by the patient. Therefore it is not possible for others to fully and completely understand what it is. The holistic patient means nurses assess the patient using their professional knowledge and experience in relation to all patient information including the patients' subjective world. This also includes the patient's physical, psychological, and social conditions, possible choices of nursing care and medical treatment, expected outcome, opinions of other professionals, values and meanings of the patient's illness and hospitalization for the family members. A nurse will start implementing the nursing care once he/she comes out with the first image of the patient and repeats updating the image when he/she obtains new information.

Building up the image of the patient by knowing him/her more, particularly based on the patient's subjective world, a nurse makes judgment on whether what he/she has found in the patient fits to implement in the nursing care of the patient. And if it is, she applies the ethical judgment whether if it is in the right direction that the patient wants. When there is no ethical dilemma, the judgment is finished. Once the target and direction for the implementation of nursing care are decided, a nurse checks if there is any restriction on when to start the care and then chooses the most effective ways of the care under the restriction. Nurses try to communicate with patients, telling them their knowledge and thoughts in order to educate and empower the patients, and also influence the patients' subjective world.

As a result of this research, we find out that those nurses who are recommended as "good nurses" did not aim simply to solve patients' problems but also to help them realize the meanings and values of their own lives with illness and health care. Knowing the patient is particularly actualized through the process of getting information about the patient and that information becomes the basis for ethical and technical decision-making. Hence it is a very important process that can determine the quality of care as a whole. The model shown in this research does not conflict with the problem-solving procedure. However, it is aimed at helping patients realize the meanings in life and to know the patients throughout the process. This model emphasizes on these factors that are crucial for the implementation of nursing care.

Japanese Relationship and Communication Style

Knowing patients is thus very important for the implementation of nursing care. Japanese nurses use some strategies to promote patients sharing information about themselves. First of all, it is essential to know Japanese relationship and communication styles in order to understand the strategies. According to Hamaguchi (1998), in Japan, a person exists in relation to the nature and other people around, i.e., a "relatum" that cannot be broken down into situation and "individuum" exists; the group or organization is considered to be a network system of relata that share an "interpersonal context" including relationships and situations and valuing things between people. Therefore Japanese culture is identified as "relationalism" (Kumon, 1982) or "contextualism" (Hamaguchi, 1998) rather than collectivism. While individual self is most valued in western societies, Japanese people in general prefer to exist harmoniously with others (Nonaka & Takeuchi, 1995).

This traditional Japanese relationship still exists today. For example, "KY" was nominated for the 2007 Japan New Words and Trends Award. K stands for Kuuki (air, atmosphere) and Y stands for Yomenai (can't read), meaning "can't read the situation" or "someone who can't read the situation," widely used among young people. KY is used to describe the situation such as "he cannot read (judge) situation," "he is not tuned in to what is going on," "he fails to sense the mood of the public," "he does not pick up the vibes." From the interviews with students from five universities in the Tokyo area, 90% of them think it is important to "read the situation," and 70% of them said they do not want to stand out from others (The Yomiuri Shimbun, 2008). The current generation who were brought up emphasizing personality and therefore valued "being-myself" yet preferred to "exist among others harmoniously" (Nonaka & Takeuchi, 1995).

On one hand characterized by respecting relationships with others, it is pointed out that Japanese, compared to Americans, have less disclosure of inner experience on all topics and with all persons (Barnlund, 1975). Barnlund explains the difference between Japanese and Americans in communicating through this phenomenon of the Japanese's idea of "public self" and "private self." The "private self" is characterized as the potentially communicable self being but usually not shared with others. The "public self" is characterized as the always available self being and easily shared with others. He also points out that Japanese have a narrow range of public self and a wide range of private self, while Americans have a wide range of public self and a small range of private self. In Japan, inner experiences are usually shared by listener's careful guessing, not by the speaker's disclosure of self. Verbal communication by Japanese is conveyed by "indirect, localized, self-controlled, situation-oriented and chain of monologues" (Nishida, 1996) to avoid outright opposition between two people and preserve harmony. For Americans, conversation with Japanese may seem endless, pointless, has a number of elusive sentences, and involves a great deal of wasted time due to a long silence (Barnlund, 1975).

Stratagems to Know the Patient's Perspective Used by Japanese Nurses

As mentioned above, in Japan, the inner experiences are often communicated nonverbally by the listener's careful guessing. Hence, it is not easy to ask for the patient's subjective world from the patient himself/herself. Japanese nurses therefore need to go beyond the normal communication style and influence the patient. Takemura and Kanda (2003) clarified the strategies that Japanese nurses use to encourage patients to talk about themselves, their feelings, perceptions, and hopes.

When the nurse attends to a patient and shows a strong interest in the patient more than his/her work requires, the patient accepts the special existence of the nurse and trusts him/her. The patient becomes able to express his/her true feelings to the nurse. One nurse stated that once she acknowledged the kind of sign that the patient was showing, she would postpone the original work plan so that she would not miss the chance of hearing the patient's true feelings. Overlooking the signs shown by patients often result in a loss of confidence in the nurse; the chance may not come around again. The point here is that when the patient selects the specific nurse to reveal his/her true heart, the nurse should not share the information with other members of the medical care team without the patient's permission; otherwise the patient perceives it as a betrayal by the nurse. In addition, it is important to prepare conditions for the patient to confide, such as talking with him/her in a private place so that the patient will know the nurse is available, and is ready to talk about his/her true feelings. The skillful nurse can bring the conversation to the point during the normal conversation. Emotional messages are often conveyed by the nonverbal signals. To those patients who are reluctant to verbalize their true feelings, the nurse must use the "considerate mode" conversation style; i.e., observe the patient closely, put himself/herself in the patient's position, imagine the world experienced by the patient, and tell the patient what he/she thinks and confirm it with the patient. If the patient does not accept the self-disclosure even after these methods are used, family members, such as a spouse can be helpful in expressing the main concern of the patient because they often share the feelings and experiences of the patient.

Three modes to know the patient. Further research shows that there are certain attitudes and views that lead to these three modes, "considerate mode," "professional role mode," and "narrative listener mode" (Takemura, 2004). Frequency and purpose in the use of each mode differ depending on the nurses.

The "considerate mode" is the manner used by Japanese when a person wants to know about another person. He/she would non-verbally guess the other party's thoughts and feelings. Japanese traditionally take a negative stance on verbal communication and value silence rather than speech; they "tend to keep the words they use to a minimum and leave much of what they wish to communicate implied rather than stated" (Nishida, 1996). Japanese patients then tend to express their feelings not by words, but by their facial expressions, eye movements, body movements, pauses or silences, and their condition and character, hoping the nurse will understand them non-verbally. Most Japanese nurses are able to avoid making patients feel uncomfortable by carefully guessing the patients' feelings and the world experienced by patients when selecting care. In addition, this mode allows nurses to provide care without feeling uneasiness towards patients. When a nurse uses the "considerate mode," a patient who is apparently being rude, incomprehensive, and trouble-some will become reasonable and excusable by guessing the reason. However, when a nurse misunderstands the world experienced by the patient, his/her surmised world of the patient and the patient's actual experienced world will be different. As a result, it will cause the discrepancies between the nurse's assumption of what the patient might need and what the patient actually needs for his/her care. It may cause the nurse to feel that his/her own efforts and expectations ended in failure.

The "professional role mode" can also be referred to as "a rational method of knowing the patient." Japanese nurses learn it through the training given during nursing educa-tion. With this mode, the nurse aims to provide appropriate nursing care to enable a patient to become an independent being again. The nurse therefore needs to know the patient. He/she will need to have the information of the patient to assess the patient's problems or to evaluate if the prob-lems are resolved. Only a little disclosure from the patient is expected, and the nurse listens to the patient with a filter of inference and judgment as a professional. The nurse also puts the patient in a nursing framework, determines the "most appropriate" care based on the framework, and provides it to the patient. Even when the nurse shows the enthusiasm for the patient, the presence of the patient becomes weak. In an extreme case, the nurse collects information of the patient for his/her own satisfaction at the provision of care, not for the patient's. In this mode, it is difficult to see what the patient really means in his/her message from the patient's framework. One nurse who previously used this mode stated, "I thought that I was listening to the patient but I wasn't. I thought that I had an interest in the patient but I hadn't. I didn't deliberate over the patient thoughts but over my own instead." In addition, the patients' response to nursing care is used in the evaluation of nursing care and in the evaluation of a nurse's competency. When the patient acts in the way that the nurse wants, the nurse is happy. When the patients show unexpected responses, the nurse may doubt of his/her competency as a nurse. This may also distort the patient's message of what it really means.

The patients' perspective, in principle, can be conveyed through verbalization of the patients' own experience. It cannot be ascertained neither by the "considerate mode," that is the traditional method of knowing a person in Japan, nor the "professional role mode" that is learned in the nursing education. Nurses in Japan, therefore, need to go beyond these communication styles. The "narrative listener mode" is not directly linked to the purpose of selecting the nursing care. With a strong interest in the patient and the patient's life, the "narrative listener" wants to know the patient and understand his/her life experience. This mode is usually used by those nurses who are recommended as "good nurses" by patients and colleagues. It is the important mode that is the key to get to know the patient's perspective. When applying this mode, the nurse temporarily puts aside his/her point of view so that he/she distinguishes it from the patient's point of view. In this way, the nurse can listen to the patient without filtering. One nurse indicated a tip for the professional role mode as, "First, listen to a patient just to know him/her. And then do it again. But this time, listen as a nurse for assessment." This mode helps know the patient's perspective and cut the chance of having an unpleasant betrayal of the nurse's unilateral expectations. In addition, the nurse does not feel threatened because he/she can be ready to deal with the patients' unexpected responses.

Four styles of conversation. So far, different ways and modes in order to know patients have been explored. For Japanese nurses particularly, conversation with patients is an important source to know the patients' subjective world. There are four different conversation styles. Our research (Takemura, 2008) concludes that there are four conversation styles: (1) conversation as a means of nursing, (2) allowing patients to talk about what they want to talk about, (3) listening to patients without judgments, and (4) engaging in casual talks. Generally, (1) and (2) are used in the professional role mode, while (3) and (4) are used in the narrative listener mode. The ability to sometimes listen to patients talk about what they want to talk about and the ability to engage in casual conversations will both influence the level of knowing the patient and the quality of nursing care in Japan.

Many nurses are keen to talk to patients in order to get information which may be useful for nursing, or to support them psychologically. In short, conversation with patients is an important means for nursing. In fact, some nurses refer to it as "getting information" when they talk to patients. Nurses are using "professional role mode" in this conversation style. The following statements are quoted from our interview in order to better understand the situation. The nurse A with 10 years of experience said that a nurse should have an intention of getting necessary information for nursing when she talks to patients:

> To talk to patients, like a casual talk, I guess there are the talks that are just a waste of time. That have nothing to do with nursing. The talks must have some intentions in the communication that have something to do with nursing. In an extreme example, a patient tells you that she has traveled to this place, traveled to that place and you listen. Conversation is going on, but it does not convey anything. It is just a waste of time. Contrarily, if she tells you that she likes to travel but now she cannot travel because of the illness and there is nothing for her to live for, or the memories of traveling with her husband comfort her life now etc., would be meaningful since you will know something precious about the patient. How you direct the conversation depends on your ability. If you are not aware of the purpose you cannot hear anything you need to hear.

Many nurses talk to patients to carry out their duties. If the nurses are able to switch between the four types of conversation it will change the way they perceive the patient or the way they carry out their duties. Six years after the first interview with nurse A, we interviewed nurse A again. Now with 16 years of experience, she has changed her conversation style to "allowing patients to talk about what they want to talk about." It has changed her way of doing work:

> I used to hear what I need to hear. But I have changed. I like to listen to patients in order to share things with them when I have time, instead of writing checkup items on the white board. I try to respond quickly to what they ask. I just listen to what patients want to tell me.

When a nurse "allows patients to talk about what patients want to talk about," the mode is still set on the "professional role mode," if she listens to the patient while making judgment as a nurse. As she puts aside the notion that she must make full use of it for the sake of nursing, the conversation style "listen to patients without judgments" turns the mode to "narrative listener mode." Nurse B with 17 years of experience confessed that when she acquired this conversation style, she came to realize that she had not listened to patients at all:

> *After many years of experience, I just couldn't have casual talks with patients as I only had the nurse perspective. For example when a patient talks about his hobbies, I try hard to extract something from there. One day I asked one of the patients with the numbness in his hand, "What did you do before?" Then he goes, "I paint." or "I keep dairy." You can just say, "Oh, very good. I painted before as well." I looked at it from nurse perspective and tried to figure out how to incorporate the patient's hobbies into his rehabilitation process.*

Nurses act as an interviewer or a listener in these three conversation styles. In Japan, nurses greet and explain things to patients, though it is rare that they talk to them on equal footing. It happens only to a few nurses who "just have some casual talks" with patients. Nurse D with 7 years experience was talking to the patient who had been hospitalized for nerve disease and respirated for years. She talked about her holiday at the beach, though it was unusual in Japan that a nurse talks to the patient about her private life. One of the researchers asked the patient how he felt about it and he replied, "I rather want to joke around than to talk about serious matters like my illness at the moment. The nurse understands my thoughts." The patient added that he enjoyed the conversation with the nurse. This nurse said that she used to care about her role as a nurse, hence communication with patients was something that she was obligated to do to. These days however, she was sometimes trying to talk to patients about casual matters:

> *I used to distinguish between my personal feelings and accepted behavior as a nurse in situations. I had the thoughts that I should ask this question as a nurse in this way in this*

situation, or I should do it this way and I should ask how the patient is feeling. But now I don't have to say, "How are you? You look worried." But I just want to talk to patients about anything other than the illness of the patient. I used to think it was a waste of time to talk about other things.

Between Modes and Conversation Styles While Holding Two Perspectives at Once

To know the patient is to know the patient's view in his subjective world and to know the patient's physical, psychological, and social situation as a whole. While nurses try to maintain both the patient's perspective and their own perspective of the patient at the same time, nurses providing care are sometimes torn by the discrepancy between these two perspectives and by giving judgment from the ethical and technical view point. It is not possible to provide the very nursing care which aims to help patients find the meanings in life without knowing "the patient's subjective world."

Our study (Takemura & Kanda, 2001) shows that nurses will not feel that they have done good nursing practice if the patients are not contented even though they practiced and applied all kinds of care. On the contrary, though, we worried that some Japanese nurses do not do their best to carry out nursing intervention for changing patients for the better, while they put so much effort on the patient's satisfaction or gaining trust. Some nurses in fact, listen carefully to the patient, stand close, and respond to whatever is needed there. However, they finish the assessment of the patient's activities of daily living half way, not even knowing what is going on in the patient's body (Takemura, 2008).

Nurse E with seven years experience talked about her experience when she reviewed the boundaries to which nurses could extend in their work and changed herself in order to do the best she could. Before the change, she used to be satisfied by what she won, for example the appreciation and trust from the patients. This is different from what she says satisfies her at her current job:

It is different. I always feel joy at nursing. I looked at it in the way that there is nothing you can do than to improve the condition of the patient. I was only seeing the surface. I was easily satisfied by the fact that I listened to patients well, helped, and stayed by the patient's side. It was the time when I was satisfied by what I had gotten from other people such as the patient trusting me or the family of the patient remembering me etc. Now I have changed. I've come to realize that a nurse's action makes a huge difference in the prognosis. I've begun to think of what I should do next to make the best of it, even if a very bad condition or bad state of disease is present. It is very different from what it was before.

In order to bring out the patient's vital force as much as possible, it is essential to know the patient's subjective world, respect the patient's will, and make full use of the power that humans can bring out when they find meanings and values in life. In addition, in order to bring out the patient's potential ability and nature, it is important to know and understand what is going on in the body of the patient, perform a careful assessment of the patient's activities of daily living, provision of nursing care based on the assessment, tell him/her about the nurse's judgment so that it might influence the patient's subjective world. Ability to switch between the three modes and four conversation styles at will and continuous effort to know the patients with both the patient and nurse perspectives will make good nursing practice come true. The three modes to know the patient and the four styles of conversation represent Japanese nurses' ways of communication. It may help to review the communication styles in order to understand the ways of knowing the patients in a different cultural context.

References

Barnlund, D. C. (1975). *Public and private self in Japan and the United States: Communicative styles of two cultures*. Tokyo: The Simul Press.

Colleen V. (1996). Disparagement of the nursing process: the new dogma? *Journal of Advanced Nursing, 23*, 120–125.

Hamaguchi, E. (1998). *The principles of Japanese research*. Tokyo: Yuhikaku Publishing (in Japanese).

Henderson, V. (1987). Nursing process: A critique. *Holistic Nursing Practice, 1*, 7–18.

Kumon, S. (1982). Organizing principles in Japanese society. In E. Hamaguchi & S. Kumon (Eds.), *Japanese groupism*. Tokyo: Yuhikaku Publishing (in Japanese).

Leddy, S. K. (1998). Processes of professional nursing. In S. K. Leddy & J. M. Pepper (Eds.), *Conceptual base of professional nursing* (4th ed.), 201–226. Philadelphia: Lippincott-Raven Publishers.

Morse, J. M., Solberg, S. M., Neander, W. L. Bottorff J. L., & Johson, J. L. (1990). Concepts of caring and caring as a concept. *Advance in Nursing Science, 13*(1), 1–14.

Nishida, T. (1996). *Communication in personal relationships in Japan.* In W. B. Gudykunst, S. Ting-Toomey, & T. Nishida, (Eds.), *Communication in personal relationships across cultures* (pp. 102–121). California: Sage.

Nonaka, I., & Takeuchi, H. (1995). *The knowledge-creating company: How Japanese companies create the dynamics of innovation.* New York: Oxford University Press.

Pesut, D. J., & Herman, J. (1998). OPT: transformation of nursing process for contemporary practice. *Nursing Outlook, 46*, 29–36.

Radwin, L. E. (2000). Oncology patients' perceptions of quality nursing care. *Research in Nursing and Health, 23*, 179–190.

Sato, T. (1986). *Nursing Process: Solving It's Practical Problems.* Tokyo: Medical Friend (in Japanese).

Sekiguchi, I. (1999). Issues of Japanese verbal communication. In I. Sekiguchi (Ed.), *Modern Japanese communication environments* (pp. 147–174). Tokyo: Taishukan Publishing (in Japanese).

Takemura, Y. (2004). Cultural traits and nursing care particular to Japan. In M. de Chesnay (Ed.), *Caring for the vulnerable: Perspectives in nursing theory, practice, and research* (pp. 235–243). Boston: Jones and Bartlett.

Takemura, Y. (2008). *Four changes to the elasticity of nurse: Succession and innovation of organizational routine as the value and knowledge of organization.* Doctoral dissertation.University of Tokyo, Tokyo, Japan (in Japanese).

Takemura, Y., & Kanda, K. (2001). The elements and the process of "good nursing practice" perceived by nurses. *Japanese Journal of Nursing Research, 34*(4), 55–65 (in Japanese).

Takemura, Y., & Kanda, K. (2003). How Japanese nurses provide care: A practice based on continuously knowing the patient. *Journal of Advanced Nursing, 42*(3), 252–259.

The Yomiuri Shimbun. (2008, January 21). 90% students object to KY. *The Yomiuri Shimbun*, p. 13. (in Japanese)

Yura, H., & Walsh, M. B. (1983). *The nursing process: Assessing, planning, implementing, evaluating* (4th ed.). Connecticut: Appleton-Century-Crofts.

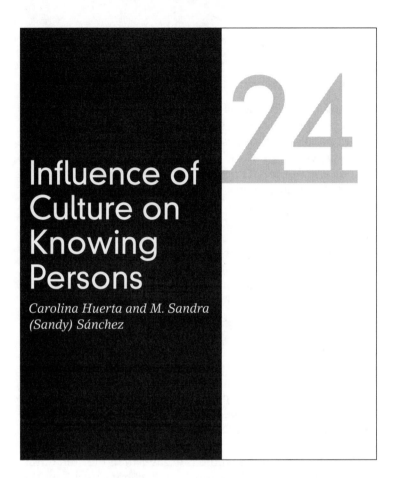

Influence of Culture on Knowing Persons

Carolina Huerta and M. Sandra (Sandy) Sánchez

Chapter Overview

This chapter focuses on the importance of knowing the person holistically as a participant in the nursing process. Carper's four fundamental patterns of knowing in nursing and the relationship between personal knowing and cultural knowing are described. Cultural knowing from both the standpoint of the client and the nurse is emphasized. Ways to increase cultural congruence between the nurse and the client are included. The impact of race and ethnicity on personally knowing a client is specifically addressed. A differentiation between race and ethnicity is included. Emphasis is placed on knowing the Hispanic client, specifically the Mexican-American client.

Culture and Knowing in Nursing

Knowing the client holistically as a primary participant in the nursing process is essential in the provision of quality client care and is a central focus of nursing practice. Given the interpersonal nature of client care, understanding the influence of culture in knowing persons is an inherent aspect of care. A full awareness of the nurse's own as well as the client's culture is critical to understanding the meaning of each person's lived experience. Making clinical judgments, thinking critically, communicating openly, and being astute contribute to knowing persons as whole(s).

Caring for clients involves complex decision-making that takes into account the entire nursing situation so that the individual can be cared for in a holistic manner. There are patterns of reasoning used by nurses in making decisions about client care: analytical, intuitive, and deductive. These patterns of reasoning are used to interpret client needs and determine actions required to address these needs. These reasoning patterns encompass *cognitive* or *Gestalt* reasoning rather than a linear approach to planning nursing care. Cognitive reasoning takes into account the totality of the client and his/her environment and makes sense of the client situation. That is, cognitive reasoning postulates, as does systems theory, that the whole is greater than the sum of the parts (Bastable, 2008). This approach to client care allows the nurse to become acculturated to the entire dynamic nursing process and enhances the appreciation of human beings as whole persons in the nursing trajectory (Locsin, 2005).

Patterns of knowing. Carper (1978) identified four fundamental ways or patterns of knowing nursing. These patterns include empirical knowing, aesthetic knowing, ethical knowing, and personal knowing or personal meaning. Her work has been used extensively to introduce nursing students to the complex knowledge that forms the basis of nursing practice (Bailey, Cloutier, & Duncan, 2007). Although empirical, aesthetic, and ethical knowing patterns are important to nursing practice and not mutually exclusive from personal knowing, personal knowing or personal meaning is paramount to nursing practice. The nurse must consider the person in his/her totality, a totality that includes the individual cultures of both the client and the nurse.

Personally knowing clients and their individual cultures is undervalued by many health care professionals. Sadly, sometimes it is not even considered, because many nurses have, for the most part, been educated or accustomed to view client care with a medical mind-set and, thus, focus on diseases, clinical manifestations, and treatments (Kardong-Edgren, 2007) instead of the unique person who happens to have a disease. Knowing the client culturally may also be devalued by nurses providing care because of their own ethnocentrism and/or cultural ignorance or blindness. *Ethnocentrism* is the belief that one's own culture is the most important or that a particular culture is superior to others. Furthermore, sometimes nurses forget their own cultural upbringing, especially regarding wellness and illness, and become *medicocentric,* i.e., they falsely believe that professional health care is the *best* health care or, worse, the *only* health care. By so doing, they discredit lay/popular health care and folk health care— and may alienate their clients in the process. While nurses should be proud of their own culture(s), whether personal or professional, they should also be able to recognize their ethnocentric or medicocentric tendencies, so that those do not get in the way of personally knowing their client and, thus, impede the provision of culturally congruent care.

Personally knowing a client is essential in the attainment of positive client outcomes. Personally knowing an individual facilitates an understanding of the impact of wellness or illness on him/her and his/her family. However, to actually know an individual culturally, nurses must first know themselves, because personal knowing requires "the qualities of self-awareness, awareness of others, and the therapeutic use of this knowledge in nurse-client interactions" (Little, 2006, p.131). In addition, personal knowing must be valued by the nurse, or it will never be implemented.

Knowing clients requires that the nurse acknowledges culture and its importance. Culture affects how individuals define and respond to health (Ángel & Worobey, 1988). "Culture is profoundly and inextricably tied to matters of health and healthcare. People learn from their own cultures how to be healthy, how to define illness, what to do to get better, and when and from whom to seek help" (Muñoz, 2007, p. 256). Culture is all around and influences every single encounter, including those between nurses and their clients. The nurse and the client each bring in their own personal and familial cultures. Because nursing care always occurs in a cultural context, personal knowing in its relationship to care-giving requires that personal ethnocentricity be identified and cultural competence be embraced.

Cultural knowing from both the standpoint of the client and the nurse provides a framework for problem-solving in all nursing situations. Knowing and appreciating the cultural backgrounds of individuals and communities involved in nursing situations are worthy endeavors that are never stagnant. The process of knowing the nurse's as well as the client's cultural identity requires an ongoing awareness that cultural identity is constantly being defined and redefined (Gray & Thomas, 2006) and, hence, is a dynamic process. The following vignette provides one example of a nursing situation in which cultural and personal knowing affect clients and their families and supports the notion that nurses must provide culturally congruent care.

> *Jesús Martínez, an 80-year-old first generation, i.e., immigrant, Mexican-American male, was diagnosed with uncontrolled diabetes, hepatic failure, and end-stage renal failure. He has been previously hospitalized numerous times and has now been admitted in critical condition to the ICU. Mr. Martínez is not expected to live much longer, and his family is aware that he is in critical condition. Neither Mr. Martínez nor his immediate family has had much formal education, and they have few financial resources. He retired from an unskilled laborer job about 15 years ago when his health started to fail. He has a wife and 7 grown children; there are 16 grandchildren and 2 great-grandchildren. His wife, children, 4 grandchildren, 2 great-grandchildren (both under the age of 5), one brother, and two sisters are at the hospital all of the time, only leaving briefly to bathe and change clothes. Mr. Martínez's primary nurse is overheard saying, "I just don't understand why all of the family, including the children, must be in the waiting room. Don't they know that the staff will call them when it's the right time?"*

The above vignette demonstrates the importance of cultural knowing. The nurse's lack of awareness and sensitivity in terms of cultural knowing is apparent. Recognition of the importance of family to Hispanic populations, especially during the last stages of life, is essential if culturally congruent care is to be provided. Ideally, nurses would recognize the need for critical reflection regarding their understanding of culture. Knowing and appreciating the cultural background of individuals affect outcomes in health care and nursing (Gray & Thomas, 2006). In order to personally and culturally know the client, then, the nurse must holistically view the individual and family, empathize with them, accept them, and, most importantly, develop cultural self-awareness.

Culture Defined

Culture is defined as the "learned, shared, and transmitted values, beliefs, norms, and life practices of a particular group that guide thinking, decisions, and actions in patterned ways" (Leininger, 1988, p. 186). Culture is much more than race, ethnicity, or religion. Culture is defined as a dynamic adaptation, a learned way of life that includes attitudes, morals, beliefs, values, ideals, knowledge, symbols, artifacts, customs, traditions, and norms of a particular group that guide behavior, make life meaningful, and are transmitted through generations (Sánchez, 2008). At best, culture is the expert cultivation of a human being in a nurturing environment. In order to culturally know people, their morality, beliefs, and attitudes assimilated as their personal lifestyle must be acknowledged. Every life event is influenced by culture, and its impact extends into the nursing arena. "The cultural context defines the [health] conditions that are recognized ... the persons who have a legitimate authority to assess" them as well as "the consequences of being defined as having a particular condition" (Mechanic, 1978, p.55).

The nursing arena has become increasingly more complex, and the role of the nurse in providing culturally competent care has expanded over time. From a practice perspective, nurses are expected to respond to the patterns brought about by globalization and the influx of immigration. Clients from diverse populations seek nursing care and present themselves with a vast array of health conditions ranging from optimum wellness to devastating illness. Nurses must adjust to the cultural diversity of their clientele if holistic, culturally congruent care is to be provided, yet they are often ill equipped to do so. Sometimes such an adjustment can be difficult because the nurses may have consciously or unconsciously acquired attitudes and beliefs towards others that are, quite frankly, distorted and inaccurate. No single culture offers the best interpretation of situations or represents the best culture of all. Nonetheless, since culture provides each person's context, and nurses are ethically obligated to be client advocates, it is imperative that nurses strive to understand their clients in order to render culturally appropriate care. Nurses are also morally obligated—and should be professionally motivated—to learn about the cultures of the most common client populations who primarily frequent the local professional health arena. It is unconscionable to do otherwise. Presuming that knowledge of the client's culture has no value in the delivery of quality nursing care is like saying that knowledge of nursing has no value in providing quality nursing care. Cultural competence is a vital nursing trait.

Cultural Awareness

Although this chapter has primarily discussed culture and cultural knowing as these concepts relate to the client receiving care, nurses also bring their own unique culture to each nursing situation. Regardless of their nationality, nurses bring their own traditions, morals, values, knowledge, belief, languages, and worldviews. Sometimes nurses fail to recognize their own culture or its impact on nursing situations, yet it is incumbent upon them to develop a clear sense of their own unique cultural identity. Doing so would contribute to an appreciation of their own culture—and perhaps that of others—and is a prerequisite to the provision of culturally congruent care and becoming culturally competent. **Cultural awareness** is acknowledging the existence of and appreciating one's own culture. Cultural awareness is the first step to cultural knowing, which requires critical self-reflection with respect to understanding oneself, one's own culture, and its impact on life. Cultural awareness is essential because beliefs guide behaviors—unless nurses know what they believe, they may not understand their own behaviors, including those involving client care, behaviors that may be health-enhancing or not. The nurse's cultural awareness leads to personal knowing and cultural knowing of the nurse and of the client.

To become culturally aware, the nurse must first conduct a cultural self-assessment, gathering data about his/her own culture. Areas that should be reflected upon include the nurse's demographics, such as name, gender, religion and/or spirituality, race, ethnicity, nationality, marital status, language(s), preferred language, formal and informal education, and occupation. Although these areas may seem rather trite and ordinary at first glance, they provide great insight when considered in the context of culture. For example, a person's name is part of self-identity. That reason alone should compel others to honor it. In addition, a person's name may, in fact, be part of his/her cultural heritage or ancestry as it may be a family name, one that has been passed from generation to generation or one that has another special cultural connection. Acknowledging or remembering that heritage may reawaken cultural pride, family connections, and the value of proper pronunciation. Once one's name is appreciated with regard to self, the nurse can more readily extend that appreciation to the names of others, including clients. Properly pronouncing names conveys respect for self, others, and culture in general.

As important as demographics are, a cultural self-assessment goes beyond those to include keen reflection or recollection of one's own lifestyle, itself a manifestation of culture. Domains to be considered are many and include general cultural life patterns; cultural values, norms, and expressions; cultural taboos and myths; cultural superstitions; worldview and ethnocentric tendencies; life-caring rituals and rites of passage; lay, folk, and professional wellness-illness cultural systems; specific cultural health beliefs and behaviors; cultural diversities, similarities, and variations; and cultural changes and acculturation. (For a more in-depth discussion of demographics or these domains, refer to Leininger's classic and timeless 1978 text or Sánchez, 2008.)

Cultural Congruence in Nursing

Nurses provide care for culturally diverse clients every day. Culturally congruent care enhances client satisfaction (Aldana, Pielchulek, & Al-Sabir, 2001) and other positive client outcomes, whereas cultural blindness creates barriers not only to accessing professional health care but also to client satisfaction (Warda, 2000). A nurse's cultural blindness can result in negative health perhaps because of barriers imposed by communication difficulties, lack of knowledge, or unwillingness to accept or appreciate another's culture. **Cultural congruence** refers to those "cognitively-based assistive, supportive, facilitating or enabling acts or decisions that are tailor-made to fit with an individual's, group's or institution's cultural values, beliefs and lifeways in order to provide meaningful, beneficial, and satisfying health care, or well-being services" (Leininger, 1991, p. 49). As such, providing culturally congruent nursing care involves much more than knowledge of a client's race or nationality. Culturally congruent care involves knowledge of the components that define the concept of culture, i.e., how an individual dresses, communicates both verbally and nonverbally, makes food choices, or worships. All of these things and more make up culture. It is quite obvious, then, that becoming a culturally aware nurse leads to personal knowing of the client.

Providing culturally congruent care requires the nurse to acknowledge his/her own worldview, or perception of the world. This worldview can be construed as a lens with which a person views the world or brings it into focus and occurs as *emic* or *etic* knowledge. **Emic knowledge** refers to the inside or personal viewpoint of the individual. That is, *emic* knowledge requires subjective understanding and assigning of meaning to situations based on an insider's understanding. *Emic* viewpoints are always culture-specific; in order to understand a situation through an *emic* viewpoint, the person must be a member of the particular cultural group. One example that comes to mind is in relation to a particular religion, one that dictates women's mode of dress. Those who do not belong to that religion may view this mode of dress as severe or outdated. Those who belong to that religious sect may consider the mode of dress as appropriate for those who share that religious culture. This viewpoint, then, is from an *emic* point of view. The other, outsider, viewpoint in this situation is an *etic* perspective or *etic* knowledge. *Etic* knowledge refers to an outsider's view in relation to a specific culture. An *etic* viewpoint refers to an objective viewpoint and may be culturally neutral or unduly critical.

Every human being is unique, and no two people regardless of their culture are exactly alike in every way, so it is probably impossible to have a fully culturally congruent client-nurse situation. Nonetheless, even if there is no such thing as 100% cultural congruence between a client and the nurse, a cultural fit is desired, one where the care rendered by the nurse is deemed appropriate and acceptable by the client. In general, client care is more culturally congruent when there are more commonalities that exist between the client and nurse. However, even when there are few commonalities, culturally congruent care can be provided when a nurse is culturally self-aware and dedicated to personally and culturally knowing the client. Developing cultural self-awareness is not difficult as there are numerous available cultural self-assessment tools, but nurses, must be willing to become culturally self-aware. They must want to be culturally competent and provide culturally congruent health care to their culturally diverse clients. If not, the gap created between the client's cultural expectations and that of the nurse's will impede the attainment of positive client outcomes that are consistent with their cultural beliefs and values.

Culturally congruent nursing care takes into consideration both the client's and the nurse's race, physical characteristics, nationality, religious affiliations, morals, beliefs, values, lifeways, social norms, ethnicity, socioeconomic status, communication patterns, and behavior. Figure 24.1 depicts

24.1

Culturally congruent care model

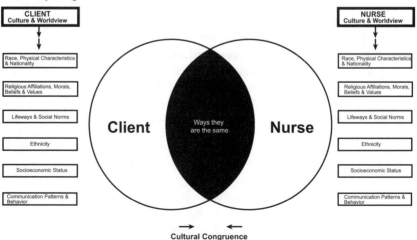

an illustration of factors influencing provision of culturally congruent care. The shaded areas refer to those commonalities shared by both client and nurse. As the circles overlap, the worldview of both the client and the nurse become more congruent. Nursing's goals are to establish cultural congruence in the care that is provided to the client and to develop cultural awareness in the nurse.

Cultural Competence: Embedded vs Subjugated Knowledge

Cultural competence in nursing facilitates positive health outcomes. Cultural competence for nurses requires that they be capable of knowing, utilizing, and appreciating cultures other than their own. **Cultural competence** is defined as "the process in which the healthcare provider continuously strives to achieve the ability to effectively work within the cultural context of a client, individual, family, or community" (Campinha-Bacote, 2003, p. 54). Cultural competence involves the nurse being culturally aware as well as learning what is culturally appropriate for the client (Sánchez, 2008) while keeping in mind that each person is unique. As with the definition of cultural congruence, cultural competence requires acceptance of the fact that people are unique and culturally diverse—and have the right to be. Each individual has his/her very own unique culture as well as an overarching culture. It is not possible to know what a person's culture is without actually getting to know the person (Sánchez, 2008), nor is it possible to know what is best for the client without openly communicating with the client and getting to personally know him/her. Disbelief in that or ignorance of that can contribute to fragmented nursing care, client dissatisfaction, and/or client alienation from the professional health care system.

According to Kleinman (1980), health and ideas about health are embedded in social and cultural contexts; that is, assessment of a client's health, his/her understanding of the illness experienced, and his/her health promotion practices require an understanding of the effects of sociocultural determinants on sickness and responses to sickness.

Ideas about health and health care are also embedded in the nurse's social and cultural context. Nurses, then, use their own embedded knowledge when they care for individual clients. **Embedded knowledge** refers to intuitive knowing and is used by nurses to know the client and recognize client needs. Embedded knowledge can enrich the nurse-client interaction, but can also be detrimental if it is faulty and results in inaccurate assumptions about the client. These inaccurate assumptions may cause a nurse to use subjugated knowledge about the client situation. **Subjugated knowledge** determines that the nurse understands the client situation more accurately than the client. The nursing assessment of the client situation is, thus, assumed to be more accurate than that of the client's understanding of the situation. A nurse's use of a subjugated knowledge approach in client care may result in an inaccurate interpretation of a client's health care situation and in poor clinical judgments (Tanner, 2006).

There are those who doubt that anyone can actually become totally culturally competent since each person has his/her own unique culture, and there is no way that nurses can learn everything about everyone else. However, most agree that even if 100% cultural competence is unlikely, the journey towards it can be amazing, especially with an open mind, the proper attitude, ongoing communication, and an appreciation for one's own as well as other cultures. For that reason, cultural awareness is the first step on that exhilarating journey towards cultural competence, one where empathy is freely dispensed, similarities are shared, diversity is celebrated, bonds are forged, and personal knowing is enhanced.

Impact of Race and Ethnicity on Personal Knowing

Knowing persons from other cultures requires an understanding of the cultural traditions peculiar to each group and subgroup, of which there are many. The reality is that the number of groups that have their own culture is not known. Although some groups and subgroups may be identified in relation to race and ethnicity, many are bound by a shared religion, nationality, region of the country in which they live, alma mater, gender, and even a profession, such as the nursing profession, to name a few.

Even though culture pertains to much more than race or ethnicity, these are two of the most common groups, and, thus, it is necessary to understand each concept. The term "race" is commonly misunderstood and misused by people who in many instances confuse it with ethnic or religious affiliation. For example, many individuals refer to "Hispanic" as a race when, in fact, it is an ethnicity. Hispanics may be of any race. They may be White (Caucasian), Black, Asian, or American Indian (Native American). It is also common to hear people whose religious affiliation is Judaism being referred to as being of the Jewish race. This erroneous categorization of people may be innocent or may be seen as racist and potentially hurtful.

Race. **Race** is defined as a category of human kind that shares certain distinctive characteristics evidenced by physical traits (Mish, 2004). This concept of race is not new but rather one first identified in the mid19th century to categorize people according to physical traits, an interest resulting from research and scientific inquiry. Unfortunately, associated with the concept of race is a focus on differences, rather than similarities, among human beings that has created "a notion of hierarchy" (Dein, 2006, p.68), especially when used in a political context.

Historically, usage of the word race refers to anthropological characteristics. That is, race refers to the physical characteristics that are shared by a particular group of people. These characteristics may relate to a shared common region or geography or to skeletal shapes, facial features, body build, hair type, or skin color. The least important characteristic is probably skin color since it can vary greatly between and among races. Yet, skin color is the one characteristic that many people think of when referring to the different races (Sánchez, 2008).

Although individuals are expected to identify their own race in terms of categories, these categories are extremely broad. These broad, imprecise categories can present problems when a person of mixed races is required to self-select racial identification on a form or application that does not provide for self-selection of more than one race. Forcing a person to select an inaccurate category only adds to the problem of pervasive and inaccurate cultural blurring. The U.S. Office of Management and Budget (OMB) census and federal forms, however, do allow individuals to identify themselves as belonging to more than one race. The U.S. Census Bureau

(2000) allows for identification of more than one race by having individuals check the box *Other* and list the name of the individual's race or races (Sánchez, 2008). Such designations foster precision and diminish false categorizations. Race is designated by the U.S. Census in terms of the following designations:

- White
- Black, African American, or Negro
- American Indian or Alaska native (with space for tribe name)
- Asian or Pacific Islander (API)
- Other (with a space for the name of the race or races)

Even when proper racial self-identification is allowed, though, identifying people by race and race alone can be construed as contributing to stereotyping, especially since so many forms and applications request racial identification. Why is that? On a health record, sometimes knowing a person's race(s) is critical because of health conditions that may tend to occur in certain races. Barring that, however, why is race important? Oftentimes, people make false assumptions or broad generalizations about another person based merely on race, sometimes even without ever meeting the person, even without personally or culturally knowing the person.

Assigning expected traits to a person based on race is flawed and leads to stereotyping or cultural cataloguing. Many textbooks and handbooks that have been written about culture for care professionals, including nursing, use a cookbook-type approach to list expected physical characteristics, individual behaviors, worldviews, communication patterns, eating styles, lifestyles, etc., for various races, ethnicities, and/or religions. While these handbooks or listings might be convenient, they tend to stereotype or reinforce negative views. Most importantly, these listings delude the reader into believing that people behave in predetermined ways instead of being unique individuals who behave in unique ways. In no way can these listings take the place of personally knowing people, who are the best sources of information about themselves. Thus, it is imperative that nurses directly discuss cultural needs with their clients, the best route to personally knowing them.

Ethnicity. Ethnicity is another way of looking at human diversity. As mentioned earlier, ethnicity is very frequently and erroneously confused with race. The word "ethnicity" comes from the word *ethnos* which literally means people or nation. It refers to people who share the same cultural identity and are classified according to common national, tribal, linguistic, or cultural origin or background (Sánchez, 2008).

There are many ethnicities that have been identified, too many to name them all. Some examples of ethnic groups, based on a person's nationality or that of his/her ancestors', include Spanish, French, Turkish, African, Cuban, English, Scottish, Mexican, Italian, Nigerian, or Irish. Although "Hispanic" is a broad ethnic term referring to people who "trace their family background to one of the Spanish-speaking nations" (Marín & Marín, 1991, p. 18), it is best to use a specific ethnicity, such as Mexican, as Hispanics vary greatly.

Because there are so many ethnic variations, it is not possible to identify a person's ethnicity based on physical appearance alone. It is something that an individual must self-identify. For example, people who identify as Cubans may present with vastly different physical characteristics based on whether they are Black, White, or racially mixed. As pointed out in the section on "Race," nurses need to understand that the terms race and ethnicity are not mutually exclusive terms. An astute nurse recognizes that clients come in wide intraethnic and intraracial variations—and that each person is unique no matter what his/her race, ethnicity, social class, or other grouping.

The confounding variable of social class frequently impacts interpretation of events surrounding client care. Social class not only affects how the client interprets events but also how the nurse interprets the same events as they occur in a nursing situation.

Knowing the Hispanic Client

Although there are many different ethnicities that could be discussed in its relation to cultural knowing, knowledge of the Hispanic client, specifically the Mexican-American client, is the focus of this discussion. That particular focus has been selected for various reasons. First, the Hispanic population is the fastest growing minority population in the United States;

second, Hispanics comprise a vastly heterogeneous population that has largely been misrepresented in the professional literature and; third, both of the authors of this chapter are most familiar with the Hispanic client due to their own ethnic and cultural heritage.

Mexican Americans (MA) are the largest Hispanic subgroup (United States Bureau of Census, 2000), comprising about 15% of the U.S. population with nearly 10% of those being MAs. Although this population continues to grow, Hispanic health research has been flawed and skewed. For example, MA men are often cast as being *macho* womanizers, when, in fact, typical MA men are hard workers who strive diligently to provide for their family's welfare. MA women, who tend to be cast as passive, submissive, and weak in the classic—but marred—MA literature, are typically strong, determined, and self-directed. They are the traditional gatekeepers of their family's health, through wellness and illness. Furthermore, even though the MA male may be the public spokesperson for the family, he usually does so only after in-depth discussions with his wife and/or other family members, discussions that may indeed have taken place in private. MAs are not fatalists but rather joyful participants in life.

In addition, much of the MA health literature presents inaccurate distinctions that blur cultural identity, insinuate intraethnic homogeneity, misuse terminology [e.g., race and ethnicity], contribute to stereotyping, and, ultimately, hinder provision of holistic culturally congruent health care. MA health research often addresses diseases, folk practices, high-risk behaviors, and migrants instead of everyday wellness and illness ideas and self-care practices of ordinary MA people, especially those occurring within the lay/popular sector. Contributing to the distortion, professional health care providers collect MA health research data within professional health care settings using structured questionnaires on atypical samples, approaches that call the data's validity into question. Even though some strides have been made, more naturalistic studies that focus on what MAs are doing to stay well or get well again within the lay/popular health care arena, where most health care occurs (Kleinman, 1980), would clarify how MAs utilize health resources.

Hispanic Self-Care Practices

Regardless of cultural affiliation, self-care represents the bulk of all health care and is the first therapeutic mode of most people in the lay health sector (Kleinman, 1980), i.e., care provided by self, family, or friends. Self-care practices include a vast array of wellness and illness behaviors, yet, oddly enough, are often not attributed to MAs. Instead, MA lay health practices have stereotypically been depicted as cryptic, primitive, or quaint as opposed to the ordinary description of mainstream everyday self-care behaviors, behaviors that probably also included home remedies (Sánchez, 2008). Such a depiction demands an explanation. Perhaps it is health professionals' unfamiliarity with cultures other than their own, i.e., cultural ignorance. Perhaps it is the health professionals' inability to see an ethnic client as an ordinary person living an ordinary, everyday life, i.e., cultural blindness. Perhaps it is that health professionals discredit ethnic self-care as *folk* care, an often devalued—and erroneously used—term. Perhaps it is that health professionals tend to forget—or perhaps fail to acknowledge—that most health care takes place *outside* of the professional arena. Perhaps it is that health professionals have deluded themselves into thinking that professional health care is *the only* health care, i.e., medicocentrism. Or perhaps it is that a client arrives at the professional sector only after self-care options have been exhausted. Who is to say? Whatever it is, cultural knowing requires that stereotypical preconceptions be discarded. Self-care behaviors of MAs and other ethnic groups should be presented in the same fashion as those of the mainstream population's, so that similarities among the groups can be illuminated instead of their differences denigrated. In fact, culturally knowing the self-care behaviors of both ethnic and mainstream aggregates is advantageous in order to understand which self-care practices are beneficial and should be reinforced—or which ones may need modification. Perhaps then it would be easier to praise ethnic and mainstream clients for their successful self-care outside of the professional arena instead of blaming them for selectively using it. The more health professionals understand about other cultures, the less xenophobia exists and harmony prevails.

Culturally Knowing the Mexican-American Client

Cultural knowing involves the personal realization that each person is unique. Cultural knowing includes understanding the high value MAs place on familism, or *familismo*. *Familismo* underlies the MA's desire to provide for the needs of family members and others who are viewed as family members though not related by blood or law, such as Godparents *(padrinos)* (Sánchez, 2008). The value of *familismo* extends to health care needs and is supported by Villarruel's claim (1995) that the primacy of caring for others is the essence of the MA family. Villarruel and Denyes (1997) suggest that a MA's care for loved ones develops as an extension of self-care—or may be even more valued as a cultural expression. As such, Villarruel and Denyes recommend that, in the MA, these intimately intertwined behaviors, i.e., self-care and care for others, be viewed as one collective concept. In addition, the MA's strong family ties and resultant family support bolster inner strength, reinforce personal responsibility, enhance confident decision-making, engender personal control and power, and, ultimately, protect health.

Personalism, or *personalismo*, is another strong MA value. *Personalismo* is the inclination to engage in personal inter-actions not only with family members or close friends but also with others, such as health professionals, who may view such social chitchat as a waste of time in an already over-scheduled and busy day. *Personalismo*, however, facilitates personal knowing, because it conveys a sense of caring about personal respect and dignity. *Personalismo* is instrumental in establishing rapport and trust, necessary ingredients for a sound nurse-client relationship. Without trust, little prog-ress can be made because the relationship will be viewed as superficial, impersonal, and noncaring. *Personalismo* is a welcoming attitude that says "You have worth," as opposed to the efficient attitude of "Let's get this thing over with." While clinical competence is definitely valued, MA clients may very well switch from health professionals who seem-ingly devalue interpersonal communication to those who value it. *Personalismo* is a time-honored tradition that enhances mutually agreed-upon, meaningful, holistic, cul-turally congruent client care. *Personalismo* opens the door to personal and cultural knowing and, hence, must be viewed as indispensable—and certainly time well spent, no matter how busy the day.

The Value of Personally Knowing the Client's Culture

According to Sánchez (1997), because of the current setup of the U.S. professional health sector, health professionals are more likely to see ill people than well. As such, health professionals may be frustrated by what may seem like a client's, especially an ethnic client's, inexcusable delay in seeking professional health care. They may very well forget to acknowledge that a huge variety of self-care practices have kept their client well up to this point and away from the professional sector. Without that cultural knowledge, the client-health professional interaction is flawed from the start. Even though a health history may be obtained, it is incomplete if it does not address the client's health definitions, health meaning, explanatory models, health expectations, or lay, folk, and professional health care practices—and an incomplete health history impedes culturally congruent care. To make matters worse, armed only with incomplete information, the culturally blind health professionals then proceed to prescribe a litany of do's-and-don't's, medications, diagnostic workups, or other treatments that may have little or no meaning to the client. Without actively including their client in the plan, they have unwittingly disrespected him/her. They bypassed a golden opportunity to culturally know their client, who still remains a virtual stranger. In addition, they are likely perceived by the client as being impersonal, uncaring, incompetent, biased, bigoted, demeaning, or, at best, oblivious. If the client refuses such a personally irrelevant protocol, the health professionals may label the client as not being "compliant," itself a lamentable word as it suggests *yielding*. Their clueless behavior, in turn, taints the client's impression of the professional health system in general. An unpleasant, unfulfilling, and perhaps adversarial cycle ensues, one that could easily have been avoided by taking the time to personally and culturally know the client.

Culturally knowing the client may have resulted in a much more positive client outcome, one based on a comprehensive health history and a *mutually* agreed upon plan that the client would *adhere* to because it was personally meaningful, relevant, and culturally appropriate (Sánchez, 1997). Such a desirable outcome would have been likely if the health professionals had removed their cultural blinders, reoriented their medicocentric mind-set, asked the client about health beliefs, meanings, behaviors, and resources, and praised him/her for self-care, i.e., engaged in cultural and personal knowing.

Being culturally competent requires that health professionals recognize that health care does not begin and end within the confines of the professional health care sector (Sánchez, 1997). In order to provide culturally congruent care, health professionals must acknowledge not only the existence of the lay and folk sectors but also their complementary roles. As such, these sectors are often used simultaneously (Eisenberg et al., 1993; Kleinman, 1980), especially for people (ethnic or mainstream) with strong cultural beliefs. Even so, less than a third of those who engage in nonprofessional health care share that information with their medical doctors (Eisenberg et al., 1993), an unfortunate reality. Hence, in order to obtain a comprehensive health history and provide culturally congruent care, health professionals must inquire about that information in a warm and receptive manner.

Summary

Health is culturally determined, uniquely perceived, and personally experienced (Sánchez, 1997), and health professionals must accept that. They must also realize that all people have a culture, whether they are from an ethnic minority or not. They all have cultural health beliefs, needs, values, and behaviors that may differ from the health professionals'.

Regardless of ethnicity, cultural health approaches are quite common among middle class population groups that revere the family (Becerra & Iglehart, 1995). Since "family practices are embedded in a cultural context that defines and determines the parameters of" (p. 50) health behavior, cultural health traditions reflect the strategic role of the family. Cultural health traditions also represent the

> *logical development of the interaction of scientific thought with cultural... attitudes over time, [they] cannot be defined neatly as the "old-fashioned" way of doing things. [Cultural*

health traditions are] not simply a collection of remedies passed down by word-of-mouth among rural villagers. [They are] evidence of a seasoned way of thinking, which incorporates that which has been most effective from earlier generations into a modern way of doing things. [They try] to preserve the best of the past in current health practices. (p. 50)

Cultural health approaches are often used along with professional methods in a complementary or integrative fashion and should not be discarded by health care professionals. Doing so would impede respect, a trusting client-provider relationship, and holistic culturally congruent client care.

Cultural knowing, then, benefits all clients, not just ethnic clients. Ethnic people are just as capable of engaging in health-enhancing behaviors as anyone else. People from the mainstream are just as likely to use home remedies as ethnics, although the specifics may vary. All people deserve holistic culturally congruent care provided by a culturally competent health provider. We are all connected!

References

Aldana, J. M., Piechulek, H., & Al-Sabir, A. (2001). Client satisfaction and quality heath care in rural Bangladesh. *Bulletin of The World Health Organization, 79*(6). Retrieved on April 28, 2008 from http://www.scielosp.org.

Ángel, R., & Worobey, J. L. (1988). Acculturation and maternal reports of children's health. Evidence from the Hispanic health and nutrition examination survey. *Social Science Quarterly, 69,* 707–721.

Bailey, P. H., Cloutier, J. D., & Duncan, C. (2007). Locating Carpers aesthetic pattern of knowing within contemporary nursing evidence, praxis and theory. *International Journal of Nursing Education Scholarship, 4*(1), 1–12.

Bastable, S. (2008). *Nurse as educator: Principles of teaching and learning for nursing practice.* Boston: Jones and Bartlett.

Becerra, R. M., & Iglehart, A. P. (1995). Folk medicine use: Diverse populations in a metropolitan area. *Social Work in Health Care, 21*(4), 37–58.

Campinha-Bacote, J. (2003). *The process of cultural competency in the delivery of healthcare services: A culturally competent model of care.* Cincinnati, OH: Transcultural C. A. R. E. Associates.

Carper, B. A. (1978). Fundamental patterns of knowing in nursing. *Advances in Nursing Science, 1*(1), 13–23.

Dein, S. (2006). Race, culture, and ethnicity in minority research: A critical discussion. *Journal of Cultural Care Diversity, 13*(2), 68–75.

Eisenberg, D. M., Kessler, R. C., Foster, C., Norlock, F. E., Calkins, D. R., & Delbanco, T. L. (1993). Unconventional medicine in the United States. *The New England Journal of Medicine, 328*(4), 246–252.

Gray, P., & Thomas, D. (2006). Critical reflections on culture in nursing. *Journal of Cultural diversity, 13*(2), 76–82.

Kardong-Edgren, S. (2007). Cultural competence of baccalaureate nursing Faculty. *Journal of Nursing Education, 46*(8), 360-366.

Kleinman, A. (1980). *Patients and healers in the context of culture: An exploration of the Borderland between anthropology, medicine, and psychiatry.* Berkeley: University of California Press.

Leininger, M. M. (1978). *Transcultural nursing: Concepts, theories, and practices.* New York: Wiley.

Leininger, M. M. (1988). Leininger's theory of nursing: Cultural care diversity and universality. *Nursing Science Quarterly, 1,* 152–160.

Leininger, M. M. (1991). *Culture care diversity and universality: A theory of nursing.* New York: National League for Nursing.

Little, M. L. (2006). Preparing nursing students to be health educators: Personal knowing through performance and feedback workshops. *Journal of Nursing Education, 45*(3), 131–135.

Locsin, R. C. (2005). *Technological competency as caring in nursing.* Indianapolis, Indiana: Sigma Theta Tau International Honor Society of Nursing.

Marín, B. V. O., & Marín, G.(1991). *Research with Hispanic populations.* Newbury Park, CA: Sage.

Marín, B. V. O., Marín, G., Padilla, A. M., & de la Rocha, C. (1983). Utilization of traditional and non-traditional sources of health care among Hispanics. *Hispanic Journal of Behavioral Sciences, 6*(1), 365–383.

Mechanic, D. (1978). *Medical Sociology* (2nd ed.). New York: Free Press.

Mish, F. C. (Ed.). (2004). *Merriam-Webster's collegiate dictionary* (11th ed.). Springfield, MA: Merriam-Webster.

Muñoz, J. P. (2007). Culturally responsive caring in occupational therapy. *Occupational Therapy International, 14*(4), 456–480.

Sánchez, M. S. (1997). Pathways to health: A naturalistic study of Mexican-American women's lay health behaviors. Dissertation Abstracts International, University of Texas at Austin. UMI No. AA19822698.

Sánchez, S. (2008). Cultural considerations. In J. Maville & C. Huerta (Eds.), *Health promotion in nursing* (pp. 96–111). Clifton Park, NY: Thomson-Delmar Learning.

Tanner, C. (2006). Thinking like a nurse: A research-based model of clinical judgment in Nursing. *Journal of Nursing Education, 45*(6), 204–211.

U.S. Census Bureau. (2000). *United States census.* Retrieved April 28, 2008, from www.census.gov.

Villarruel, A. M. (1995). Mexican-American cultural meanings, expressions, self-care and dependent-care actions associated with experiences of pain. *Research in Nursing & Health. 18*(5), 427–436.

Villarruel, A. M., & Denyes, M. J. (1997). Testing Orem's theory with Mexican Americans. *Image: Journal of Nursing Scholarship. 29*(3), 283–288.

Warda, M. (2001). Mexican-Americans' perceptions of culturally competent care. *Western Journal of Nursing Research, 22,* 203–224.

Glossary

Cognitive or Gestalt Reasoning: takes into account the totality of the client and his environment and makes sense of the client situation.

Culture: learned, shared, and transmitted values, beliefs, norms, and life practices of a particular group that guide thinking, decisions, and actions in patterned ways.

Cultural Awareness: acknowledging the existence of and appreciating one's own culture. Cultural awareness is the first step to cultural knowing, which requires critical self-reflection with respect to understanding oneself, one's own culture, and its impact on life; reflection on one's or someone else's cultural customs, beliefs, norms, life practices; prerequisite to cultural competence and provision of culturally congruent care.

Cultural Competence: "the process in which the healthcare provider continuously strives to achieve the ability to effectively work within the cultural context of a client, individual, family, or community" (Campinha-Bacote, 2003, p. 54).

Cultural Congruence: those "cognitively-based assistive, supportive, facilitating or enabling acts or decisions that are tailor-made to fit with an individual's, group's or institution's cultural values, beliefs and lifeways in order to provide meaningful, beneficial, and satisfying health care, or well being services" (Leininger, 1991, p. 49).

Cultural Knowing: knowing yourself or someone else culturally; what cultural concepts are pertinent and meaningful.

Cultural Sensitivity: being tuned into the importance of culture, yet not being completely aware of specific details.

Embedded Knowledge: intuitive knowing; used by nurses in recognizing client needs.

Emic **Knowledge:** the personal, or insider's, viewpoint in relation to a specific culture.

Ethnocentrism: the belief that own culture is the most important or that a particular culture is superior to others.

Etic **Knowledge:** an outsider's viewpoint in relation to a specific culture.

Folk Health Care: wellness or illness health care provided by unlicensed, nonprofessional health care specialists.

Lay/Popular Health Care: wellness or illness health care rendered by self, family, friends; unlicensed, nonprofessional health care providers; the most frequently used sector.

Medicocentrism: the belief, by health professionals, that professional health care and its practices are superior to lay/popular or folk health care.

Professional Health Care: wellness or illness health care provided by people who have received formal education and/or state or national licensure or certification.

Race: a category of humankind that shares certain distinctive characteristics evidenced by physical traits.

Subjugated Knowledge: determines that the nurse understands the client situation more accurately than the client.

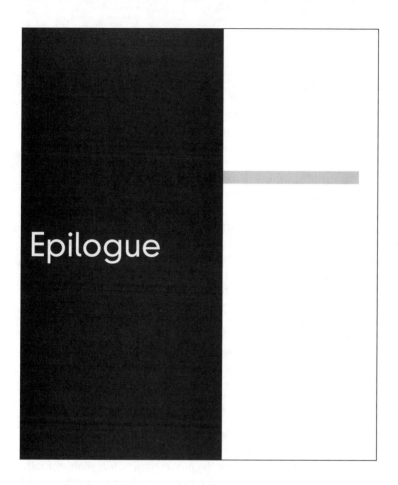

Epilogue

Moving Forward in a Contemporary Practice of Nursing

And so we have come to a pause, a temporary resting place in which to gather our thoughts and savor the new ideas and understandings that have come to us. Commonalities well up in each chapter and are very similar to what Fleck (1935/1979) would have called a "thought collective" — a gathering in of likeminded individuals who participate in the discovery and integration of knowledge. A name for a thought collective in this day and era might be the idea of a discipline, that group of scholars so ably represented in this book, who have come together to share their knowledge for the common good.

505

Fleck held that there is no new knowledge; rather, there is a gradual accretion and building of knowledge. In this sense, we all stand on the shoulders of those who have gone before—an eloquent testimony to their courage and caring that we see embodied in the thoughts of those within these chapters; the ontology giving meaning and life to the epistemology. Fundamental to the premise of this book is that we all contribute to a transformation rather than to a Kuhnian type overthrow of current knowledge paradigms. Change occurs from the inside out, and so in this book, the changes that are described are drawn from inside practice, inside the discipline, and inside Nursing. In all there is a current of change—away from the source of what no longer fits, to a way of knowing, being, and doing in nursing that transcends the constraints of the unexamined routines of practice and embedded thought of other disciplines.

In the prologue to this book, the traditional nursing process was introduced as an embedded routine of practice that no longer is a fit for nursing. Lawler, Rafferty, and Traynor (2002) archly noted,

> *Much of the discourse about "individualized" care, however, has been filtered through nursing process rhetoric which is, in itself, an inherently positivistic and economically driven construct, and which does not allow for embodiment or lived experience more generally. (p. 179)*

We agree. This book has called for a contemporary process of nursing based on knowing persons on which to ground practice—not the rote, linear, traditional nursing process. Advocating a practice that is based on knowledge implies the truth, the trustworthiness, and the morality of the activities by those who practice knowing the person distinctly as critical to professional practice. The epistemology of knowing in Nursing is predicated on the understanding that to know is to establish the truth. The weight of knowing persons brings great responsibility, and the nursing scholars within these pages have risen to the call.

Inherent in these chapters is the re-visioning of knowing that is able to advance nursing as a discipline whose epistemology is shaped by its past, but whose future is informed by all that is available, including knowledge from other disciplines. For example, the idea of embodied knowing encompasses a form of sentience that is beyond words. Recent research by scientists has shown that the human heart has its own knowing, responding and informing the brain. The grateful heart whose resonance helps heal the body also can be dynamically measured several feet away (HeartMath.org). One of the editors of this book has completed phase one of an interdisciplinary research study that suggests *stored* human intention can actually *change* physical matter (Pajunen, Purnell, Tiller, & Dibble, 2009), with futuristic implications that emphasize how essential informed caring intention is for healing now. There are myriad other research studies on the fringes of what is considered traditional and conventional science. These help inform and affirm how and what we know in practice—indeed, in all of our life relationships: the inner cosmos and outer cosmos are not only connected, but also constitute a grand unity. When we reflect on this grandeur, knowing really becomes another way of seeing.

So our call for a contemporary process of nursing is not a call to do away with what has transpired before, but to honor, acknowledge, reaffirm, and move forward strengthened by the knowledge that is part of our nursing heritage. Our call for inclusiveness in disciplinary knowledges may not be without difficulty, not unlike differentiating between the blurred edges of medicine and nursing in many arenas of practice. It is here that we must turn to our conception of what is this practice we call nursing. Boykin, Parker, and Schoenhofer (1994) call for an explicit conception of nursing grounded in caring; this is where we begin, and this is the place to where we return.

This book is just a beginning. Those many distinct ways of knowing that are not specifically addressed in these chapters—ways such as narrative knowing, woman's knowing, and intuitive knowing—these we cherish for another time and another volume. Thank you for journeying with us.

Marguerite J. Purnell, PhD, RN, AHN-BC and
Rozzano C. Locsin, RN, PhD, FAAN
Coeditors

References

Boykin, A., Parker, M., & Schoenhofer, S. O. (1994). Aesthetic knowing grounded in an explicit conception of nursing. *Nursing Science Quarterly, 7*, 158–161.

Fleck, L. (1979). *Genesis and development of a scientific fact.* Chicago: The University of Chicago Press. (Original work published 1935).

Heart Math.org http://www.heartmath.org/research/science-of-the-heart.html Accessed January 9, 2009

Lawler, J., Rafferty, A. M., & Traynor, M. (2002). Knowing the body and embodiment: Methodologies, discourses and nursing. In *Exemplary research for nursing and midwifery* (pp. 166–187). New York: Routledge.

Pajunen, G. A., Purnell, M. J., Tiller, W. A., & Dibble, W. E. (2009). *Altering the acid-alkaline balance of water via the use of an intention-host device.* In press.

INDEX

O

T